The Racehorse: A Veterinary Manual

PIETER H. L. RAMZAN, BVSc(Sydney), MRCVS

Rossdales Veterinary Practice
Beaufort Cottage Stables
Newmarket, Suffolk, UK

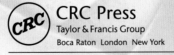

CRC Press
Taylor & Francis Group
Boca Raton London New York

CRC Press is an imprint of the
Taylor & Francis Group, an **informa** business

CRC Press
Taylor & Francis Group
6000 Broken Sound Parkway NW, Suite 300
Boca Raton, FL 33487-2742

© 2014 by Taylor & Francis Group, LLC
CRC Press is an imprint of Taylor & Francis Group, an Informa business

No claim to original U.S. Government works

Printed on acid-free paper
Version Date: 20140219

Printed and bound in India by Replika Press Pvt. Ltd.

International Standard Book Number-13: 978-1-4822-2191-6 (Hardback)

This book contains information obtained from authentic and highly regarded sources. While all reasonable efforts have been made to publish reliable data and information, neither the author[s] nor the publisher can accept any legal responsibility or liability for any errors or omissions that may be made. The publishers wish to make clear that any views or opinions expressed in this book by individual editors, authors or contributors are personal to them and do not necessarily reflect the views/opinions of the publishers. The information or guidance contained in this book is intended for use by medical, scientific or health-care professionals and is provided strictly as a supplement to the medical or other professional's own judgement, their knowledge of the patient's medical history, relevant manufacturer's instructions and the appropriate best practice guidelines. Because of the rapid advances in medical science, any information or advice on dosages, procedures or diagnoses should be independently verified. The reader is strongly urged to consult the drug companies' printed instructions, and their websites, before administering any of the drugs recommended in this book. This book does not indicate whether a particular treatment is appropriate or suitable for a particular individual. Ultimately it is the sole responsibility of the medical professional to make his or her own professional judgements, so as to advise and treat patients appropriately. The authors and publishers have also attempted to trace the copyright holders of all material reproduced in this publication and apologize to copyright holders if permission to publish in this form has not been obtained. If any copyright material has not been acknowledged please write and let us know so we may rectify in any future reprint.

Except as permitted under U.S. Copyright Law, no part of this book may be reprinted, reproduced, transmitted, or utilized in any form by any electronic, mechanical, or other means, now known or hereafter invented, including photocopying, microfilming, and recording, or in any information storage or retrieval system, without written permission from the publishers.

For permission to photocopy or use material electronically from this work, please access www.copyright.com (http://www.copyright.com/) or contact the Copyright Clearance Center, Inc. (CCC), 222 Rosewood Drive, Danvers, MA 01923, 978-750-8400. CCC is a not-for-profit organization that provides licenses and registration for a variety of users. For organizations that have been granted a photocopy license by the CCC, a separate system of payment has been arranged.

Trademark Notice: Product or corporate names may be trademarks or registered trademarks, and are used only for identification and explanation without intent to infringe.

Library of Congress Cataloging-in-Publication Data

Ramzan, Pieter H. L., author.
  The racehorse : a veterinary manual / Pieter H.L. Ramzan.
    p. ; cm.
  Includes bibliographical references and index.
  Summary: "Written by one of the UK's leading equine veterinary practitioners, this textbook is dedicated wholly to the veterinary management of the racehorse. The Racehorse: A Veterinary Manual brings together all the major orthopaedic and non-orthopaedic conditions likely to be encountered in racehorse practice and concisely details state-of-the-art best practice for diagnosis and management strategies. The book spans the full range of fields relevant to the clinician including topics as diverse as rehabilitation, respiratory medicine, exercise physiology, pre-purchase and herd health. Well-illustrated and comprehensive, it succeeds in being both practical and firmly evidence-based, making it an invaluable resource for clinicians worldwide as well as a useful reference work for many non-veterinarians in the racing industry"--Provided by publisher.
  ISBN 978-1-4822-2191-6 (alk. paper)
  I. Title.
  [DNLM: 1. Horse Diseases. 2. Horses. 3. Veterinary Sports Medicine--methods. SF 956]

SF951
636.1089--dc23
                                                                2014006005

Visit the Taylor & Francis Web site at
http://www.taylorandfrancis.com

and the CRC Press Web site at
http://www.crcpress.com

CONTENTS

Preface		viii
Abbreviations		x
Acknowledgements		xii
PART 1	**Injuries and Conditions of the Musculoskeletal System**	**01**
CHAPTER 1	**Injury management and rehabilitation**	**3**
	Introduction	3
	Acute care and wound management	6
	Management of joint disease	15
	Rehabilitation	21
CHAPTER 2	**Regional musculoskeletal conditions**	**31**
	The foot	31
	The fetlock and pastern	50
	The metacarpus/metatarsus ('cannon')	92
	The carpus	108
	The upper forelimb	124
	The tarsus (hock)	136
	The upper hindlimb	152
	The pelvis	168
	The neck and back	179
	Other musculoskeletal conditions	190

PART 2	**Other Body Systems**	**199**
CHAPTER 3	**Respiratory conditions**	**201**
	Upper airway obstructions	201
	Lower airway disease	222
CHAPTER 4	**Cardiovascular conditions**	**235**
	Heart murmurs	235
	Arrhythmias	236
	Jugular thrombosis/thrombophlebitis	237
	Exercise-related sudden death (cardiopulmonary failure)	239
CHAPTER 5	**The head**	**241**
	Dentistry	241
	Wounds	244
	Eyes	246
	Airways	248
	Other	251
CHAPTER 6	**Gastrointestinal conditions**	**255**
CHAPTER 7	**Urogenital conditions**	**265**
	Urinary tract problems	265
	Female reproductive system	265
	Male reproductive system	268
	Intersex disorders	270
CHAPTER 8	**Neurological conditions**	**271**
	Vertebral column conditions	271
	Viral infections	273

CHAPTER 9	**Skin conditions**	**277**
	Injuries	277
	Infections	278
	Other conditions	282
CHAPTER 10	**Miscellaneous conditions**	**291**
CHAPTER 11	**Infectious diseases**	**293**
PART 3	**Training and Management**	**301**
CHAPTER 12	**Selection of the racehorse**	**303**
	Overview	303
	The vetting procedure	304
	Pre-purchase radiography	306
	Pre-purchase ultrasonography	311
	Assessment of airway function	311
	Public auction vetting: the yearling	312
	Public auction vetting: the 'breeze-up' 2 year old	312
	Public auction vetting: the horse-in-training	313
	Conformation	313
	Heart size	315
	Genetics of selection	315
CHAPTER 13	**Exercise physiology and training**	**317**
	Overview of exercise physiology	317
	The racehorse as athlete	317
	Adaptations to training	318
	Fundamentals of training	319

	Training aids	320
	Fitness testing	322
	Track types	323
CHAPTER 14	**Nutrition**	**327**
	Principles of feeding	327
	Key nutrients	327
	Basic feed types	329
	Supplements	330
	Assessing nutritional problems	330
	Poor appetite/condition	331
	Feeding for performance	332
CHAPTER 15	**Ergogenic aids**	**333**
	Overview	333
	Nutritional aids	333
	Non-nutritional aids	335
CHAPTER 16	**Blood analysis**	**337**
	Blood constituents	337
	Sampling	339
	Effects of training	339
	Interpretation	340
CHAPTER 17	**Herd health**	**343**
	Biosecurity	343
	Housing and air hygiene	345
	Lower airway disease	345
	Musculoskeletal injuries	346

CHAPTER 18	Transport	349
	Overview	349
	Effects of transport	349
	Veterinary management for long-distance transport	351

Part 4	Appendices	353
APPENDIX 1	Normal clinical parameters	355
APPENDIX 2	Drug administration reference table	356
APPENDIX 3	Guide to best practice for humane destruction in emergency situations	358
APPENDIX 4	Blood reference ranges	360
INDEX		361

PREFACE

The Thoroughbred racing industry is now more than ever a globalized affair. Transport and communication links that have made the world a smaller place for travel and business have had an equally profound effect on racing and breeding activities, as well as the veterinary advances that support them. While regional variations in disease and injury will always exist, clinicians in Europe, the Americas, Asia, Africa and Australasia largely face the same challenges in respect of maintaining the health and well-being of racehorses under their care.

The primary aim of this book is to provide a practical and objective source of veterinary information, pertinent to the Thoroughbred racehorse, that is accessible to both the racehorse and non-racehorse clinician. It is also hoped that others within the industry interested in veterinary matters will find it a useful reference work. While there are several excellent texts available on equine orthopaedics and sports medicine, information relating to racehorses is fragmented and sometimes contradictory. Many conditions are poorly serviced by the literature, and descriptions of even those common to other equine disciplines frequently fail to take account of practicalities of management peculiar to the racing industry. Racing practice is a very particular blend of population medicine and highly focused individual care and is a specialism in its own right.

I was very conscious throughout this project of the need to create a text based more on evidence than anecdote. The great challenge, of course, is that much of what we do as equine clinicians is derived empirically; indeed, there is no scientifically validated 'best' way to manage respiratory disease or for that matter most orthopaedic injuries. On the other hand, one would be unwise in the pursuit of objectivity to discount the value of shared experience and by doing so exclude knowledge that has accumulated over generations in one of the hotbeds of equine veterinary endeavour. But rather than simply transcribe the received wisdoms of Newmarket racing practice, every effort has been made to build the text from a scientific base by reviewing not just the published equine literature but much relevant work from human sports medicine. The reader should also be reassured that as far as possible the text has been made relevant to all the major racing jurisdictions, not just the United Kingdom and Europe.

This work seeks to draw together those conditions that might reasonably be encountered in the day-to-day management of a racing yard and arms the practitioner with information necessary for clinical problem solving. Orthopaedic injury necessarily accounts for the major part of the book. Advice on rehabilitation periods and prognosis is undoubtedly of particular interest to the user and these have been defined as tightly as possible in order to be of practical benefit. As very little published information exists on likely return to racing following most injuries (in relation to uninjured cohorts), categories from excellent to poor have been used for prognosis. Where more specific figures exist these have been included in the relevant chapters. Also of enduring interest to clinicians and trainers are recommendations for withdrawal times of medications prior to racing. In this, however, it is not possible to provide guidelines, due to the shifting goalposts of testing procedures, regulatory advice and individual variability in pharmacokinetics. Here the reader is referred to drug detection times published by regulatory boards and current advice from local veterinary clinicians.

Preface

The chapters on non-orthopaedic conditions are also intended to be racehorse specific. This has influenced not just the choice of conditions included, but in many cases extends to describing key diseases as they might be presented to a front-line clinician. A practical approach to diagnosis and management as viewed from the stable door is the objective, rather than comprehensive coverage of medical and surgical procedures. Likewise, the scope of the chapter on infectious diseases is restricted to conditions of primary importance to the movement of horses (intra- and internationally) for which testing may be undertaken.

Inevitably in a book of this type there will be omissions both intentional and unintentional; however, an honest attempt has been made to compile a clinically relevant text for the racehorse and I hope that in these efforts I have done justice to the subject.

Piet Ramzan

ABBREVIATIONS

ACS/IRAP	autologous conditioned serum/interleukin-1 receptor antagonist protein
ADAF	axial deviation of the aryepiglottic fold/s
AF	atrial fibrillation
AHS	African horse sickness
AHSV	African horse sickness virus
AI	artificial insemination
AL-DDFT	accessory ligament of the deep digital flexor tendon ('inferior check' ligament)
AL-SDFT	accessory ligament of the superficial digital flexor tendon ('superior check' ligament)
APC	atrial premature complex
APJ	articulating process joint
AST	aspartate aminotransferase
AV	atrioventricular
BAD	branchial arch defect
bpm	beats per minute
BWT	body weight
C3	third carpal bone
CAD	cricoarytenoideus dorsalis (muscle)
CdCL	caudal cruciate ligament
CEM	contagious equine metritis
CFT	complement fixation test
cfu	colony-forming units
CHO	carbohydrate
CK	creatine kinase
CNS	central nervous system
CO_2	carbon dioxide
CP	crude protein
CrCL	cranial cruciate ligament
CSA	cross-sectional area
CT	computed tomography
DDFT	deep digital flexor tendon
DDSP	dorsal displacement of the soft palate
DIPJ	distal interphalangeal joint
DIT	distal intertarsal joint
DM	dry matter
DMSO	dimethyl sulphoxide
DSL	distal sesamoidean ligament
DSP	dorsal spinous process
ECG	electrocardiogram/electrocardiography
EEE	Eastern equine encephalitis
EHV	equine herpesvirus
EI	equine influenza
EIA	equine infectious anaemia
EIPH	exercise-induced pulmonary haemorrhage
ELISA	enzyme-linked immunosorbent assay
epg	eggs per gram
EPM	equine protozoal myeloencephalitis
EPO	erythropoietin
ESWT	extracorporeal shockwave therapy
EVA	equine viral arteritis
FEC	faecal egg count
FPJ	femoropatellar joint
GA	general anaesthesia
GAG	glycosaminoglycan
GGT	gamma-glutamyl transpeptidase
GnRH	gonadotropin–releasing hormone
GPS	global positioning system
HA	hyaluronate/hyaluronic acid
HBOT	hyperbaric oxygen therapy
hCG	human chorionic gonadotropin
HR	heart rate
HR_{max}	maximal heart rate at exercise
IFAT	indirect fluorescent antibody test
IM	intramuscular
IRU	increased radiomarker uptake
IV	intravenous
JE	Japanese encephalitis

Abbreviations

LFTJ	lateral femorotibial joint	PRP	platelet-rich plasma
		PSB	proximal sesamoid bone
Mc3	third metacarpal bone (forelimb 'cannon')		
MFC	medial femoral condyle	RBC	red blood cell
MFTJ	medial femorotibial joint	RLN	recurrent laryngeal neuropathy
MPA	methylprednisolone acetate		
MRI	magnetic resonance imaging	SA	sinoatrial
MSM	methylsulfonylmethane	SDFT	superficial digital flexor tendon
Mt3	third metatarsal bone (hindlimb 'cannon')	SIJ	sacroiliac joint
MVE	Murray Valley encephalitis	SLB	suspensory ligament branch
MVEV	Murray Valley encephalitis virus	STIR	short tau inversion recovery
NMES	neuromuscular electrical stimulation	T3	third tarsal bone
NO	nitric oxide	TA	triamcinolone acetonide
NSAID	non-steroidal anti-inflammatory drug	TENS	transcutaneous electrical nerve stimulation
OA	osteoarthritis	TMT	tarsometatarsal joint
OCD	osteochondritis dissecans		
OCL	osseous cyst-like lesion	VEE	Venezuelan equine encephalomyelitis
		VHR_{max}	speed at maximal heart rate
P1	first phalanx	VPC	ventricular premature complex
P2	second phalanx		
P3	third phalanx	WBC	white blood cell
PCR	polymerase chain reaction	WEE	Western equine encephalitis
PCV	packed cell volume	WNV	West Nile virus
PI	palatal instability		
PIPJ	proximal interphalangeal joint ('pastern' joint)	YO	year old
POD	palmar/plantar condylar osteochondral disease		

Radiographic projections

CdCr	caudocranial	DLPaMO	dorsolateral–palmaromedial oblique
CdL-CrMO	caudolateral–craniomedial oblique	DLPlMO	dorsolateral–plantaromedial oblique
		DMPaLO	dorsomedial–palmarolateral oblique
CdM-CrLO	caudomedial–craniolateral oblique	DMPlLO	dorsomedial–plantarolateral oblique
		DPa	dorsopalmar
CrCd	craniocaudal	DPl	dorsoplantar
D35°PrDDiO	dorso(35°)proximodorsodistal oblique	DPr-PaDiO	dorsoproximal–palmarodistal oblique
D45°PrL-PlDiO	dorso(45°)proximolateral–plantarodistal oblique	LM	lateromedial
		ML	mediolateral
D50°Pr45°L-PaDiMO	dorso(50°)proximo(45°)lateral–palmarodistomedial oblique	PaPr-PaDiO	palmaroproximal–palmarodistal oblique
D60°Pr-PaDiO	dorso(60°)proximal–palmarodistal oblique		

ACKNOWLEDGEMENTS

I am indebted to Luca Cumani and the team at Bedford House Stables for much of what I have learnt about the racehorse during my time in Newmarket. Luca's exacting standards and drive have underpinned the professional development of myself and several colleagues, and instilled in a cadre of younger trainers an intelligence in their approach to veterinary work that will prove an enduring legacy. Working with this next generation has also enriched my professional life and I particularly wish to thank Marco and Lucie Botti, David and Jennie Simcock, Ed Walker, Matt Cumani, Ed Vaughan, Charlie Henson and Guillermo Arizcorreta for having made my job a pleasure and not a chore; the future of Thoroughbred racing in Europe is in safe hands. Thanks also to Mario Baratti, Danny Planas, Gavin Moody, Dermot Barry and all the other assistant trainers, farriers, head lads and lasses at the front line of veterinary care with whom I work on a daily basis.

Thanks to Ian and Karen Cox, who set me on this path of a lifetime spent with horses. Also to Ian Gollan, Bruce Campey and Michael Yates, who were instrumental in shaping my choice of career, and to the late Ken Ferguson and his partners Keith Jones and Alistair Lees for their encouragement in its early stages.

I thank Mike Shepherd, whose unrivalled work ethic and good humour are a great tonic to those around him, and all my colleagues past and present in Newmarket from whom I have both learnt and drawn inspiration, particularly Rob Pilsworth, Peter Rossdale, Neil Steven, Lewis Smith, Andrew McGladdery, Deidre Carson, Marcus Head, Sarah Powell and Celia Marr. Thanks also to all the support team (secretaries, nurses, laboratory, pharmacy and yard staff) at Beaufort Cottage Stables and Rossdales Equine Hospital and Diagnostic Centre, who have assisted me over the years; although too numerous to list individually, all have contributed to a great collaborative environment that continues to foster veterinary excellence. Thanks to Lorraine Palmer for her help on perennial research projects, Mary Black for holding many a horse and to Sarah Powell, Lewis Smith, Emily Haggett, Marcus Head and Josie Meehan for image contributions. Also thanks to Jill Northcott, Peter Beynon and Kate Nardoni for their assistance during the production of this book, to Rob Pilsworth and Scott Pierce for taking the time to review it, and to Ray Wilhite for anatomical illustrations.

Finally, and most importantly, to Sarah for her patience, selflessness and support throughout the course of this project.

Dedication

It is only fitting that I dedicate this book to my parents, who have seen so little of me these past years and to whom quite simply I owe everything.

Part 1
INJURIES AND CONDITIONS OF THE MUSCULOSKELETAL SYSTEM

CHAPTER **1**   Injury management and rehabilitation

CHAPTER **2**   Regional musculoskeletal conditions

CHAPTER 1
INJURY MANAGEMENT AND REHABILITATION

INTRODUCTION

All athletes, whether equine or human, are susceptible to a range of orthopaedic injuries during training and competition. By definition, training for any athletic pursuit involves progressive overloading of the musculoskeletal system in readiness for competition, during which limits of fitness and strength are tested.

In common with all sports, horseracing has a range of discipline-specific injuries that may occur in the training population. These are a function both of the biomechanical demands of racing and the physical characteristics of the racehorse, and although injury patterns may vary with training style or local conditions, the genetic and physical uniformity of the Thoroughbred population ensures a similar spectrum of pathology regardless of geographical location. Many of these injuries are unique to racehorses, while others can be found in the wider equine population.

Most racehorse injuries occur during training rather than racing. The majority of these result simply in temporary interruption or modification to exercise rather than in curtailment of career; the proportion of injuries that result in fatality is very small. The overall prevalence of injury in horseracing compares favourably to that seen in some human athletic populations (e.g. military recruits and track and field athletes); however, the consequences of injury at high speed can be much more serious in horses. Key responsibilities of the racehorse clinician include early recognition of pathology and risk management to safeguard the musculoskeletal health of the individual racehorse and prevent catastrophic injury.

Causes of injury

Musculoskeletal injuries can involve bone, joints and soft-tissue structures such as tendons, ligaments and muscles. Injuries may arise from a single acute overloading event but far more commonly they are the result of cumulative damage built up over a period of weeks or months. This applies particularly to bone injuries (including fracture); the great majority of serious fractures that occur in racehorses are associated with pre-existing pathology.

Bone is a dynamic, living tissue that adapts architecturally ('remodelling') to the loads imposed on it throughout training. Below a certain threshold this adaptation is a healthy and necessary process that involves both bone resorption and laying down of new bone. However, when training volumes are excessive or do not allow for recovery, the process may become maladaptive such that bone repair cannot keep pace with deterioration. Accumulated microdamage caused by continued cyclical loading at predilection sites may lead to development of cortical cracks and, ultimately, complete fracture in some circumstances. Bone weakened in this manner may also be susceptible to failure when high strains are imposed upon it during high-intensity (fast gallop/racing) exercise or when muscular fatigue forces the affected bone to take a greater share of the impact load. These stress fractures may be encountered across a spectrum of severity from subclinical to catastrophic.

Epidemiology

The majority (approximately 80%) of musculoskeletal injuries occur in training rather than at the racetrack. The risk of fracture, however, is much greater when a horse is racing than training because of the greater intensity of workload experienced on the racetrack. When training and racing are both considered, the overall fracture incidence rate is approximately 1/100 horse months (i.e. 1 fracture/month for every 100 horses in training). More than 75% of horses sustaining non-fatal fractures will race again; stress fractures involving the front cannon, pelvis and tibia are the most common individual injuries in flat racing, with osteochondral injuries of the middle carpal and fetlock joints also being important.

Less than 5% of musculoskeletal injuries (and <10% of fractures) are fatal. The majority of catastrophic injuries predominantly involve the fetlock or its support structures, and most occur in the forelimb. Risk of fatality is greater in jump racing than flat racing and reflects the increased likelihood of falling, as well as the longer distances raced (*Table 1.1*). Not all fatalities are the result of fracture, with up to 20% caused by cardiovascular or respiratory incidents.

Risk factors

Individual susceptibility

- Genetic susceptibility to injury likely to be a factor, but has not been quantified and heritable basis unknown.
- Certain conformational faults are associated with greater risk of some injuries (Chapter 12, p. 313); dependent on severity.
- Early-life factors (nutritional imbalances, restricted exercise) may affect soundness in training.

Age

- 2 YO more likely (approximately 3 times) to sustain musculoskeletal injury than older horses (training and racing); largely due to first exposure to conditioning programme rather than immaturity.
- Risk of musculoskeletal injury declines with age, but risk of catastrophic fracture increases.

Training and speed

- Likelihood of injury is lower with appropriate conditioning.
- Different injury types often associated with particular stage of training/level of exercise intensity.
- Injury patterns and rates vary between trainers.
- Cumulative fast exercise without sufficient allowance for rest and repair (particularly if over short period of time) increases risk of catastrophic injury.
- Horses also at greater risk if they have undertaken no fast work in the 30-day period prior to a race engagement (bones poorly conditioned).
- Training to fatigue is a risk factor for injury: muscle activity normally serves to dampen loading forces on limb and when muscles fatigue, greater strains are experienced by bones/joints/tendons/ligaments.

Track surface and condition

- Loads imposed on limb are the primary factor involved in development of acute and fatigue injuries.
- Track surface, type and condition affect magnitude and rate of loading.
- Vertical load at foot impact determined by compactability/hardness of surface.
- Equally important: horizontal shear stress caused by deceleration of hoof within track surface. Surfaces with high cohesion (shear strain) restrict hoof slide; low cohesion limits support during propulsion phase.
- Deceleration is more rapid on harder tracks, resulting in higher peak impact force and higher frequency vibrations through hoof and limb: greater risk of injury.
- Soft/deep track surface: lower peak forces but more tiring (and slower) ground and, when very deep, may result in greater strains in flexor tendon during late stance phase.
- Hoof–track interaction can also be influenced by shoe type.

- Turf: greater risk of fracture and tendon strain with firmer ground. Most common catastrophic racing injury on turf is proximal phalangeal (P1) fracture.
- Dirt: risk of fracture increases with muddier conditions. Most common catastrophic injury on dirt and synthetic tracks is biaxial sesamoid bone fracture.
- Overall risk of fatal injury is consistently lower on turf tracks than on synthetic or dirt tracks.
- Track maintenance and firmness is at least as important a risk factor for injury as track surface type.

Track geometry

- Influence of track geometry: strain is greatest on outside leg in turns. Greater strains with smaller turn radius, but can be limited by banking (optimal camber not known, but 6% is current preferred maximum).
- Uphill tracks may increase risk of hindlimb stress injury: greater peak forces in hindlimb and increased stride frequency (more loading cycles).

Orthopaedic medications

- Most serious racetrack fractures arise from pre-existing pathology.
- Inappropriate use of analgesic/anti-inflammatory measures (systemic and intra-articular medications, shockwave, cold therapy) may impair recognition of early warning signs of impending injury and permit pathology to progress closer to catastrophic failure during racing or fast work.

Risk management and prevention

Musculoskeletal injury has welfare and career implications for affected individual horses as well as economic impact on yard and owners of lost training days and racing opportunities. Halting the progression of injury at an early pathological stage can shorten rehabilitation periods and reduce the incidence of catastrophic fractures. As there is currently no practical screening tool for fracture detection that can be universally applied to the population at large, trainer and veterinary education and vigilance is of great importance. While total mitigation of risk is unrealistic, minimizing injury rates and reducing the severity of those injuries that do occur should be achievable with consideration of the following:

- Applying safer exercise regimes to optimize bone conditioning and readiness for high-intensity work.
- Exercise regimes that allow for individual variation in maturity and response to training: avoid imposing inappropriate training goals.
- Regular assessment of conditions and safety of local training tracks.
- Recognition that conditioning response differs between track types; reduction in workload when changing to new surface is advisable.
- Greater vigilance at stages of training considered 'high risk' for particular injuries.
- Familiarization with features of individual horses' action throughout the training season permits recognition of new/uncharacteristic lameness.
- 'Risk assessment' of lameness through targeted application of diagnostic blocking +/− imaging where necessary.

Table 1.1 **Fatalities per 1,000 starts**

	UK	USA	AUSTRALIA
Flat racing	0.4–0.9	1.4–1.9	0.33–0.44
Hurdle racing	4.9	3.1	6
Steeplechasing	6.7		8.3

- Many fetlock condylar fractures can be detected before serious (surgical) injury occurs through use of flexed dorsopalmar radiographic projection (**Figures 1.1a, b**) or MRI.
- Avoid non-targeted intra-articular or systemic analgesic medications that may mask impending injury.
- Pre-race inspections.

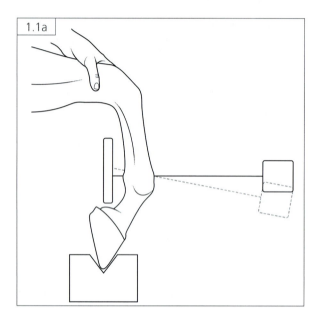

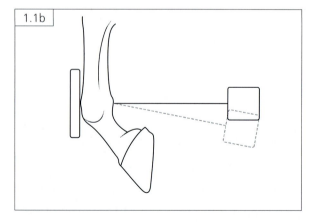

Figs. 1.1a, b Radiographic positioning for flexed dorsopalmar (forelimb) (a) and plantarodorsal (hindlimb) (b) fetlock projections.

ACUTE CARE AND WOUND MANAGEMENT

Injury management on the track
Assessment

The clinician attending an injured horse on the track must rapidly assess and manage both the injury and the immediate situation to ensure the safety of the rider, other personnel, the public and other horses. If not already aware, ground staff should be notified to implement closure of the track and mobilization of horse recovery transport if required. The injured horse is often excitable and may be unaware of its injury, and immediate administration of a sedative will facilitate safe assessment/stabilization.

Determining whether an injury is catastrophic or potentially treatable is generally straightforward (see Appendix 3: Guide to best practice for humane destruction in emergency situations). The clinician's primary responsibility is the welfare of the horse and if assessment determines the presence of an injury that is incurable, causing excessive pain and for which no other options of treatment are available at the time, immediate euthanasia on humane grounds may be warranted. Informed consent for euthanasia should be obtained from the trainer/owner but unnecessary delay avoided. At a race meeting, euthanasia should preferably be conducted behind screens or vehicles. In the case of a catastrophic injury an insured horse should be positively identified and an independent postmortem examination undertaken to document findings.

If uncertainty exists over the severity or potential to treat an injury, a second opinion should be obtained or the horse stabilized and removed to appropriate premises such as a surgical facility for further assessment. Euthanasia may be conducted at the request of the owner at any point regardless of injury status; however, connections should be advised that to do so without meeting recognized criteria for immediate humane destruction might invalidate any potential insurance claim. In cases requiring life-saving surgical or medical intervention, economic considerations are a matter for negotiation between the insurance company and the owner (not the veterinary surgeon).

Stabilization

Fracture management takes priority over dressing of skin wounds. Fractures should (if appropriate) be stabilized to prevent further injury and permit the horse to be safely transported using the guidelines shown in *Table 1.2*.

Commercially available dorsal splints (Kimzey Leg Saver) are applied over a light dressing and are rapidly applied to fetlock injuries in the field. Although this type of splint provides dorsopalmar rather than mediolateral stabilization (therefore considered more ideal for pastern rather than condylar fractures of fetlock), little difference is noted in practice and they are satisfactory for use in all fetlock injuries.

Transport

- Once fracture has been stabilized, analgesic medication +/− sedative drugs may be administered to facilitate transport.
- Consider local stabling for unstable pelvic fractures at risk of catastrophic internal haemorrhage (poor candidates for long-distance transport).
- Transport vehicle should be brought as close to horse as possible to minimize distance walked.
- Low-loading horse ambulance with ramp is preferable; horse can be walked forward off ambulance on arrival at destination.

Table 1.2 Guidelines for stabilizing fractures for transport or to prevent further injury

Fetlock/pastern (forelimb)	Dorsal splint (Kimzey Leg Saver) for alignment of bony column (cannon/P1/P2), or immobilizing (Robert Jones) bandage with palmar and lateral splints.
Fetlock/pastern (hindlimb)	Dorsal splint (Kimzey Leg Saver) or Robert Jones bandage with plantar and lateral splints. Only partial alignment of bony column possible due to reciprocal apparatus of hindlimb, and horse may resent movement.
Mid-forelimb fracture (mid-cannon to lower forearm)	Robert Jones bandage with lateral and caudal splints. Splints extend from ground to top of elbow (lateral splint to above shoulder for injuries of forearm).
Mid-hindlimb fracture (cannon and hock)	Robert Jones bandage with lateral and caudal splints (to top of hock).
Elbow	Robert Jones bandage with caudal splint from ground to elbow. Stabilizes carpus and allows weight bearing.
Tibia (only if complete/unstable fracture)	Robert Jones bandage with lateral splint from ground to hip.
Fractures above shoulder or stifle	Splinting is contraindicated in most cases.

- Horse facing forward (for hindlimb fractures) or backward (forelimb) offers little practical advantage for injury stabilization.
- Adjustable partitions useful to support both flanks during transit.
- Non-slip floors (or wood shavings).

The recumbent horse

Management of the recumbent horse can be challenging. Several diverse conditions can cause a horse to fail to rise, and examination may be complicated by limited resources in the field and close proximity of the public. The circumstances leading up to recumbency and observation of the horse's ability to make attempts to rise may assist assessment.

Background
- Obtain information on nature of fall or incident.
- Recumbency in jump racing after a fall is relatively common and when in the latter stages of a race is often simply caused by horse being 'winded'. These horses lie still with laboured breathing and generally rise uneventfully within 20 minutes.
- Failure to rise when encouraged to do so (when breathing has normalized) or further collapse indicates a condition more complicated than simple hypoxia/exhaustion.
- When exhaustion is considered an unlikely cause of collapse, possible musculoskeletal injury should be investigated.
- When a recumbent horse is encountered in a stable or field there is generally little background information available; possibility of illness as well as injury should be considered.

Initial examination
- Demeanour, consciousness (pupillary and withdrawal reflexes), mucous membrane colour, pulse and respiration rate give some indication of nature/severity of problem.
- Poor mucous membrane colour/rapid pulse (HR >60 bpm) and deteriorating vital signs may indicate catastrophic internal bleeding.

Musculoskeletal examination
- Assessment of musculoskeletal integrity, particularly that of pelvis and back, can be difficult in a recumbent horse.
- Assess neck, back, uppermost side of pelvis and all four distal limbs (without moving horse) for obvious fracture or instability.
- Tightness of gluteal/caudal thigh muscles may indicate exertional rhabdomyolysis.
- Using ropes, horse may be rolled onto opposite side and assessment of limbs/pelvis undertaken as above. This may stimulate attempts to rise.
- Rectal examination of pelvis for obvious instability or internal haematoma indicating fracture.
- If limbs/pelvis appear intact, horse may be encouraged to rise.

Examination: neurological
- Neurological reflexes tested to identify site of any neurological dysfunction.
- Reflexes typically subdued in a stressed/recently exercised horse; full assessment may be hindered during initial 30 minutes to 2 hours following incident.
- If fully conscious but unable to move hindlimbs +/− forelimbs: vertebral fracture with spinal involvement likely.
- Spinal injury in cranial neck: only able to raise head; exaggerated withdrawal reflex all four limbs.
- Spinal injury C6–T2: only able to raise head and neck; absence of forelimb withdrawal reflex.
- Spinal injury caudal to T2: can dog-sit; loss of skin sensation over trunk (if T2–L4: exaggerated hindlimb withdrawal reflex).

Management
- 'Winded' horse: nasal insufflation with oxygen.
- Catastrophic limb or vertebral fracture: immediate euthanasia.
- Comatose/semi-comatose: may recover if not deteriorating; fixed/dilated pupils associated with poor prognosis and warrants euthanasia.
- When the reason for recumbency remains uncertain following preliminary investigation and the condition is not deteriorating, anti-inflammatory drugs (corticosteroids and NSAIDs) should be administered and removal to a quieter location (drag mat and transport) recommended.
- Euthanasia if still recumbent and para- or tetraplegic after 1–2 hours.

Skin wounds

The approach to treatment of skin wounds is determined primarily by anatomical location, severity and involvement of adjacent/underlying structures. Choice of wound repair and bandaging is often geared towards minimizing interruption to training.

Assessment of wounds
- Determine proximity to important underlying structures (joints/tendon sheaths/tendons).
- Injury to deeper structures may not always be visible through skin wound when limb is in weight-bearing position: wound should also be explored with limb flexed.
- Suspected synovial involvement warrants synoviocentesis.
- Exploration of wound +/– ultrasonography/radiography to ensure no foreign body present.

Management
- Primary wound closure through suturing/stapling results in faster healing and better cosmetic outcome.
- 'Clean' wounds: 'golden' period for primary wound closure is approximately 4 hours (>4 hours: significant bacterial contamination and greater likelihood of eventual wound breakdown).
- Small (<1 cm) cuts/abrasions/flaps on lower leg are generally not repaired: clean wound and wet poultice for initial 12–24 hours plus continued exercise.
- Larger cuts: irrigate and full or partial primary closure (staples/sutures).
- Falling/stumbling/road injuries: partial- or full-thickness abrasions over front of fetlock or carpal regions (**Figures 1.2a, b**). Skin loss usually prevents primary closure and most important consideration is to rule out synovial involvement. Fetlock wounds: initial wet poultice then bandage for exercise. Carpal and proximal limb wounds may be left unbandaged. May require antibiotic therapy.
- Wound cleansing/irrigation: may use tap water, tap water saline, dilute (0.1–0.2%) povidone–iodine or chlorhexidine (0.05%).
- Sutures are preferred for areas under high tension (greater strength).

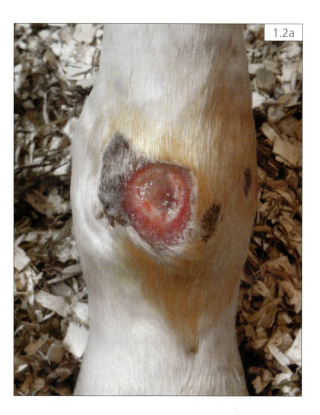

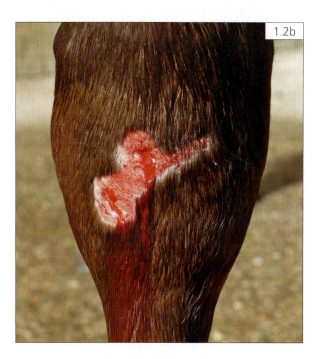

Figs. 1.2a, b Examples of road wounds to the hind fetlock (a) and carpus (b).

- Staples can be applied quickly and often without need for administering drugs; are preferred for low-tension wounds.
- Puncture wounds may be troublesome as infection is seeded in deeper tissues and little opportunity for drainage.
- Major wounds sometimes best treated under general anaesthesia (GA): permits better debridement, irrigation and repair.

Wound dressings and exercise
- Bandaging assists healing by minimizing wound movement and contamination and providing conditions (warm, moist) conducive to repair.
- Acute phase: antiseptic contact dressings can reduce surface contamination and assist healing.
- Frequency of dressing change dependent on amount of exudate.
- Once healthy granulation tissue bed has formed, little need for antibiotic therapy.
- Exercise during healing phase: dependent on severity of initial injury, type of repair and desire to avoid wound breakdown.
- Horses with wounds at 'high stretch' sites may require removal from ridden exercise until sutures/staples removed at 10–14 days.
- Horses with many other repaired wounds, including those on the upper limb, can remain in work with little risk of wound breakdown.

Proud flesh
- Infilling of wound cavity with granulation tissue is normal part of repair process.
- Infection/wound movement inhibits wound edge contraction and stimulates granulation tissue production.
- Wounds on lower limb more prone to development of proud flesh due to greater contamination and relative lack of supportive tissue underlying the skin.
- Non-healing wounds should be investigated for possible presence of foreign body, bone sequestrum or infection.
- Treatment: topical corticosteroid cream plus bandaging +/− antibiotic therapy until granulation tissue back to level of surrounding wound edge.
- Topical astringents such as zinc sulphate useful for limiting granulation tissue proliferation (used in preference to caustic agents such as copper sulphate/silver nitrate, which can harm wound edges and delay healing).
- Initial debulking by surgical trimming useful in some circumstances (granulation tissue is free of sensory innervation and can be excised without analgesia).

Bone sequestration
- Thin outer lining of bone (periosteum) supplies blood to outer cortex and serves as an osteogenic organ to assist healing, particularly following fracture.
- Damage to periosteum (direct cortical trauma/ local infection) can cause disruption to blood supply of underlying bone, resulting in separation of an avascular bone sequestrum from the underlying parent bone.
- Occurs most commonly in cannon (metacarpal/ metatarsal) region (poor protective covering of soft tissue).
- Causes non-healing wound +/− draining tract +/− lameness.
- Diagnosis is by radiography: signs typically delayed >2 weeks following initial injury (**Figure 1.3**).
- Treatment: antibiotic therapy (2–4 weeks oxytetracycline) resolves most cases.
- Surgical debridement often advocated as treatment of choice, but rarely necessary and post-surgical wound management can interfere with training.

Wounds involving tendon/ligament
Assessment
- Most commonly involve the hindlimb and are sustained during racing.
- Deep wounds overlying tendons/ligaments should be assessed clinically/ultrasonographically to determine the extent of the injury.
- Injury to tendon may not be immediately apparent at level of wound until the limb is raised/flexed.
- Concurrent involvement of digital tendon sheath possible with injuries in the fetlock region.

Management

- Suspected tendon laceration: leg should be dressed and splinted with fetlock in slight flexion for transport to surgical facility.
- Tendons heal at a slow rate and repair never results in re-creation of completely normal tendon tissue.
- Repair of wounds involving paratenon/tendon often complicated by independent movement of tendon through granulation tissue; immobilization (casting) may be beneficial.
- Partially lacerated tendon: limb immobilization for up to 6 weeks.
- Lacerated tendon: limb immobilization +/− suture repair of tendon.
- Superficial injuries to tendons/ligaments require less recuperation time than comparable tendon strain (p. 24).
- Rehabilitation guided by ultrasonographic reassessment.
- Prognosis for return to full athletic function is considerably better for hindlimb than for forelimb: complete laceration of hindlimb superficial digital flexor tendon (SDFT) does not preclude return to training.

Interference injuries

Traumatic skin/soft-tissue injuries sustained at exercise have characteristic features depending on the type of interference; individual management is determined principally by the severity/depth of the injury. Sporadic/accidental injuries may be attributed to deep track surface, freshness of horse or inattentive rider, while recurrent injuries may arise from conformation faults, poor shoeing or lameness.

Overreach

- Occurs when back of forelimb struck by back foot.
- Typically involves a single heel (injuries to back of fetlock/pastern or cannon uncommon).
- Varies in depth/severity: superficial grazes to deep flap wounds.
- Most commonly: superficial flap of skin/hoof at heel bulb coronet (**Figure 1.4**). Often deeply embedded with dirt and may be lame if infected or when exercised on deep track.

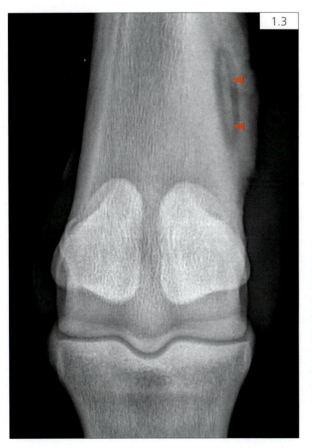

Fig. 1.3 Radiograph (DPa) showing typical bone sequestrum (arrowheads) of the forelimb cannon bone.

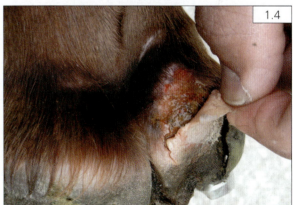

Fig. 1.4 Typical overreach injury.

- Management: initial wet poultice to clean site, thereafter keep open. Flap may be excised if pocketing dirt. Antibiotic therapy if local infection develops.
- Prevention (if recurrent problem): overreach boots +/– altered shoeing (change in forelimb breakover achieved by either using rolled toe shoe or shoeing front feet with aluminium plates and hind feet with steel shoes).

Brushing
- Cuts/abrasions/knocks on inside of pastern/fetlock caused by interference with opposite limb (**Figure 1.5**). Usually sustained at faster paces.
- When on forelimb: usually with base narrow/toe out conformation.
- When on hindlimb: often result of a close/'plaiting' hindlimb action or bilateral hindlimb lameness.
- Prevention (forelimb): exercise bandages/shoeing to redirect breakover laterally.
- Prevention (hindlimb): exercise bandages/change of shoeing: 3/4 shoe (less shoe to catch) or lateral trailer (pivots toe laterally)/management of concurrent lameness. Hindlimb interference may diminish with strengthening through training/maturity.

Medial fetlock interference injury
- Single/repetitive blunt injury to inside of forelimb fetlock may cause acute inflammation and lead to persistent subcutaneous thickening/acquired bursa over the medial sesamoid bone (**Figure 1.6**).
- Subsequent prominence of site may predispose to further recurrent trauma.

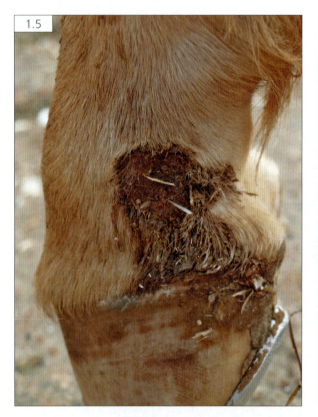

Fig. 1.5 Brushing injury of the hind pastern.

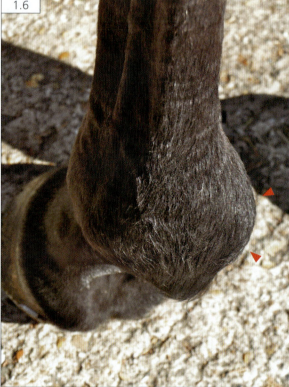

Fig. 1.6 Medial fetlock interference injury. Note the prominence of the medial sesamoid region (arrowheads).

- Varies in severity: may initially be intensely painful to palpate but lameness generally mild.
- Exposed position of palmar nerve over sesamoid bone makes it susceptible to trauma: focal neuritis.
- Usually occurs with base narrow/toe out conformation.
- Can be differentiated from more serious injuries (suspensory ligament branch [SLB] desmopathy, sesamoid bone fracture) on clinical grounds and response to treatment.
- Management: systemic/topical anti-inflammatory +/− antibiotic medication. Slow resolution of swelling is typical.
- Exercise bandages may prevent recurrence of trauma in some cases.
- Long-standing seromas can be treated with intrabursal steroid administration.

'Speedy' cuts

- Short lacerations on inside of one or both hocks/hind cannons (**Figure 1.7**) caused by front foot/same side or opposite hindlimb.
- Generally require only topical wound management and do not interfere with training.

Scalping

- Injury to front of hind pastern caused by striking the front foot.
- Prevention: subtle alteration of breakover of front feet or hind feet often sufficient to prevent limbs meeting during exercise. Change in forelimb breakover achieved by either using rolled toe shoe or shoeing front feet with aluminium plates and hind feet with steel shoes.

Tendon knock/bandage 'bow' or 'bind'

- Subcutaneous swelling over back of forelimb tendon bundle noted after exercise or when bandages removed.
- May result from blunt trauma or tight/slipped bandage.
- Clinically may resemble SDFT tendinitis in acute phase and ultrasonography may be warranted to assess integrity of tendon (typically reveals thickened subcutaneous/peritendinous tissues) (**Figure 1.8**). Focal damage to tendon may occur but is rare.

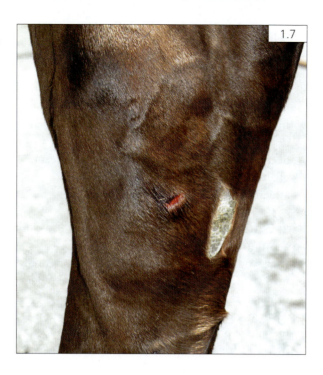

Fig. 1.7 'Speedy' cut on the inside of a hock.

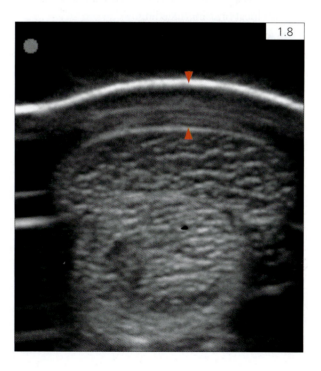

Fig. 1.8 Ultrasonogram (transverse) of a tendon knock/bandage 'bow' or 'bind'. Note the thickening of subcutaneous tissues (arrowheads).

- Self-resolving, although systemic and topical anti-inflammatory measures may assist return to normal appearance; rest not usually required. Tendon damage may necessitate rehabilitation depending on severity.
- In rare cases of severe bandage 'bow' (prolonged or overtight bandage application), avascular necrosis of tendon +/− overlying skin may occur: guarded to poor prognosis for return to full athletic function.

Kick wounds

Assessment
- Kick wounds sustained at exercise most commonly involve the forearm (**Figure 1.9**), point of shoulder or upper hindlimb.
- Many occur during warm-up exercise and by time of presentation the horse will have exercised (therefore possible to judge presence of orthopaedic injury).
- Most are benign and of little concern.
- Skin wounds usually small (<5 cm) and associated with local bruising/bleeding.
- Synovial involvement is rare.
- Wounds directly overlying bone may require radiographic assessment depending on presence of lameness.

Management
- Wound closure generally not required due to small size and location in area of high mobility.
- Antibiotic +/− anti-inflammatory therapy if local infection develops.
- Horses with uncomplicated wounds can generally remain in ridden exercise.
- Injuries at sites with little muscle protection may result in local bone sequestration or (rarely) cortical fracture: inner aspect of radius/tibia most susceptible.
- Possibility of fracture should be investigated if degree (or persistence) of lameness inconsistent with local infection.
- Radiological evidence of fracture propagation may not be apparent until 1–2 weeks post injury.
- Suspected fracture: stable rest (+/− hand walking to manage any concurrent cellulitis) until confirmation.

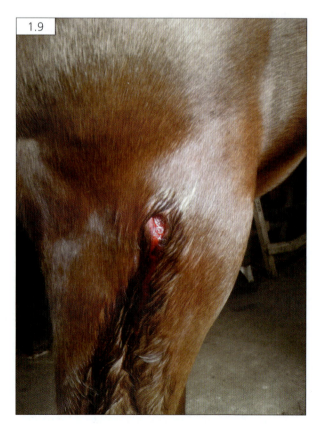

Fig. 1.9 Typical kick injury to the elbow.

Synovial infection

Infection within a synovial space (joint or synovial bursa) is potentially a life-threatening condition. Unless recognized and treated promptly and aggressively, persistent infection of the synovial space or irreversible destruction of articular tissue may occur, leading to lameness that may be incompatible with athletic or non-athletic future. Wounds in the region of synovial cavities or lameness that might be attributable to synovial sepsis should be investigated without delay. Infections resulting from direct wound contamination usually involve mixed bacterial species, while iatrogenic infections (following intra-articular injection) most commonly involve *Staphylococcus aureus*.

Assessment
- Acute-onset, moderate–severe lameness.
- Not invariably associated with obvious wound or history of trauma.
- Marked effusion of affected joint +/− localized cellulitis usually noted.
- Infection of anatomically well-protected joints/bursae (e.g. navicular bursa) may be associated with little palpable abnormality.
- Synoviocentesis: collection of synovial fluid sample for cytological analysis +/− through-and-through needle lavage to assess wound communication.
- Synovial sample: total white blood cell (WBC) count >10 x 10^9/l (10,000/µl), total protein >50 g/l (5 g/dl) and toxic/degenerative cytological change strongly indicative of infection.

Management
- Hospitalization and prompt treatment improves outcome.
- Large-volume lavage of synovial cavity (frequently under GA) plus antibiotic therapy (systemic/regional perfusion) to clear bacterial contamination and debris.
- With appropriate management, prognosis for survival to discharge is good (>80%) and return to athletic use fair (>50%).
- Poorer prognosis with concurrent bone/tendon/ligament involvement.

MANAGEMENT OF JOINT DISEASE

Applied anatomy
Joints facilitate the transfer of load between bones. In most cases this involves repetitive movement in one or more planes; in order to minimize wear and distribute load evenly, a near frictionless environment is required.

Joint stability
Excessive or abnormal movements are limited passively by the geometric 'fit' between adjoining bones as well as the support structures such as the joint capsule, collateral ligaments and surrounding tendons. Active stability is provided by muscular activity and mediated by proprioceptive nerve endings. In a healthy joint the intrasynovial pressure is usually subatmospheric (influenced by synovial fluid volume and degree of extension/flexion), which also assists stability.

Joint capsule
The joint capsule is a dense fibrous structure lined with synovial membrane that in addition to stabilizing the joint acts as a seal for joint fluid. The capsule forms a sleeve around the joint and is anchored on adjoining bones through specialized fibrocartilaginous attachments. Thickness varies with location and function, with most joint capsules incorporating some stabilizing ligaments.

Cartilage
Articular (hyaline) cartilage lines the articulating surfaces of opposing bones and along with lubricating synovial fluid serves to provide frictionless movement. Articular cartilage varies in structure both between different joints and different weight-bearing locations within individual joints, but is essentially a high water-content matrix of collagen fibrils and proteoglycans. Cartilage is avascular and the cartilage cells (chondrocytes) that produce matrix receive their nutrition by diffusion from synovial fluid within the joint.

Synovial membrane
Secretory lining on the inner surface of the joint capsule; covers all internal joint surfaces apart from articular cartilage. Produces hyaluronic acid and other components of synovial fluid; mediates nutrient exchange between blood and joint.

Synovial fluid

Synovial fluid acts both as a lubricant to facilitate frictionless joint movement and as a transport medium for nutrition of articular cartilage. It is a filtrate of plasma and derives its viscosity from hyaluronic acid; volume and viscosity vary between joints.

Joint pain

Pain perception from the joint comes from several sources. The joint capsule is richly innervated both superficially and deeply with low-threshold mechanoreceptor nerve endings; mechanical stimuli and increased intra-articular pressure (from joint distension) can therefore contribute to the development of lameness. Higher threshold mechanoreceptors are found near the bony insertions of articular ligaments. Synovial and capsular pain receptors (nociceptors) have a high threshold for pain perception in normal joints, but the chemical stimuli associated with osteoarthritis (OA) and synovitis can reduce this tolerance. Pain in many equine orthopaedic conditions arises from the highly innervated subchondral bone rather than the joint itself: loading of the joint leads to raised intra-osseous fluid pressure (and therefore pain) at sites of osteochondral damage.

Joint injury and repair

Damage to articular cartilage can arise from a single traumatic event, however OA in the racehorse is more typically the result of chronic repetitive overloading and an imbalance between damage and repair. Degradation of matrix causes swelling and softening of cartilage and loss of normal mechanical function, leading to fibrillation/erosion and associated changes in underlying subchondral bone. This is sometimes accompanied by an inflammatory response with excessive joint fluid of reduced viscosity. Secondary interruption to normal functioning of the synovial lining of the joint can lead to chronic joint effusion.

Articular cartilage has no direct blood supply and therefore a limited ability to repair itself. Return to full structural integrity and normal function depends on depth, severity and location of injury. Partial-thickness injuries generally do not heal. Full-thickness defects may benefit from the blood supply of underlying bone, but typically repair with fibrocartilage (mechanically inferior to articular cartilage).

Chronic joint injury may result in proliferation of soft tissue and bone at joint margins (osteophytes/'bone spurs'), in part as a response to joint instability. These changes may predispose to fragmentation or chip fracture of articular margins.

Management of joint disease

The diagnosis and severity of injury largely determine appropriate management. The approach to acute injuries (synovitis, osteochondral fragmentation) or those associated with risk of fracture may differ considerably from that taken with chronic/long-standing joint disease. Goals of treatment include returning affected joint/s to normal function as rapidly as possible, optimizing the long-term health of joint/s by limiting progression of disease, and managing pain/lameness to permit continuation of training. The main methods available to achieve this are described below.

Exercise modification

The diagnosis and chronicity of injury determine whether exercise modification is required, and the optimum rest/rehabilitation period. In many cases of low-grade or chronic joint pathology rest is neither curative nor desirable. Continued training in some circumstances may be aided by the use of treadmill or swimming exercise, or tracks with surface/geometry considered sympathetic to the particular injury.

Physical therapy

Acute synovitis may benefit from cold therapy and topical anti-inflammatory measures. Physical therapy is generally of little use in chronic joint conditions; however, regular cold therapy is widely used and is possibly beneficial to recovery from fast exercise.

Surgery

The majority of racehorse joint disease is manageable non-surgically. Surgery is not the leading intervention for OA but may be advocated in the treatment of conditions such as chronic proliferative synovitis and certain types of osteochondral fragmentation/fracture in which conservative therapy has proven unrewarding. In these cases debridement of osteochondral defects may improve the prognosis for future soundness. Possible surgical techniques of future interest include cartilage repair and grafting. Arthroscopy may also be useful as a diagnostic procedure in some circumstances.

Intra-articular therapies

Joint disease is often best managed by delivering medication directly to the target site. While intra-articular medications are not considered to 'heal' cartilage, they may be disease or symptom modifying; interference with the inflammatory cascade can break the cycle of cartilage degeneration (and therefore limit joint pain). The goal of intra-articular therapy is long-term preservation of athletic function through protection of cartilage; elimination of lameness is also important to normalize gait and limit overloading of other limbs. Although the relationship between observable lameness at a trot and action/performance at faster paces is not currently known, in the absence of evidence to the contrary it is presumed that managing such lameness is beneficial at some level to the athlete with joint pathology. Most of the available intra-articular therapies exert an influence on cartilage metabolism that persists beyond the time that the product is actually present in the joint.

Objective risks associated with intra-articular medication include introduction of infection into the joint (synovial sepsis) and, in the case of corticosteroids, laminitis. These risks are very low (combined incidence 0–0.04%) in the racing Thoroughbred with appropriate technique/dosing. Some medications may be associated with occasional inflammatory joint 'flare' and justify combination therapy to prevent occurrence. Of greater importance is the potential to mask warning signs of impending fracture through elimination of lameness, and in certain circumstances medication should be used only after undertaking a 'risk assessment' for potential fracture propagation (particularly with fetlock disease).

The main classes of intra-articular medication in common use are corticosteroids, sodium hyaluronate (hyaluronic acid/hyaluronan) and autologous biological ('regenerative') products (*Table 1.3*). Clinical presentation, diagnosis, regulatory constraints and cost are key factors in the choice of appropriate therapy for the individual. Indications for treatment range from reduction of acute inflammation or assisting post-surgical rehabilitation, to controlling chronic lameness in full work. Treatment is often empirical and even in horses with similar pathology there may be considerable individual variation in response; post-medication exercise protocols and interval to remediation should reflect this. A 24-hour rest (stable rest/walk) period following any intra-articular medication is recommended and may prolong the effects of medication.

Table 1.3 Intra-articular medications used for management of joint disease

PRODUCT		ACTION	USE AND EFFICACY
Corticosteroids	Triamcinolone acetonide (TA), methylprednisolone acetate (MPA), betamethasone, dexamethasone.	Strongest anti-inflammatory agents available for intra-articular use and have greatest potential to modify lameness. Anti-inflammatory effects include reduced vascular permeability (joint filling), reduced migration of inflammatory cells and inhibition of pro-inflammatory enzyme release. Relatively short half-life within joint space but can exert prolonged effect on synovial lining and cartilage. TA: may be chondroprotective; no detrimental effects with normal use. Very low risk of laminitis with total body dose of <40 mg. MPA: longest acting but can potentiate cartilage degeneration.	TA: 6–10 mg/joint. Duration of therapeutic effect typically 4–8 weeks. Betamethasone and dexamethasone: less potent and limited efficacy for lameness. MPA efficacious but used infrequently because of prolonged detection time.

(continued overleaf)

Table 1.3 *(continued)*

PRODUCT		ACTION	USE AND EFFICACY
Hyaluronic acid (HA)	Non-sulphated glycosaminoglycan found in synovial fluid and cartilage. Primary function is joint lubrication (determines visco-elasticity of synovial fluid).	Half-life within joint is short (few days in normal joint, few hours in arthritic joint) but exerts prolonged effect on joint health. Primary effect on cartilage and synovial metabolism rather than as replacement for endogenous HA; anti-inflammatory effects and inhibits cartilage degeneration. Correlation between molecular weight/concentration/volume and clinical effect is uncertain; currently not possible to differentiate between products clinically.	Typically used in combination with intra-articular corticosteroid (TA). Efficacy in pain management/improving function: delayed peak effect in humans at 4–8 weeks. Cost-effectiveness (based on clinical effect) questionable.
Autologous biological products ('regenerative therapies')	Autologous conditioned serum/interleukin-1 receptor antagonist protein (ACS/IRAP): disease-modifying OA product; harvested blood incubated with glass spheres, which stimulate leucocytes to produce anti-inflammatory cytokines and growth factors. Platelet-rich plasma (PRP): concentrated platelet (and growth factor)-rich portion of plasma. Mesenchymal stem cells.	ACS/IRAP: disease-modifying protective and anti-inflammatory activity. PRP: growth factors proposed to enhance tissue repair.	ACS/IRAP: variable treatment frequency (single course or regular treatments). Limited analgesic effect but may reduce joint inflammation. PRP: variable treatment frequency. Efficacy undetermined. Both products have benefit of being free of prohibited substances (if peripheral blood also clear at time of harvesting). Scientific validation and standardization of protocols needed. Favourable clinical reports (equine and human) but randomized clinical trials required. Stem cells: efficacy undetermined.
Other disease-modifying OA drugs	Glucosamine. Pentosan polysulphate (frequently in combination proprietary products +/− HA).	Possible disease-modifying protective and anti-inflammatory activity.	Variable treatment frequency. Favourable clinical reports (equine) but randomized clinical trials required.
Anabolic steroids	Stanazolol.	Upregulates collagen synthesis, chondrocyte and osteoblast proliferation and has anti-inflammatory effects *in vitro*	Low-dose (5 mg; 2% of intramuscular 'anabolic' dose) medication administered out of training +/− rest period. Favourable clinical reports (equine) but randomized clinical trials required. Use should adhere to regulatory controls.

There is no single intra-articular therapy that is most appropriate for all joint conditions. Corticosteroids (most commonly triamcinolone acetonide) are the mainstay of intra-articular therapy for OA, frequently used together with sodium hyaluronate (HA): this combination is generally considered to give the best short- to medium-term control of lameness while optimizing joint/cartilage health.

Systemic medications

Systemic medications may be used as an adjunct to other OA therapies (*Table 1.4*). NSAIDs have an established role in managing lameness; however, long-term use or administration without risk assessment for further injury is discouraged. Other systemic medications are proposed to assist cartilage repair; however, strong evidence of efficacy is generally lacking and clinical effect likely to be small.

Table 1.4 Systemic medications used in the management of joint disease

PRODUCT		ACTION	USE AND EFFICACY
Non-steroidal anti-inflammatory drugs (NSAIDs)	Class of drugs with similar action that includes phenylbutazone, meloxicam and aspirin (acetylsalicylic acid).	Inhibit inflammatory pathways. Efficacy greater for pain than inflammation/filling. Aspirin: poor analgesic with short half-life; proposed to improve blood supply in sclerotic bone conditions (decreases platelet aggregation) but little/no supporting evidence.	Useful in acute synovitis; more effective in inflamed than normal tissues. Long-term use discouraged as may mask signs of injury and accelerate cartilage degeneration.
Corticosteroids	Dexamethasone most commonly used for orthopaedic disease.	Potent inhibitor of multiple inflammatory pathways.	Single administration (IV/IM) during acute phase of injury; useful drug for reducing synovitis but poor analgesic.
Polysulphated glycosaminoglycans (GAGs)	Disease-modifying osteoarthritis medication. Derived from bovine trachea.	IM administration results in therapeutic concentrations in joint. No direct analgesic effect. Inhibits inflammatory cascade of OA; also chondroprotective (stimulates HA and collagen production).	Weekly administration (IM) after initial loading course. Reduces severity of experimental OA signs in humans/horses. Clinical effect undetermined.
Pentosan polysulphate	Disease-modifying OA medication. Derived from beechwood hemicellulose.	IM administration results in therapeutic concentrations in joint. No direct analgesic effect. Anti-inflammatory and chondroprotective effects (stimulates HA and proteoglycan production).	Weekly administration (IM). Clinical effect undetermined.
Hyaluronic acid (sodium hyaluronan)	Produced through microbial fermentation.	IV and oral forms. Possible anti-inflammatory effects in joint have been demonstrated after IV/oral administration.	Regular (weekly) IV administration or daily oral use. Clinical effect likely to be small.
Tiludronate	Bisphosphonate drug.	Systemic administration (IV infusion). Acts on bone turnover and has disease-modifying effect in sclerotic and osteopenic bone conditions.	Single or periodic administration. Duration of effect on bone turnover likely to be months. Efficacy undetermined for most equine conditions. Some evidence of increased risk of bone weakening/fracture with prolonged bisphosphonate use in humans.

Nutraceuticals (oral joint supplements)

Nutraceuticals (*Table 1.5*) are dietary supplements with little primary nutritional value that are proposed to assist cartilage healing either through provision of 'building blocks' of cartilage metabolism or interference with the inflammatory cascade of OA. Long-term daily supplementation with products containing one or more of these nutrients is common. Considered safe to use; however, strong supporting evidence of efficacy (humans/equine) is lacking for all products, bioavailability of some products in horses is doubtful and any clinical effect is likely to be small. Use should be considered on cost–benefit grounds.

Topical anti-inflammatory medications

Topical products used to cool or tighten the lower leg are in common use (p. 28). Topical anti-inflammatory drugs intended to achieve therapeutic levels within the joint are a more specific treatment and limited at present to diclofenac. Efficacy with daily/twice daily application appears to be similar to oral NSAID therapy. Topical therapy merits consideration as a management option for OA, but is not in widespread use at present.

Table 1.5 Nutraceuticals used in the management of joint disease

PRODUCT	DESCRIPTION	USE AND EFFICACY
Glucosamine	Precursor of chondrocyte GAG; proposed to have chondroprotective and anti-inflammatory effects. Derived from shellfish/animal/fungal sources.	Conflicting evidence of efficacy in humans; some modification of OA symptoms demonstrated. Biological rationale for use but currently limited evidence of efficacy in horses.
Chondroitin sulphate	'Building block' of cartilage. Derived from bovine trachea.	Conflicting evidence of efficacy in humans; less support for use than glucosamine. Clinical effect likely to be small.
Hyaluronic acid (sodium hyaluronan)	Produced through microbial fermentation.	Limited evidence of efficacy in modifying synovitis/OA.
Avocado/soybean lipids (unsaponifiables)	Anti-inflammatory and possible regenerative effect on cartilage.	Some evidence of efficacy in modifying OA symptoms/disease in humans and horses.
Green-lipped mussel lipids	Contains omega-3 fatty-acids, vitamins and minerals.	Biological rationale for use but limited evidence of efficacy. Clinical effect likely to be small.
Methylsulphonylmethane (MSM)	Proposed to be a source of biologically active sulphur.	Limited evidence of efficacy. Any clinical effect likely to be small.

REHABILITATION

The goal of any rehabilitation programme is to return the racehorse to optimal athletic function while avoiding unnecessary loss of training time and conditioning or risking reinjury. The duration and type of rehabilitation required to return the injured structure to near-normal function differ for bone and soft-tissue injuries. In many instances, more than one approach to treatment may be available for consideration and individual factors such as stage of season and career goals may influence management decisions. Favoured rehabilitation periods for most racehorse injuries have evolved through experience rather than scientific validation and the recommendations in Chapter 2 should be considered as guidelines only.

Prognosis

Prognosis is defined as the prediction of likely outcome of an injury and is derived from both general knowledge of that injury from the larger population and specific clinical details of the individual case being considered. Prognosis is dynamic and may be influenced by factors arising throughout treatment or rehabilitation.

Despite the inherent flaws associated with attempting to predict individual outcome based on population averages, it is useful to categorize prognosis so that trainers/owners can make informed management decisions. The evidence base available to racehorse clinicians to formulate strong guidelines on likelihood of favourable outcome with any particular course of action is very limited; most interventional studies involve small numbers of horses and do not utilize controls. The prognosis recommendations in Chapter 2 therefore draw on relevant published work and clinical experience and, where available, more specific outcome figures are included in the text. These should be considered guidelines only and subject to the circumstances of the individual case as determined by the treating clinician. The likelihood of expected return to full use (if so desired) is categorized in *Table 1.6*.

Table 1.6 **Categorization of the likelihood of expected return to full use following injury**

PROGNOSIS	DESCRIPTION	EXPECTED RETURN TO FULL USE (%)
Excellent	Full recovery to normal function can be expected.	>80
Good	Expect improvement; most recover to full function.	70–80
Fair	Expect improvement; significant chance of insufficient recovery/recurrence/ongoing problems.	60–70
Guarded	Not possible to predict with certainty whether full or partial recovery to full use will occur; recurrence or need for ongoing attention may be expected.	40–60
Poor	Unlikely to recover fully regardless of management; may deteriorate.	<40

Exercise

Rehabilitation typically involves a rest period of variable length to allow initial repair processes to occur, followed by a gradually increasing level of loading exercise to encourage damaged tissue to remodel/strengthen back to optimal function. Many injuries heal satisfactorily when some daily light exercise is permitted rather than complete stable confinement. The need for an initial period of inactivity is determined by injury type/severity and should be prescribed on an individual basis. Horses with mild lameness or stress injuries detected early in the pathological process can often be removed from cantering/fast exercise and safely walked or trotted throughout rehabilitation, while to do so for other injuries might compromise quality or speed of healing.

Stable rest

Stable rest is widely used for the initial post-injury period, although it is not always necessary or ideal for healing of many injuries. Feed energy intake should be reduced and precautions taken to minimize the risk of colonic impaction (Chapter 6, p. 258). It is preferable to feed haylage and avoid straw bedding.

Complete immobilization may be desired for some fractures at high risk of catastrophic displacement. Horses may be tied up to prevent lying down/rising and limit the strains that this imposes on the hindlimbs, although fatigue sometimes results in attempts to lie while restrained, which is also not without risk. In rare circumstances it might be desirable/possible to support the injured horse in a sling for the initial weeks following fracture, although substantial nursing input is required for these cases. When horses are tied up for orthopaedic injury, they should be permitted to feed with their heads down to lower the risk of pleuropneumonia (Chapter 3, p. 233). Regular blood sampling to monitor inflammatory markers is recommended when patients are receiving anti-inflammatory/analgesic medication that can mask pyrexia.

Walking

Some daily low-loading exercise has advantages over complete inactivity for the repair of many musculoskeletal injuries. Choice of in-hand walking or horse-walker exercise is dependent on the type of injury and the horse's temperament. Low-dose sedative medication (acepromazine) may be used to ensure overactivity is avoided.

Paddock turnout

For most injuries controlled exercise is preferable to unrestricted turnout, as even in small pens horses are capable of abrupt motion that can overload the repairing limb. If turnout is utilized during rehabilitation, it should generally not commence until the period when trotting exercise would have resumed. However, when the primary objective is removal from training loads rather than rehabilitation (such as for carpal immaturity), paddock turnout at an earlier stage of the rehabilitation programme is permissible.

Treadmills

Treadmill exercise is useful for the rehabilitation of many injuries. Exercise duration and speed can be tightly controlled and the intensity of workload increased according to the planned programme without the variability and risks inherent to training on the track. A safe and regular treadmill belt surface and an ability to train to faster paces without the weight of a rider avoids unnecessary and irregular loading of the limb and has the potential to improve outcomes of some injuries.

Swimming

Swimming is a cross-training aid that permits low-level aerobic exercise without limb loading (Chapter 13, p. 321). While it permits activity and some retention of fitness during rehabilitation of some injuries, swimming is not appropriate in all circumstances (e.g. considered to be detrimental for AL-SDFT desmopathy). The effect of swimming on the healing of many conditions such as those involving the back/pelvis is undetermined.

Water treadmill/water walker

Water treadmill use in rehabilitation is common but effects on fitness are limited and there is little current evidence of improved healing of orthopaedic injuries.

Rehabilitation: stress fractures
Classifying injuries

Stress fractures may become clinically apparent at any point on the spectrum of severity from early microfailure to complete cortical disruption. As a general rule, injuries that are detected at a more advanced pathological stage (such as when the fracture line has breached the cortex) require longer out of training than those detected at an early 'stress reaction' stage. The severity of the injury also determines the need for surgical fixation or limb immobilization. An important part of planning rehabilitation, therefore, is accurate classification of injury.

Radiography is an inferior technique for classifying stress injuries, as bone changes may either be too subtle for radiographic detection or lag behind the onset of clinical signs by some weeks. Bone scan (gamma scintigraphy) is a technique with good sensitivity for the detection of injury, but is also unsatisfactory for staging progression. MRI is the 'gold standard' modality for injury classification; however, it is currently only feasible to perform standing MRI of the lower limb (fetlock/cannon/lower carpus).

The diagnosis and classification of injuries higher in the limb therefore relies on clinical findings aided by combinations of radiography, ultrasonography or bone scan. This does not generally allow the precise staging of pathology that is possible in human athletes; additionally, humans can communicate the presence and quality of pain experienced during recuperation, permitting appropriate adjustment of exercise intensity. Racehorse clinicians are restricted by the insensitivity of available imaging modalities, and recuperation programmes for many injuries are empirical. As a general rule, however, initial lameness and the rapidity with which it diminishes (with rest) correlate well with the length of rehabilitation required. A broad guide to injury classification is shown in *Table 1.7*.

Table 1.7 **Classification of stress injury severity**

GRADE	LAMENESS*	RADIOGRAPHY	BONE SCAN
1	None/subtle	Normal	Mild IRU
2	Mild–moderate	Normal	Moderate IRU
3	Moderate–marked	Periosteal/endosteal reactive change	Moderate–marked IRU
4	Moderate–marked	Periosteal/endosteal reactive change +/– cortical fracture line	IRU involving more than one cortex
5	Severe	Complete fracture of one/both cortices	Not required

* Unilateral lameness may not always be a feature (due to bilateral pathology).
IRU, increased radiomarker uptake.

Rehabilitation

Recommendations are influenced by grade and location of injury. Stress fractures at anatomical sites that are considered high risk for either catastrophic deterioration or recurrence of injury must be treated more conservatively than injuries at 'low-risk' sites. Some stress fractures (e.g. humeral injuries) may propagate at low levels of exercise and the relative proportion of time spent in stable confinement or walking should be determined on an individual basis. General recommendations are:

- Mild stress injuries (grades 1 and 2):
  - Stable confinement until sound at trot.
  - Return to walking as soon as possible.
  - Monitor soundness at each 'step-up'.
  - Total time out of cantering exercise: 6–8 weeks.
- Moderate stress fractures (grades 2 and 3):
  - 3–4 weeks stable confinement.
  - 3–4 weeks walking.
  - Monitor soundness at each 'step-up'.
  - Total time out of cantering exercise: 9–12 weeks.
- High-risk fractures (graded severe plus potential for catastrophic propagation):
  - Fetlock: consider surgical fixation or bandage immobilization depending on fracture type.
  - Following surgical fixation: 4–8 weeks stable rest/4–6 weeks walking is typical.
  - Pelvis/tibia: consider tying up for initial 4–6 weeks to minimize risk of fracture propagation when moving or rising in the stable. Further 4–6 weeks stable rest/6–8 weeks walking.

Monitoring healing

Monitoring of healing to ensure that it is safe to step a horse back into faster work is desirable, particularly if recuperation times have been minimized due to training targets. Unfortunately, accurate monitoring of bone strength is not possible in the racehorse. Radiography is of little use for most stress injuries, and bone scan activity usually remains elevated after effective healing has taken place. MRI can be used to determine reduction of inflammatory change in the case of fetlock injuries, but is not widely applicable. Therefore, the only practical way to monitor progress is regular clinical evaluation to ensure that lameness does not recur when exercise intensity increases.

During the early rehabilitation period ultrasonographic or radiographic imaging may assist managerial decisions such as appropriate timing to let a cross-tied horse down or resumption of walking or ridden exercise. It is only useful when obvious bone callus or a cortical fracture is present and progression (smoothing) of periosteal modelling can permit estimation of the stage of healing.

Nutrition

Providing the rehabilitating horse is fed a balanced diet with sufficient trace elements and an appropriate calcium–phosphorus ratio, there is little nutritional advantage to be gained from any form of supplementation in respect of bone healing. Carbohydrate (starch) intake should be reduced and free-choice forage made available. Excessive body weight (BWT) gain should be avoided as this may increase loading on the limb (and the need for conditioning) on return to exercise.

Rehabilitation: tendons

The SDFT plays a crucial role in the loading of the forelimb during locomotion, acting both to limit hyperextension of the fetlock at faster paces and as an elastic energy store that contributes to overall efficiency of movement. The repair tissue that replaces the torn collagen type I fibrils of a strained tendon has poorer elastic strength and capacity for repetitive loading under high strains than undamaged tendon. Successful return to injury-free training following a tendon strain is a direct function of how closely the mechanical properties of the recovered tendon approach those of 'normal' tendon. This is determined by the extent of original injury as well as the quality of its repair. Tendon tissue is slow to heal and it is considered that gradual loading as the tendon strengthens encourages remodelling and fibre alignment. Most horses with significant SDFT strains should not return to fast work for 9–12 months following injury.

Classifying injuries

Objective assessment of lesion severity is of use in determining a rehabilitation programme and prognosis. The full extent of the injury is best assessed after the initial swelling subsides (1–3 weeks after the initial signs). The entire tendon should be scanned and cross-sectional areas of tendon and lesion measured at each of seven zones (each approximately 4 cm) from the accessory carpal bone to the fetlock. Tendon echogenicity and fibre alignment are graded in each zone.

Classification of injury: the percentage of tendon volume affected is derived from summation of the lesion cross-sectional area at seven zones throughout the cannon (*Table 1.8*).

Management: acute phase

Management in the initial days aims to limit inflammatory response and minimize the overall extent of injury:
- Topical cold therapy 2–3 times daily.
- +/– initial single administration of systemic corticosteroid to reduce swelling.
- Systemic NSAIDs throughout first week as required.
- Stable bandage (changed twice daily) to limit filling in leg.
- Stable confinement +/– limited hand walking.
- If severe loss of tendon integrity with sinking of fetlock, immobilizing (Robert Jones) bandage may be required during initial weeks.

Management: rehabilitation phase

Gradual reintroduction to controlled exercise is preferable. If turnout is desired, this should only follow on from the walking/trotting phase and should initially be in a small paddock. Treatment protocols are empirical, but the key points are:
- Severity of injury determines recuperation time, but in general at least 6 months out of cantering required.
- Monitoring of healing by serial ultrasound examinations (every 3 months or as required).
- Quality of fibre pattern alignment is an important prognostic indicator for likelihood of reinjury on return to fast work.
- Decrease or stability in size of tendon/size of lesion and increase in echogenicity are main determinants of progress.
- Enlargement of the tendon (by >10%) between scans may indicate excessive loading for the stage of healing and the exercise level should be reduced.
- Training programmes that minimize peak strains/high impact loading in the injured tendon may improve chance of successful return to racing: treadmill (reduced load bearing) and inclined/uphill (lower speeds and SDFT strain) training.

Table 1.8 Classification of equine tendon injury

Mild injury	0–15% tendon volume	<10% lesion size at maximum injury zone
Moderate injury	16–25% tendon volume	10–40% lesion size at maximum injury zone
Severe injury	>25% tendon volume	>40% lesion size at maximum injury zone

Adapted from Smith RKW, McIlwraith CW (2012) Consensus on equine tendon disease: building on the 2007 Havemeyer symposium. *Equine Vet J* **44(1)**:2–6.

Additional interventions

Additional therapies (*Table 1.9*) aimed at reducing the likelihood of tendon reinjury are varied and frequently marketed aggressively. Quality scientific evidence to support these interventions is generally lacking and these therapies should be considered purely as an optional adjunct (rather than an alternative) to a controlled exercise programme.

Table 1.9 Some additional therapies for superficial digital flexor tendon injuries

THERAPY	ACTION	EFFICACY
Intralesional injection: stem cells	Injection of mesenchymal stem, stromal or progenitor cells proposed to improve qualities of healed tendon.	Preliminary evidence of reduced reinjury rate; validation required.
Intralesional injection (other): platelet-rich plasma, insulin-like growth factor-1, poly-sulphated GAG, hyaluronic acid	Various therapies proposed to optimize quality of healing or speed maturation of healing tissue.	Little/no quality evidence of efficacy.
Tendon splitting	Scalpel/needle lancing of core lesion during acute phase may limit physical/enzymatic damage to adjacent tendon tissue.	Little/no quality evidence of efficacy.
Surgery: desmotomy of accessory ligament of the SDFT (AL-SDFT or 'superior check' ligament)	Sectioning of AL-SDFT reduces future load bearing in the SDFT.	Does not reduce risk of reinjury in most cases. Results in redistribution of load-bearing forces: considerable risk of suspensory ligament injury on return to training. Consider for recurrent or severe tendinitis only.
Thermocautery (bar/pin firing)	Intended to cause counter-irritation and stimulate inflammatory response +/− formation of supportive scar tissue.	Not shown to reduce risk of reinjury and ethical concerns limit use.
Pulsed magnetic field therapy	Proposed to modulate inflammation/stimulate cellular repair.	Current evidence does not support use.
Therapeutic ultrasound	Thermal (heating from sound wave absorption) and non-thermal (cavitation) effects.	Conflicting evidence (human studies). No clinical efficacy demonstrated in horses.
Therapeutic laser therapy ('low level'/'cold'/'Class III' laser therapy; 'high-power'/'Class IV' laser therapy).	Potential modulation of inflammatory response and cellular repair.	Conflicting evidence (human studies). No clinical efficacy demonstrated in horses. Possible biological rationale for use.

The exercise programme shown in *Table 1.10* can be used as a general guide, with progression of exercise determined on an individual basis by ultrasonographic re-examinations. A shorter rehabilitation programme may be considered for subtle/mild injuries for which the risk of any reinjury with more rapid return to training is deemed acceptable. In these cases ultrasonographic monitoring throughout the rehabilitation period is the best guide to determining the readiness for increased loading on an individual basis. With satisfactory clinical and ultrasonographic progress, a return to trotting at 8–10 weeks, cantering at 16–20 weeks and fast work at approximately 6 months may be possible.

Table 1.10 **Recommended exercise programmme for superficial digital flexor tendon rehabilitation**

WEEK	EXERCISE	WEEK	EXERCISE
0	Stable confinement	23	30 min walk/15 min trot
1	Stable confinement	24	30 min walk/15 min trot
2	Stable confinement	25	30 min walk/15 min trot
3	10 min walk	26	30 min walk/15 min trot
4	15 min walk	27	25 min walk/20 min trot
5	20 min walk	28	25 min walk/20 min trot
6	20 min walk	29	25 min walk/20 min trot
7	25 min walk	30	25 min walk/20 min trot
8	25 min walk	31	20 min walk/25 min trot
9	30 min walk	32	20 min walk/25 min trot
10	30 min walk	33	15 min walk/30 min trot
11	35 min walk	34	15 min walk/30 min trot
12	35 min walk	35	Resume cantering
13	40 min walk	36	
14	40 min walk	37	
15	40 min walk/5 min trot	38	
16	40 min walk/5 min trot	39	Build up cantering
17	40 min walk/5 min trot	40	
18	40 min walk/5 min trot	41	
19	35 min walk/10 min trot	42	
20	35 min walk/10 min trot	43	
21	35 min walk/10 min trot	44	Resume fast work/galloping
22	35 min walk/10 min trot		

Shading: ultrasonographic re-examination recommended.

Physical therapy

Physical therapies may be used to limit inflammation and further tissue damage during the acute phase following injury, to modulate the healing response in order to optimize the return to full normal function, and to manage acute and chronic pain. Many physical therapies are widely used in human and equine sports rehabilitation (*Table 1.11*); however, the majority are ineffectual or have anecdotal support only.

Cold therapy

By reducing blood flow (through vasoconstriction) and tissue metabolism, cooling can reduce the local swelling (oedema/haematoma) that occurs in the acute phase following injury. It is most effective when utilized within the first 24–48 hours and should be applied for 15–30 minute periods 2–4 times/day. Regular post-exercise cold therapy is also useful as a management aid for horses in fast work to minimize joint/soft-tissue inflammation.

Effective application of cold therapy to the lower limb is easily accomplished. Ice baths, purpose-designed cooling units and cold-water spas can be very effective at deep cooling of the lower limb. Reusable ice boots/gel wraps can also be efficient cooling aids; however, it is important that they conform to the leg. Cold water hosing is relatively inefficient.

Heat therapy

Heat increases local circulation through vasodilation. For this reason it is usually avoided in the acute phase following injury, but may be beneficial during the repair phase that follows to increase metabolism and speed healing. Relief of muscle spasm is another application.

Table 1.11 **Physical therapies used in equine sports rehabilitation**

THERAPY	DESCRIPTION	USE AND CLINICAL EFFECT	RESEARCH SUPPORT OF EFFICACY
Massage	Increases range of movement of joints and may have a role in restoring flexibility and function after injury.	Limited evidence that it may reduce muscle soreness after fatiguing exercise; optimal timing for assisting recovery unknown.	Uncertain.
Manipulative therapy/ chiropractic	Proposed to improve vertebral symmetry and restore normal joint motion and back/pelvic kinematics.	Little equine research. Some support for treatment of human back pain; however, clinical effect (reduced pain/return to normal function) is limited.	None/weak.
Extracorporeal shockwave therapy (ESWT)	Pressure wave generated by mechanical concussion, with release of kinetic energy at interfaces of different tissue densities. Proposed to upregulate healing, particularly at ligament/bone interfaces.	Little strong/consistent evidence that ESWT improves outcome in most equine/human orthopaedic conditions. Most useful in management of insertional tendinopathies; may induce neovascularization and repair. Short-term analgesic effect reported. Denervation through long-term use is a possible explanation for some reports of clinical efficacy.	Uncertain.

Table 1.11 *(continued)*

THERAPY	DESCRIPTION	USE AND CLINICAL EFFECT	RESEARCH SUPPORT OF EFFICACY
Electrotherapy (TENS: transcutaneous electrical nerve stimulation; NMES: neuromuscular electrical stimulation)	Direct application of electrical current to skin to stimulate nerves or neuromuscular units.	Used in human medicine primarily as adjunct to drug administration for management of acute and chronic pain. Current evidence is insufficient to support use.	None/weak.
Therapeutic ultrasound	Ultrasound generates acoustic energy that is absorbed in tissues through which sound waves pass. Can generate heat; also non-thermal effects such as cavitation and thought to have positive effects on blood flow and tissue metabolism. Depth of penetration up to 10 cm for 1 MHz.	Little evidence of efficacy in management of musculoskeletal pain and soft-tissue injury. Low-intensity pulsed ultrasound (daily) shortens healing time of acute, non-surgical fractures in people. Use in stress fractures and following surgical repair is not considered beneficial.	None/weak.
Acupuncture	Proposed to achieve physiological effects through stimulation of specific points by variety of means (needles/pressure/electricity/laser).	Large placebo effect in human trials. Positive effects (such as analgesia) generally of small magnitude.	None/weak.
Therapeutic laser therapy ('low level'/'cold'/Class III laser therapy; 'high-power'/Class IV laser therapy).	Potential modulation of inflammatory response and cellular repair.	Conflicting evidence (human/laboratory studies); short-term analgesia demonstrated with treatment within possible effective dosage window (600–950nm). No clinical efficacy demonstrated in horses.	Uncertain.
Pulsed magnetic field therapy	Proposed to enhance blood flow and tissue metabolism, with resulting analgesic effect and reduction in healing times.	Current evidence is insufficient to support use.	None/weak.
Vibration therapy	Mechanical vibration platforms proposed to have effect on bone mineral density and theoretical positive effect on bone strength, fracture healing and proprioceptive repair.	May have role in human geriatric medicine. Current evidence is insufficient to support use in human/equine athletes.	None/weak.
Hyperbaric oxygen therapy (HBOT)	Increased oxygenation of tissues proposed to have physiological effects that may lead to enhanced healing.	Some evidence that healing of certain conditions (arterial ulcers, osteomyelitis) is improved with HBOT. Current evidence is insufficient to support its use for musculoskeletal injury.	None/weak.

Research support definitions: **strong**, studies generally support effectiveness; **uncertain**, some positive findings are available, but confirming research needed; **none/weak**, little or no positive data available.

Heat can be applied through direct conduction by using hot packs/wheat bags; care should be taken to avoid burns when doing so. Depth of penetration of heat with direct conductive methods is limited to approximately 1 cm. Infrared lamps are also used for radiant heating. For heating of the deeper tissues (up to 10 cm), therapeutic ultrasound is required; heating is greatest at tissue interfaces and in tissues with a high collagen or protein content.

Topical therapy

A wide variety of topical liniments, cooling gels, osmotic sweats and clays are used on the lower limb to manage inflammation. Use of these products is supported by empirical evidence only, but many appear to have a positive effect in reducing heat or swelling. Protocols for application vary between products but can be classified as open or bandaged. Common ingredients of many anti-inflammatory preparations include menthol, witch hazel distillate (*Hamamelis virginiana*), peppermint oil, eucalyptus oil, salicylate and aloe vera. Menthol is an active ingredient that elicits a strong perception of cooling (mediated by stimulation of thermosensitive nerves) and through inhibition of nerve conduction also acts as an analgesic. Witch hazel has anti-inflammatory effects but is less potent than corticosteroids. Dimethyl sulfoxide (DMSO) is frequently used as a skin penetration enhancer in compounded preparations for delivery of anti-inflammatory medication (usually corticosteroids) into deeper tissues. Other ingredients have little or no support for efficacy but are generally considered benign. Use of some products (including kaolin clay) should be avoided on broken or infected skin.

Capsaicin is a naturally occurring irritant compound that can be found in low- and high-concentration topical products. It appears to act through initial irritation/hypersensitivity, which is followed by a longer period of desensitization, particularly when used over a long period. Efficacy is likely to be restricted to the skin.

Counter-irritation

The principle underlying the use of counter-irritation is that provocation of an inflammatory response may assist or revitalize healing processes in the limb. Counter-irritation may take the form of topical 'blisters', cryotherapy (freeze firing), or thermocautery (pin or bar firing). Blistering is most commonly used for dorsal metacarpal disease, splints and curbs and involves the use of an irritant or caustic skin dressing/paint (iodine/cantharadin/mercuric iodide-based) that is applied to effect depending on the product. The result is usually a superficial dermatitis and associated cellulitis, with thickening of the limb that may persist for weeks. Cryotherapy (freeze firing) is the application of a liquid nitrogen-cooled probe to the skin; local hair depigmentation (or loss) and temporary desensitization of the skin result after a mild inflammatory reaction. Pin or bar firing involves the invasive cautery of skin +/– underlying tendon or bone. Another counter-irritation technique is direct (needle) scarification of the cannon, typically used for the treatment of dorsal metacarpal disease (+/– infiltration of corticosteroid).

There is little evidence base for the efficacy of any counter-irritation method in assisting the quality or speed of healing, and in particular support for the use of firing as a preferred treatment for superficial digital flexor tendinitis has diminished with evidence that healing may be compromised. Any observed benefits of blistering/firing can usually be attributed to the enforced rest that accompanies these interventions. There is limited anecdotal support for the use of thermocautery in selected cases of splints or curbs where prolonged rest has been ineffectual.

CHAPTER 2
REGIONAL MUSCULOSKELETAL CONDITIONS

THE FOOT

Applied anatomy (Figure 2.1)

The hoof capsule (comprising wall, sole and frog) is a specialized structure of keratinized horn that encases the distal extremity of the limb. Germinal cells at the coronary band continually produce hoof tissue that grows down the wall to be worn away and lost at the ground surface; wall growth is affected by many factors but typically occurs at a rate of 8–10 mm/month. The hoof wall is thickest at the toe and becomes progressively thinner towards the heels. On the sole, the white line is the junction between the soft inner horn of the hoof wall and the solar horn. The frog is a wedge of more pliable horn that is bordered on each side by a deep groove (sulcus).

Suspended within the hoof capsule by a system of interlocking lamellae is the distal phalanx (P3 or pedal bone). Enzyme-mediated remodelling of these lamellae permits the continuous 'ratcheting' downward of maturing keratin while maintaining the strong bond between P3 and hoof. At the back of the foot, between P3 and the frog and heels, lies the loosely collagenous digital cushion. When foot strikes ground, the thinner wall at the quarters allows expansion of the heels; the digital cushion, along with collateral cartilages, acts as a 'shock absorber' to dampen downward movement of the middle phalanx (P2).

The distal interphalangeal joint (DIPJ), or 'coffin' joint, is a hinge joint between P2 and P3 and the boat-shaped navicular bone, which is maintained behind them by a sling of ligaments. This joint is encased

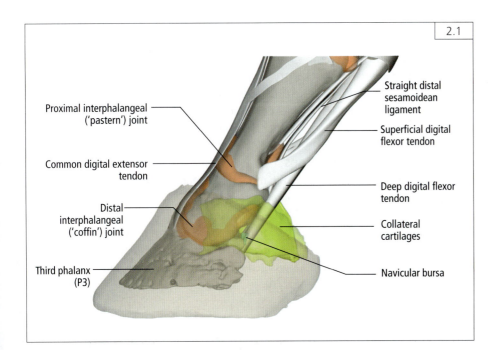

Fig. 2.1 Major structures of the foot.

within the hoof capsule; however, the dorsal pouch extends above the coronet. The common digital extensor tendon passes down the front of the lower pastern over this synovial pouch to insert on the extensor process of P3. The DIPJ is capable of movement in several planes including rotation and sliding; however, its primary action is flexion/extension, being stabilized by articular congruity, collateral ligaments and the deep digital flexor tendon (DDFT). At the back of the foot, the DDFT passes around the palmar/plantar face of the navicular bone then fans out into its insertion on the underside of P3. The DDFT is separated from the navicular bone by the navicular synovial bursa.

Synovial communications
DIPJ and navicular bursa: there is good diffusion of treatment drugs (in therapeutic quantities) in normal horses.

Examination
Feet should be observed both weight bearing and raised for symmetry of size and shape (with opposite foot) and dorsopalmar and mediolateral balance. Dynamic foot balance is assessed by observing how the feet strike the ground at a walk and trot (should land level). Digital pulse and foot warmth relative to the opposite limb and assessment of shoe fit, nail holes and hoof capsule defects may assist diagnosis.

Palpation of the coronet and heels may elicit a focal pain response in cases of infection. DIPJ effusion is best noted by palpation of the dorsal pouch (above the coronet) with the limb weight bearing, and should be compared with the opposite foot. Pain on deep palpation of the flexor tendon at its most distal extent between the heels may indicate navicular bursa pathology.

Response to careful and systematic application of hoof testers to all regions of the sole and frog will usually localize pain arising from infection or bruising. Comparison with the opposite foot and determining repeatability is advisable before commencing to explore the foot invasively. Removal of the shoe is necessary for assessment of the white line and the sole should be cleaned (wire brush) in preference to paring before exploration.

Bruised foot ('corn')
Bruising of the heel angle ('seat of corn') is largely a problem of front feet and predominantly affects the medial side of the foot. The condition is manifested by increased sensitivity to pressure on the affected heel angle and is typically associated with evidence of acute/chronic bruising or localized infection at the white line. Bruising of other parts of the sole is less common and when it occurs is usually the result of direct trauma (stone bruise).

Cause
- Loading forces concentrated by shoe, particularly if shod close +/− collapsed heels.
- Uneven footfall (secondary to mediolateral foot imbalance) may contribute.
- Toe out conformation: lateral toe strikes ground first then medial heel, predisposing to shunted heel/bruising.
- Damage at white line frequently predisposes to secondary infection at site.

Risk factors
- Bruised foot is the most common cause of foot lameness in training.
- Risk factors include foot conformation (low/collapsed heels; mediolateral imbalance) or inappropriate shoeing (shod too close on inside bar).

History
- Acute onset forelimb lameness.
- Most commonly arises when due for re-shoeing (rather than when freshly shod).

Signs
- Mild–moderate lameness; usually better on grass/soft surface.
- Unilateral/bilateral.
- Focal pain response to hoof testers.
- +/− increased digital pulse (usually mild).
- Signs generally milder than with subsolar abscess (p. 36).

Diagnosis
- Clinical findings usually definitive.
- Appearance of affected heel angle: can range from normal to thin/flat-soled, with normal or discoloured/disrupted white line (**Figure 2.2**).
- Diagnostic blocking if required: lameness abolished with blocking of relevant (medial or lateral) palmar digital nerve.

Management
- If no infection, avoid unnecessary paring of foot otherwise thinning of sole/prolapse of sensitive solar corium may result, delaying recovery.
- Poultice if cannot distinguish from infection (typically 12–24 hours).
- Re-shoeing to minimize pressure on affected site ('seating-out') +/− set full/wide at the quarters.
- Specialist shoes (¾ plate/¾ bar/heart bar) sometimes required for troublesome cases.

Prognosis
- Excellent. Return to ridden exercise usually possible within 1–3 days.

Dorsopalmar foot imbalance (collapsed/flat heels)

This condition involves low/collapsed heels +/− an overlong toe. It can affect both front and hind feet but secondary lameness is most common in the front feet. Typically bilateral but may be unilateral. May be associated with a simple imbalance of the hoof capsule or a more profound alteration of the hoof–pedal bone (P3) relationship (flat/negative solar angle of P3). Usually worsens with time in training unless preventive measures are taken. Low heels cause greater loading of the back of the foot during stance (and on toe at breakover). This predisposes to subsolar bruising (+/− laminar tearing at the toe). A small proportion of affected horses suffer from recurrent foot lameness.

Cause
- Thoroughbreds are predisposed due to conformation and hoof quality.
- Deformation of hoof occurs with loading during fast exercise.
- Long-term foot management (inappropriate dressing of heels) contributes to loss of balance.

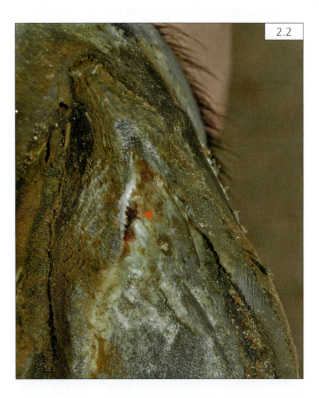

Fig. 2.2 Bruised foot. Note the haemorrhage (arrowhead) at the white line of the medial bar.

Risk factors
- Dorsopalmar foot imbalance is very common.
- Risk factors include shoeing practices (frequency of shoeing/overdressing of heels/shoeing close at heels to avoid lost shoes) and training itself (fast work linked to lowering of heel angle).
- Individual susceptibility may have a genetic component.

History
- Typically develops over months/years.
- More rapid loss of foot shape may occur in a shorter period (weeks) with inappropriate foot care in susceptible horse; commonly during rest period from training.

Signs
- Broken-back hoof–pastern axis.
- May develop secondary lameness (Bruised foot, p. 32).

Diagnosis
- Clinical findings are definitive (**Figure 2.3**)
- External appearance of hoof is poor guide to alignment of internal structures.
- Diagnostic blocking: lameness usually abolished with palmar digital nerve block.
- Imaging rarely needed but recommended if lameness is persistent or recurrent.
- Radiography: may reveal 'reverse rotation/inclination' of P3; palmar processes of P3 closer to solar margin than the toe is (on LM projection) (**Figures 2.4a, b**).
- MRI: occasionally justified in poorly responsive cases to rule out other injuries. Signs of laminar disruption and concussive strain involving the P3/navicular bone are typical.

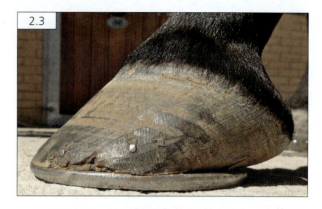

Fig. 2.3 Dorsopalmar foot imbalance: low heels and broken back hoof–pastern axis.

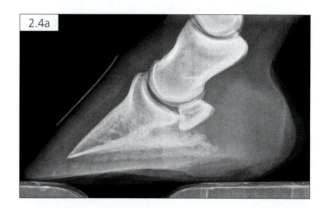

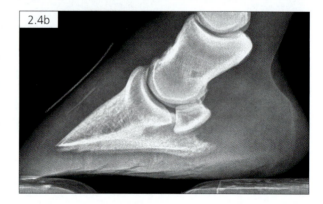

Figs. 2.4a, b Radiographs (LM) of both front feet of a horse. (a) Normal P3–solar relationship. (b) Reverse inclination/rotation of P3.

Management
- Balance between practicalities of shoeing for continued training/racing (avoiding pulled shoes) and prevention of longer-term deterioration in shape of foot; not always compatible.
- General rule: style of shoe used should be the simplest that successfully keeps horse sound in short/medium term. May require experimentation over several shoeings.
- Many cases manageable with correct trimming (to prevent excessive length of toe and crushing of heel tubules) combined with shoes that distribute load better through back of foot (more length at heel) and ease breakover.
- Bar shoes (straight/egg bar/heart bar) +/− sole packing for more troublesome cases.
- Flat- or reverse-inclination of P3: if poor response to above, may be appropriate to wedge heels (5–6°) with a wedge-shoe or pads. Can sometimes yield good medium-term soundness, although subsequent increased pressure on coronet of heels may reduce rate of heel growth.
- Biotin supplementation: small improvements in hoof growth/quality with long-term (months) daily supplementation (20–60 mg/day).
- Problematic cases may benefit from being rested barefoot in deep bedding to encourage heel growth when out of training.

Prognosis
- Condition not reversible but progression can usually be halted.
- Most cases can be kept sound in training with appropriate management.

Quarter crack

These are longitudinal cracks of variable length in the hoof wall (**Figure 2.5**) that can develop anywhere from the medial or lateral quarter to the heel. They may be full or partial thickness; involvement of sensitive tissue is common due to the thin hoof wall at the quarters. Cracks usually originate in the upper half of the hoof wall or close to the coronet. They are most common in the front feet.

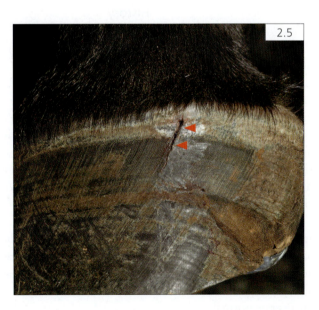

Fig. 2.5 Quarter crack. Note the fresh crack extending to the coronary band (arrowheads).

Cause
- Typically arise from stresses in the hoof capsule.
- Occasionally secondary to hoof wall defects arising from previous injury/scarring to the germinal cells at the coronet, such as following deep overreach injury.

Risk factors
- Uncommon condition.
- Mediolateral foot imbalance or poor forelimb conformation (toe out) may predispose.

History
- Acute onset of quarter crack +/− lameness.

Signs
- Lameness (if present) is usually mild–moderate in severity.
- Other signs include increased digital pulse, pain on palpation of coronet above the crack and bleeding at top of crack/coronet after exercise.

Diagnosis
- Clinical findings definitive.

Management
- Lameness and assessment of instability/depth (hoof testers) guide management in acute phase.
- Fresh cracks extending to sensitive tissue should be poulticed to resolve infection before considering repair.
- Address any underlying foot imbalance.
- Primary goal is stabilization of hoof capsule to prevent progression (and resolve lameness). Usually achieved with bridging acrylic hoof patch +/− bar shoe.
- Type of repair dependent on location/length of crack. If at caudal heel: bar shoe +/− floating of heel (to remove from load bearing) may be more appropriate than patching.
- Once crack stabilized, may resume normal training.

Prognosis
- Minimal interruption to training with appropriate management. May recur if underlying foot imbalance present.

Subsolar abscess
Localized infection under the sole causes acute and often marked lameness. Depending on location, severity and management, infection either remains subsolar or tracks up the white line to emerge at the coronet. Most common in the front feet.

Cause
- Usually secondary to repetitive bruising (p. 32).
- Can arise from direct penetration of sole (p. 38).
- Less commonly with compromise to white line (p. 56).

Risk factors
- Any age/stage of training.
- Foot imbalance (mediolateral or dorsopalmar) and poor shoeing predispose.

History
- Acute-onset lameness.

Signs
- Moderate–marked unilateral lameness; worse on the turn.
- Increased digital pulse/warmth of foot.
- Moderate–marked focal pain response to hoof testers.
- +/− focal swelling/pain at coronet (if infection about to burst out proximally).

Diagnosis
- Clinical findings usually definitive.
- Evidence of infection can usually be found on inspection of solar surface of foot (**Figures 2.6a–d**).

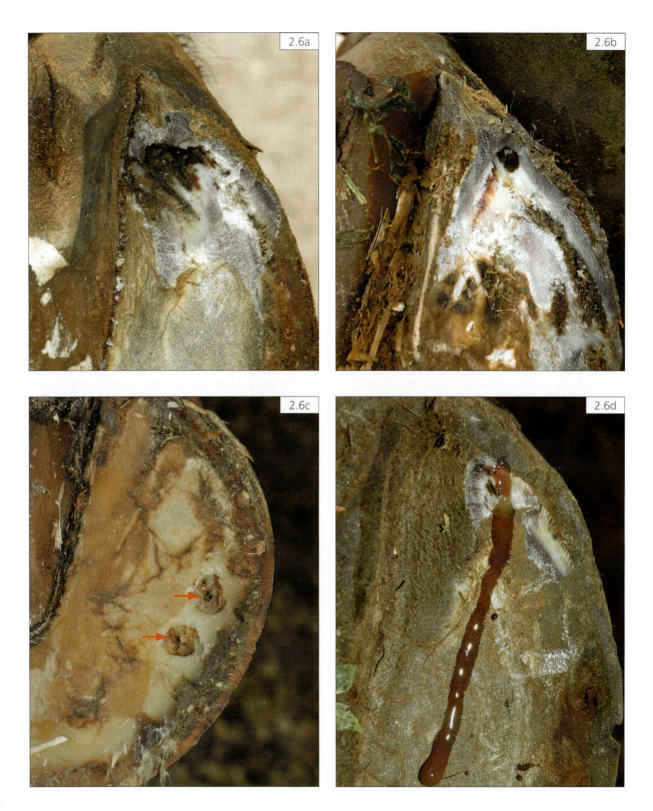

Figs. 2.6a–d Subsolar abscess. (a, b) Infected 'corn'. (c) Solar penetration from shifted shoe: two nail holes that have been explored to establish drainage (arrows). (d) Drainage established from the medial solar angle.

Management
- Infection usually self-limiting but drainage is desirable to speed recovery.
- Shoe should be removed and sole pared in area of greatest response to hoof testers.
- If focal defect found, establish drainage with loop knife.
- Osmotic poultice as required (until infection has subsided) +/− stand foot in shallow tub of salt water/diluted disinfectant once/twice daily.
- +/− poulticing over coronet if indicated.
- Stable rest +/− walking until infection resolved.
- Drying of sole (24 hours) prior to reshoeing.
- If sensitive sole becomes exposed/prolapsed, lameness may continue beyond resolution of infection and is best resolved with shoeing.

Prognosis
- Most cases resolve rapidly following drainage and can be reshod within 2–5 days.
- Rarely, long-standing/deep abscessation may result in focal infection of the adjacent portion of the pedal bone (Septic pedal osteitis, p. 39).

Foot penetration/puncture
Foot penetration by foreign objects typically affects the sole; less commonly the frog. Effects of penetrating injury are determined by location and depth; a subsolar abscess (p. 36) is a common outcome. Shifted shoes are the most frequent cause and bleeding indicates penetration of sensitive corium. Penetration by other objects (building nails/screws) is rare but when it occurs is often in the frog or sulci. These are potentially more serious injuries, as infection of deep vital structures of the foot (navicular bursa/DIPJ/digital tendon sheath/DDFT) may result.

History
- Acute-onset lameness or penetrating object detected.

Diagnosis
- Clinical findings (length/orientation of penetrating object) generally sufficient to determine risk to deep structures of the foot.
- If object is no longer in foot, paring of sole/frog and use of hoof testers to locate entry point.
- Penetration of the frog often difficult to find because of the soft horn and absence of bleeding.
- Radiography: risk assessment in cases where object still in place.
- MRI: useful modality in challenging cases, particularly in subacute phase to detect DDFT involvement or sequestration of flexor aspect of P3. Not definitive for detection of synovial sepsis in acute phase.
- Synoviocentesis: (DIPJ +/− navicular bursa +/− digital tendon sheath) indicated if synovial sepsis suspected.

Management
- Spread shoe/shoeing-nail penetration: any solar defect (including toe clip) from which bleeding is noted is best opened with a loop knife to establish drainage and the foot poulticed. Care taken to avoid prolapse of sensitive corium.
- Systemic +/− regional antibiotic perfusion may be warranted if concern over potential for infection of P3.
- Suspected synovial penetration: referral to hospital facility. Synovial involvement is an emergency that requires early diagnosis and aggressive and appropriate management (navicular bursoscopy, lavage +/− debridement) for good outcome.

Prognosis
- Shoeing-nail penetration: minimal interruption to training (typically 2–5 days).
- Synovial sepsis following frog penetration: poor prognosis for return to full athletic soundness (<30%) and high mortality rate unless early surgical intervention (regardless of structure involved).

Nail bind ('quicked' hoof)
Nail bind is lameness/inflammation arising from close proximity of a shoeing nail to sensitive tissue of the foot. It does not always result in secondary infection and may occur in any foot.

Risk factors
- Any age/stage of training.
- Horses with thin-walled feet or boxy feet at greater risk.

History
- Lameness in immediate (within 1–2 days) post-shoeing period.

Signs
- Mild–moderate lameness.
- Increased digital pulse/warmth of foot.
- Hoof tester pain response focal to a single nail.
- Clench of suspect nail may be high on hoof wall.

Diagnosis
- Clinical findings strongly indicative.

Management
- Mild lameness: remove affected nail.
- Moderate lameness (or no improvement following nail removal): removal of shoe and treatment as for subsolar abscess (p. 36).

Prognosis
- Minimal interruption to training with appropriate management.

Septic pedal (P3) osteitis
Septic pedal osteitis is infection of P3. Usually focal and limited to the solar margin of the bone. Occasionally associated with sequestrum formation. May affect any foot.

Cause
- Occurs secondary to infection within the hoof capsule in proximity to P3.
- May follow long-standing subsolar abscess where effective drainage has not been established. May also following deep foot penetration (nail).

Risk factors
- Any age/stage of training.
- Inappropriate or delayed treatment of subsolar abscess or foot penetration.

History
- Persistent/recurrent foot lameness (over weeks) following subsolar abscess.

Signs
- Same as for subsolar abscess (p. 36).

Diagnosis
- Radiography: signs of bone infection may not be visible for 1–3 weeks after initial injury/infection. Focal radiolucent defect of P3 in region of solar defect (**Figure 2.7**).

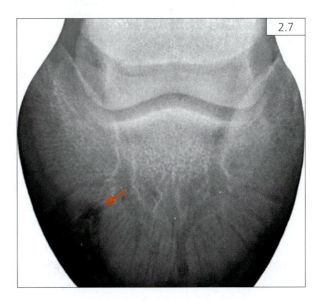

Fig. 2.7 Radiograph (D60°Pr-PaDiO) of hindlimb septic P3 osteitis. Note the poorly defined irregular lysis of the lateral solar margin (arrow) underlying a wider radiolucent area (excavated sole).

Management
- Mild clinical/radiological findings: antibiotic medication (2–4 weeks; oxytetracycline preferred) may resolve infection and avert need for surgery.
- Most cases with advanced radiological findings require open debridement: standing surgical procedure accessing infected solar margin of P3 through sole. Post-surgery hospital shoe/plate permits daily antiseptic dressing until the solar defect heals.
- Maggot debridement therapy is a treatment option for surgical cases.

Prognosis
- Good prognosis for return to full soundness.
- Non-surgical cases: return to training determined by level of soundness.
- Surgical cases: return to ridden exercise generally possible in 6–10 weeks.
- Recurrence of infection following surgery in a small proportion of cases.

Pedal bone (P3) fracture
Fractures involving P3 occur in several configurations. The causes and management vary according to injury type (*Table 2.1*).

Table 2.1 **Types of pedal bone (P3) fracture**

FRACTURE TYPE	DESCRIPTION	CAUSE
Palmar/plantar process ('wing') fracture	Oblique or sagittal fracture of wing to medial or lateral solar margin (**Figure 2.8**). Often articular. Predominantly in forelimb. Most common configuration in racehorses. Fractures of left forelimb lateral or right forelimb medial wing most common when racing counterclockwise.	Usually an acute exercise-related overloading injury.
Sagittal/parasagittal fracture	Midline/near-midline fracture (**Figure 2.9**). Invariably articular. Forelimb or hindlimb.	Typically due to direct trauma (such as kicking wall for hindlimb fracture) but may also be exercise-related.
Extensor process fracture	Fragmentation of extensor process (insertion of common digital extensor tendon) at dorsoproximal aspect of P3 (**Figure 2.10**). Invariably articular. Fragment size varies. Predominantly in forelimb.	Likely to be stress injury but acute injuries also occur.
Frontal fracture	Rare. Frontal fracture line extending for variable distance along dorsal aspect (**Figure 2.11**). Non-articular. Predominantly in forelimb.	Cause unknown; likely to be acute overload/traumatic event such as a fall.
Solar margin fracture	Fragmentation of dorsal solar margin of P3 (**Figure 2.12**). Fragments typically small/thin. Predominantly in forelimb. May not be clinically active at time of detection; of questionable importance other than as marker of possible prior foot pain.	Associated with flat feet +/− chronic foot soreness and likely to arise from repetitive concussion.

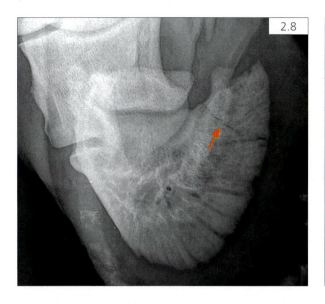

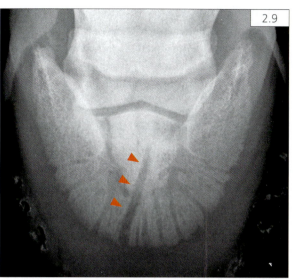

Fig. 2.8 Radiograph (D50°Pr45°L-PaDiMO) of a P3 wing (non-articular) fracture. Note the radiolucent fracture (arrow) through the lateral wing.

Fig. 2.9 Radiograph (D60°Pr-PaDiO) of a P3 sagittal (articular) fracture (arrowheads).

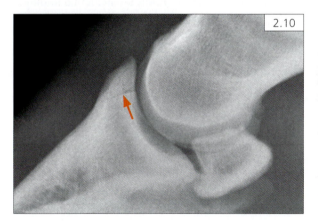

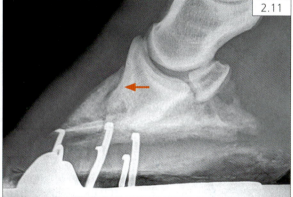

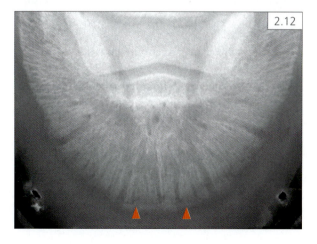

Fig. 2.10 Radiograph (LM) of a P3 extensor process (articular) fracture. Note the non-displaced fracture line (arrow).

Fig. 2.11 Radiograph (LM) of a P3 frontal (non-articular) fracture. Note the radiolucent fracture line (arrow) in the frontal plane, with displacement.

Fig. 2.12 Radiograph (D60°Pr-PaDiO) of a P3 fracture. Note the solar margin fracture (arrowheads).

History
- Acute-onset lameness.
- May initially be mistaken for other causes of foot pain; investigation usually prompted by failure of lameness to resolve with poulticing/reshoeing.

Signs
- Clinical findings non-specific for fracture configuration but as a general rule greater severity of lameness with articular fractures.
- Sagittal/parasagittal fractures are articular: severe acute lameness.
- Wing fractures: mild–moderate lameness, may be intermittent.
- +/– increased digital pulse (usually mild).
- Variable response to hoof testers but often resent strong percussion of hoof wall or sole.
- +/– effusion of DIPJ depending on injury type.

Diagnosis
- Clinical findings non-specific and generally do not permit differentiation from other causes of foot lameness.
- Diagnostic blocking: lameness usually improved by blocking of foot (but may not be completely abolished).
- Radiography: in acute phase, fracture line usually narrow and multiple projections may be required for detection. Wide/irregular lucency or fragment with rounded/sclerotic margins implies longer-standing injury.
- Bone scan: may be required (rarely) if radiography not diagnostic. Intensity of IRU diminishes with time from injury but can persist for many months.

Management
- Conservative management in most cases: stable rest (8–12 weeks) followed by walking.
- Bar shoe +/– quarter clips recommended during rest phase (also for return to training for wing fractures).
- Sagittal fractures with articular incongruity: surgical (lag screw) fixation may give best chance of long-term athletic soundness.
- Majority remain visible radiologically long term: return to exercise dictated by clinical rather than radiological improvement.

Prognosis
- Prognosis for return to full use:
  - Non-articular (wing) fractures: excellent (80–90%).
  - Articular wing fractures: good (approximately 70%).
  - Articular sagittal/parasagittal fractures: good (>70%).
  - Extensor process fractures: fair (approximately 60%).
  - Frontal fractures: fair.
- Overall prognosis best for hindlimb fractures.

Pedal bone (P3) cyst

Osteochondrosis lesion that typically becomes clinically active in early training. Most common location is in the proximal portion of P3 on the midline, but dorsopalmar position, size and communication with DIPJ vary. Usually unilateral and solitary and predominantly in forelimb. Prevalence unknown but almost invariably associated with lameness (rarely an incidental finding).

Cause
- See Osteochondrosis (Other musculoskeletal conditions, p. 192).

Risk factors
- Rare condition.
- Risk factors for development of condition unknown.

History
- Found in any age of horse, but most commonly first detected at yearling/2 YO stage when exercise increases.
- Acute or intermittent lameness in early cantering phase of training.
- Often initially mistaken for foot bruise/infection.

Signs
- Clinical findings and diagnostic blocking pattern similar to other foot conditions.
- Mild–moderate unilateral lameness, often transient/intermittent.
- Increased digital pulse; variable or negative response to hoof testers; +/– effusion of DIPJ.

Diagnosis
- Diagnostic blocking: lameness usually abolished/improved by blocking of DIPJ or palmar digital nerve block.
- Radiography: upright pedal (D60°Pr-PaDiO) and weight-bearing DPa projections; usually smooth-margined circular lucency +/− surrounding sclerosis a variable distance from the joint margin (**Figures 2.13a, b**).
- Presence of arthritic change or irregular density/thickness of subchondral bone (DIPJ) may be strong indicators if cyst not radiologically evident (**Figure 2.14**).
- MRI: diagnostic modality of choice for both diagnosis and surgical planning.

Management
- Surgical debridement of the cyst offers best chance of return to athletic soundness, but individual circumstances (surgical access) frequently mean surgery reserved for cases responding poorly to conservative management.
- Conservative management: satisfactory for paddock or non-racing use; return to full athletic use also possible. May also be treatment of choice for cases in which MRI findings indicate active inflammation of P3/'immaturity' of cyst in a young horse. Stable rest/walking for 10–16 weeks +/− intra-articular medication (corticosteroid +/− hyaluronic acid). Periodic intra-articular medication often necessary on return to training.

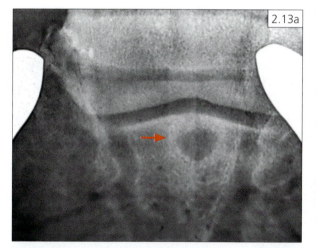
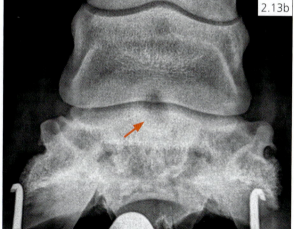

Figs. 2.13a, b Radiographs (DPr-PaDiO, standing DPa) of a P3 subchondral bone cyst. Note the circular radiolucency (arrow) in dorsal P3.

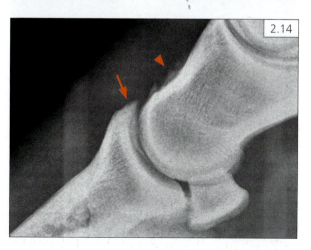

Fig. 2.14 Radiograph (LM) of DIPJ osteoarthritic change. Note the lysis of the extensor process (arrow) and modelling of dorsal P2 (arrowhead).

Prognosis
- Conservative management: prognosis for return to full racing soundness guarded.
- Surgery: good–excellent prognosis for athletic soundness.

Navicular bone fracture
Rare and sporadic cause of lameness. Configuration of fracture typically oblique and sagittal (either side of midline) but may involve lateral or medial wing. Rarely, avulsion fractures of distal border. More common in forelimb than hindlimb.

Cause
- Forelimb fractures: sustained at exercise and presumed to be acute overload injury.
- Hindlimb fractures: often attributed to direct trauma such as kicking a wall.

Risk factors
- Rare condition.
- Risk factors unknown.
- Role of pre-existing navicular pathology not known.

History
- Acute and usually severe lameness.
- First noted either in stable or following/during exercise.

Signs
- Moderate–marked unilateral lameness.
- Signs referable to foot may be subtle/mild: slightly increased digital pulse +/− inconsistent response to hoof testers +/− effusion of DIPJ.

Diagnosis
- Radiography: upright P3 and skyline navicular projections most useful (**Figures 2.15a, b**).
- Should be differentiated from bipartite/tripartite navicular bones: these are congenital, are generally not associated with severe lameness and are often bilateral.

Management
- Sagittal fractures: although return to racing has been reported with conservative management, expectations should be for paddock soundness only.
- Stable rest (8–12 weeks) with bar shoe/wedged heel prior to walking/restricted turnout.
- Surgical repair (lag screw fixation) of sagittal fractures for paddock salvage or light ridden use has been reported but is rarely considered.

Prognosis
- Forelimb fractures: guarded to poor prognosis for return to racing regardless of management.

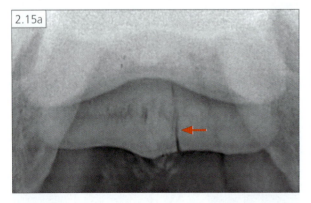

Fig. 2.15a Radiograph (PaPr-PaDiO) of a navicular bone fracture (forelimb). Note the parasagittal fracture (arrow); increased density of the navicular bone is also present.

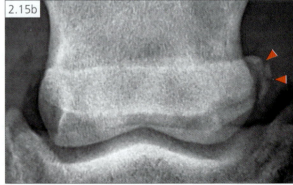

Fig. 2.15b Lateral fragmentation (arrowheads) of hindlimb navicular bone.

- Hindlimb fractures: more favourable prognosis for return to racing than forelimb injuries (conservative management).

White line disease ('seedy toe')

A disease of the white line in which progressive disruption of the horny layers (beginning at the solar margin and tracking proximally) causes separation within the hoof wall. Usually seen at the toe; width of involved tissue varies, but typically 2–3 cm. Most common in forelimb and usually unilateral, but may affect more than one foot.

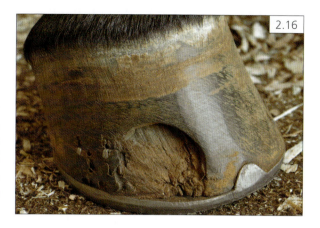

Fig. 2.16 Seedy toe. Dorsal hoof wall defect following resection of underrun horn.

Cause
- Opportunistic fungal +/– bacterial invasion of white line.
- Mechanical (e.g. poorly balanced feet) or environmental factors make the white line vulnerable to infection.
- Slowly progresses up hoof wall, largely without causing signs of inflammation as it is confined to inert keratin.

Risk factors
- No strong associations with type of bedding and occurs in both wet and dry environmental conditions.
- Incidence increases with age.

History
- Often first detected at routine shoeing.

Signs
- Usually no external sign of disease on hoof wall.
- Area of discoloured/widened white line +/– hollow cavity beneath the hoof at toe, extending for variable distance up dorsal wall (**Figure 2.16**).
- +/– mildly increased digital pulse.
- Lameness usually only a feature with extensive lesions or secondary infections.

Diagnosis
- Clinical findings definitive.
- Radiography: sometimes useful in advanced cases to plan treatment. LM projection to highlight proximal extent of gas shadow.

Management
- Dictated by severity and stage of season.
- Treatment involves resection of the dorsal hoof wall overlying the hollow lesion back to bordering healthy tissue, cleaning/disinfecting exposed tissue and supporting hoof capsule.
- Topical treatment without resection of little use.
- Support: bar shoe +/– prosthetic hoof filler +/– natural-balance or square toe shoe to move breakover back.
- Extensive lesions best addressed out of season, as radical hoof wall resection may cause short-term lameness and interrupt training.
- Oral biotin supplementation.

Prognosis
- Recurrence is common.
- Interference to training is usually minimal: occasional episodes of foot soreness/infection.

Laminitis

Laminitis is an important and potentially life-threatening disease in which breakdown of the bond between P3 and the inner hoof wall occurs. Severity varies depending on degree of initial compromise to this bond, and ranges from mild inflammation or realignment of P3 within the hoof capsule through to catastrophic loss of support of P3 or even shedding of hoof. Duration of acute phase of disease may be days/weeks, and recovered but seriously affected horses may display chronic or recurrent laminitis long term. Initial severity of damage and point at which P3–hoof connection is stabilized determine the degree of short- and long-term disability.

Cause
- Complex cascade of events that involves vascular, enzymatic, inflammatory or metabolic factors to varying degrees.
- Vascular system of equine foot may predispose to laminitis due to presence of arteriovenous 'shunts', which allow blood to bypass the sensitive structures of the foot under certain circumstances (thus depriving lamellae of blood supply).
- Normal growth of hoof wall past P3 is facilitated by enzymes: inappropriate activation of these enzymes by inflammatory mediators is involved in breakdown of the bond between dermal and epidermal lamellae.
- Developmental phase of laminitis: damage can occur 48–72 hours before clinical signs become apparent.
- Weakened P3–hoof bond: weight bearing (+/– pull of DDFT) rotates/displaces P3 towards (and sometimes through) sole, with subsequent acute/chronic damage to blood supply and sole.
- Usually worse in forelimbs because of greater load, although all four feet can be affected.

Risk factors
- Racehorses are at lower risk of developing laminitis than the general horse population, but when it does occur is frequently serious.
- Supporting limb laminitis: most important type of laminitis seen in racehorses. Severe unilateral lameness (due to infection/orthopaedic injury) may result in heavy loading of supporting limb: causes arterial compression and subsequent lack of blood supply to the hoof. May develop insidiously as initial lameness masked by that of opposite limb. Occurs in weeks/months after initial insult and affects 10–20% of horses at risk. Greater risk with full limb casts/transfixation pin casts/greater BWT/longer duration of casting.
- Colitis/pneumonia/endotoxaemia: severe systemic infections requiring hospitalization may trigger the inflammatory cascade that results in loss of basement membrane integrity in hooves.
- Corticosteroid-induced laminitis: corticosteroids may have an insulin-mediated effect on basement membrane; high systemic doses are considered a risk factor for laminitis, although direct link is tenuous. Racehorses less susceptible than other breeds; typical total body doses of ≤40 mg triamcinolone acetonide for orthopaedic medications carry negligible risk of laminitis.
- Carbohydrate-overload laminitis: exceeding the foregut's capacity to digest starch (grain) or sugars found in pasture can lead to changes in hindgut microbial populations. Subsequent release of endotoxin can cause enzymatic breakdown of basement membrane. Rarely a cause of laminitis in racehorses.

Signs
- Lameness/foot soreness involving front (+/– hind) feet, variable severity (mild to marked); worse on hard surface.
- Obel grading system:
  - Grade 1: alternately lifting feet; not lame at the walk.
  - Grade 2: stiff and resists turning at the walk and lame at the trot.
  - Grade 3: lame at the walk; stilted gait; resists lifting feet.
  - Grade 4: will not move unless forced.
- Increased digital pulses/warm feet.
- Hoof tester pain response greatest over sole near apex of frog.
- Depression around coronet +/– convexity of sole may indicate 'sinking' of P3.

Diagnosis
- Clinical findings usually indicative.
- Radiography (LM projection): allows assessment of P3–hoof alignment/displacement. Serial radiography can be used to monitor progression.

Management
- Level of intervention determined by severity.
- Remove/treat inciting cause.
- Distal limb cold therapy may be useful during prodromal phase.
- Mechanical support of feet to stabilize P3: redistribute loading away from dorsal laminae and reduce tension in the DDFT.
- Foot support options depend on individual circumstances: simplest (mild cases) is barefoot on soft/conforming bedding +/− solar and frog supports (lily pads) through to full sole support systems/foam pads or shoeing with raised heels (glue-on shoes preferable).
- Analgesia: NSAIDs to effect.
- +/− acepromazine (0.02–0.06 mg/kg IM 2–3 times/day, or oral dosing to achieve mild sedation) for possible vasodilation and to limit movement.
- Mild laminitis: stable confinement/deep bedding/phenylbutazone until clinical improvement.
- Failure to control pain/'sinking' of P3 with penetration of sole/recurrent severe abscessation/loss of hoof capsule may warrant euthanasia.

Prevention
- Supporting limb laminitis: preventive measures at time of initial surgery/treatment of at-risk horses; pain management plus heel wedges (20°)/solar support/caudal breakover on supporting limb. Forced walking may be desirable for some conditions (e.g. cellulitis/lymphangitis).
- Endotoxaemia cases: continuous distal limb cold therapy (1°C; preferably to mid-cannon level) during risk period for endotoxaemia limits delivery of trigger factors to lamellae by reducing blood flow to foot. Thought to be beneficial primarily during developmental phase. Anti-endotoxic medical therapy.

Prognosis
- Prognosis for survival +/− return to athletic use is correlated to severity of pain and speed of progression.
- Mild cases with no/little P3 rotation: good prognosis for return to full soundness.
- 'Sinking' of P3 associated with high mortality.
- Degree of P3 rotation is not a reliable predictor of survival, but has implications for long-term soundness.

Keratoma

A keratoma is an aberrant, firm, slow-growing keratinous mass that develops within the foot between the hoof wall and P3. It causes lameness due to impingement on the internal structures of the foot. Usually in forelimb, solitary and unilateral and generally found under dorsal hoof. Pressure from enlargement of the mass may cause gradual deformation of the hoof wall, deviation of the white line and/or focal resorption of P3. Disruption of the white line may predispose to secondary infections.

Cause
- Underlying cause not known but thought that previous trauma to hoof or chronic irritation may contribute.

Risk factors
- Rare condition.
- Any age/stage of training.
- Risk factors unknown.

History
- Chronic/recurrent foot lameness.
- May initially be mistaken for other causes of foot pain (bruising, subsolar abscess).

Signs
- Mild–moderate lameness.
- +/− mild increase in digital pulse.
- Focal deviation of white line is common.
- Distortion/buttressing of hoof wall in long-standing cases.

Diagnosis
- Clinical findings and diagnostic blocking pattern similar to other foot conditions.
- Radiography: usually diagnostic, although some lesions are not visible. DPr-PaDiO projection: smooth-edged radiolucent defect in P3 margin (differentiate from normal 'notch' or crena at the toe of P3) +/− new bone on mid-dorsal margin of P3 on LM projection (**Figure 2.17**).
- CT (**Figure 2.18**): diagnostic modality of choice to assist surgical planning, as allows superior visualization of sensitive/insensitive laminar tissue (compared with MRI).

Management
- Surgical removal is treatment of choice.
- Surgical approach dependent on location of lesion: partial- or full-length hoof wall resection.
- Post surgery: application of hospital plate that stabilizes the hoof and permits daily dressing.
- Return to training is dependent on healing of hoof wall/solar defect; 2–4 months out of ridden exercise is typical.

Prognosis
- Prognosis for return to full use is good–excellent (>80%) with surgical removal.
- Recurrence is uncommon.
- Conservative management usually unsuccessful due to continued growth of mass and recurrent lameness.

Thrush
Thrush is an infection of the frog/sulci in one or more feet caused by anaerobic bacteria that break down hoof horn and progressively invade sensitive tissue.

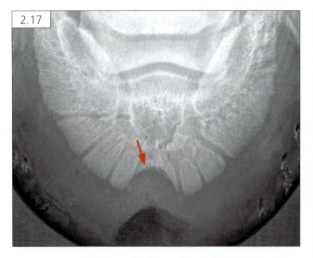

Fig. 2.17 Radiograph (D60°Pr-PaDiO) of a keratoma. Note the smooth-margined radiolucency at the dorsal solar margin (arrow). Should be differentiated from normal crena of P3.

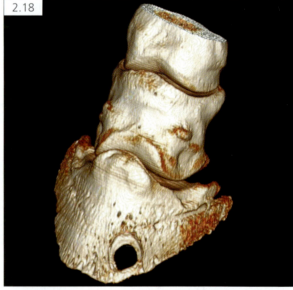

Fig. 2.18 CT image of a keratoma. Note the space-occupying lesion in the dorsal wall of the foot.

Cause
- The bacteria responsible (most commonly *Fusobacterium necrophorum*, one of the causes of foot rot in sheep) are opportunistic invaders and are found in normal faeces and soil.

Risk factors
- Predisposing factors include conditions that lead to deep frog clefts (sheared heels, boxy foot), poor foot care/trimming and damp stable environment.
- Commonly seen in horses being stable rested.

History
- Usually detected at shoeing.
- May present with acute or chronic foot lameness.

Signs
- Black, foul-smelling discharge from sulci or frog.
- Frog horn usually underrun (**Figure 2.19**).
- +/– mild increase in digital pulse.
- +/– subtle lameness.
- Advanced infection or infections in feet with sheared heels may extend into sensitive tissue between bulbs of the heel, causing soreness/filling of the lower pastern.

Diagnosis
- Clinical findings definitive.

Management
- Trimming of frog/sulci to expose underrun/infected tissue to air.
- Topical application of copper sulphate crystals, bleach (10% hydrogen peroxide solution) or povidone–iodine (10% solution) daily until healthy.
- Address any foot imbalance/hygiene factors thought to be causative.

Prognosis
- Excellent; does not interfere with training.
- Resolves in days/weeks with appropriate management.

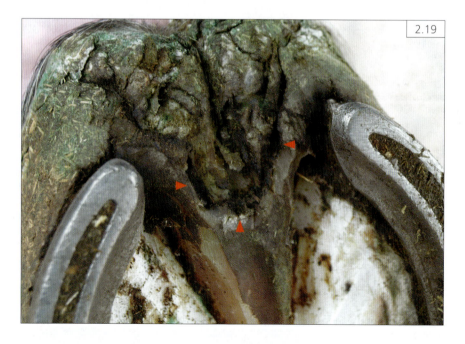

Fig. 2.19 Thrush: underrun horn of frog (arrowheads).

THE FETLOCK AND PASTERN

Applied anatomy

The fetlock joint is the articulation between the third metacarpal/metatarsal ('cannon', Mc3/Mt3) bone and the first phalanx ('long' pastern bone, P1) (**Figures 2.20a, b**). It is a high motion joint, subject to large forces during fast exercise and, in combination with the flexor tendons/suspensory apparatus, plays an important role in the energy efficiency of equine locomotion. Movement of the joint is primarily extension (during weight bearing) and flexion (during limb protraction). At maximal loading the fetlock hyperextends, with the back of the fetlock being capable of striking the ground.

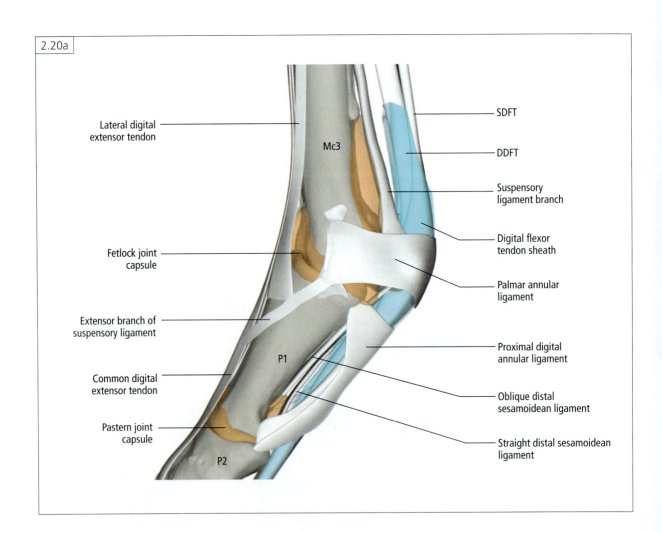

Fig. 2.20a Major structures of the fetlock and pastern (lateral view).

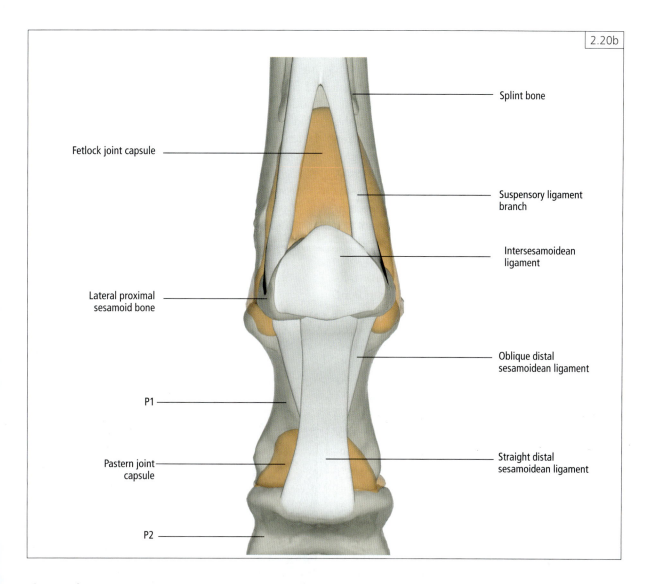

Fig. 2.20b Major structures of the fetlock and pastern (palmar view) with flexor tendons removed.

The distal condyles of the cannon bone are separated by a prominent sagittal ridge that articulates with a corresponding central groove in P1. Together with strong collateral ligaments, this ridge restricts rotational motion (although at full loading there is some lateral torsion of P1 relative to the cannon). The paired proximal sesamoid bones (PSBs), each interposed in the suspensory apparatus, sit at the back of the joint and serve to provide strength to the suspensory ligament and flexor tendon unit, which would otherwise be weak in compression. The suspensory ligament splits into two branches in the mid-cannon region, each branch fusing with its respective PSB and being continued functionally by the distal (straight, oblique, cruciate and short) sesamoidean ligaments below the back of the fetlock; weaker extensor branches run forward on the pastern to join the common digital extensor tendon. The thick intersesamoidean ligament forms a groove between the sesamoid bones over which the flexor tendons run at the back of the joint, constrained by the proximal annular ligament. Both the SDFT and the DDFT broaden at this point in their course to apply greater surface contact with the suspensory apparatus.

At the level of the fetlock, the SDFT forms a ring (manica flexoria) around the DDFT then it bifurcates below the fetlock into its terminal branches, which insert above and below the proximal interphalangeal joint (PIPJ, 'pastern' joint). Emerging from this bifurcation the DDFT continues down into the back of the foot. High at the back of the pastern, deep to the flexor tendons, the distal sesamoidean ligaments (straight, oblique and cruciate) attach the base of the sesamoids and intersesamoidean ligament to P1 and P2, thus stabilizing the PIPJ. The PIPJ is a relatively low-motion articulation between P1 and P2 and is the site of few problems in the racehorse.

The fetlock joint has both dorsal and palmar/plantar pouches. The palmar/plantar pouch ('articular windgall') is found between the back of the cannon bone and the suspensory ligament branches (SLBs). Close to this pouch is another synovial space, the digital tendon sheath ('tendinous windgall'/'windpuff'). The tendon sheath surrounds the flexor tendon bundle from the lower quarter of the cannon through the back of the fetlock and into the mid-pastern. By contrast, the PIPJ is a relatively low volume articulation and is constrained by collateral ligaments and the flexor tendon bundle/ tendon sheath. There are no direct communications between any of these synovial structures.

Examination

Synovial effusion of the fetlock joint or digital tendon sheath is usually readily apparent with the limb weight bearing. Observation of the limb from in front or behind the horse may reveal prominence of a SLB or sesamoid bone. It is useful to determine whether soft-tissue thickening is solely medial or lateral, confined to the fetlock or above, or extending below the fetlock into the pastern.

With the leg raised in passive flexion, careful palpation of the structures around the fetlock joint is undertaken to determine the presence of any repeatable pain response. Key sites are the dorsoproximal aspect of P1, the SLB/sesamoid bone interface, the medial and lateral distal cannon, the sesamoid/base of the sesamoid regions and the flexor tendon bundle. Pain responses should be compared with the opposite limb. Forced flexion of the joint allows assessment of synovial pain and any restriction of range of motion.

Proximal phalangeal fracture

P1 fracture is one of the most important injuries affecting the racehorse fetlock. Several configurations of P1 fracture occur; most common is the 'split pastern' (mid-sagittal fracture). May affect the forelimb or hindlimb. Classification of fracture type is determined by length, plane and direction of fracture line and the presence of comminution:

- Incomplete mid-sagittal fracture: fracture line propagates from the sagittal groove (typically dorsal half of groove) extending for a variable length down into P1. May be 'short' or 'long' (**Figures 2.21, 2.22a, b, 2.23**).

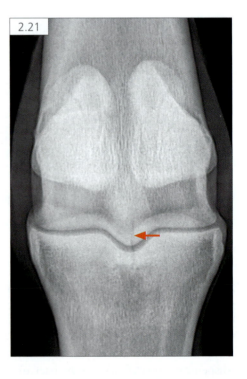

Fig. 2.21 Radiograph (DPa) of a short incomplete sagittal P1 fracture. Note the short linear lucency (arrow) at the proximal articular margin of P1.

Regional Musculoskeletal Conditions

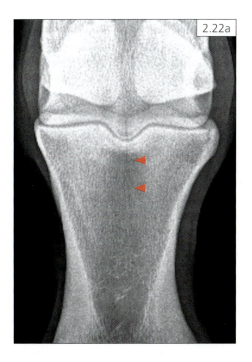
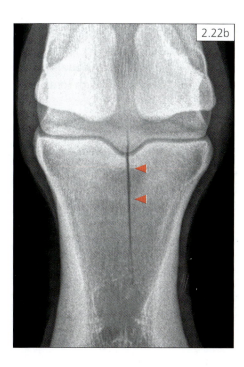

Figs. 2.22a, b Radiographs (DPa) of long incomplete sagittal P1 fractures. Note the faint (a) and clear (b) linear lucencies (arrowheads) in P1.

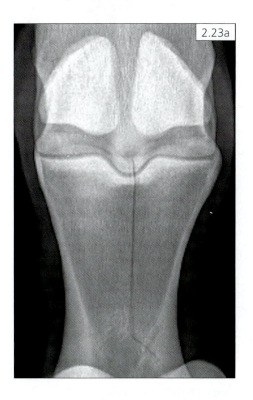
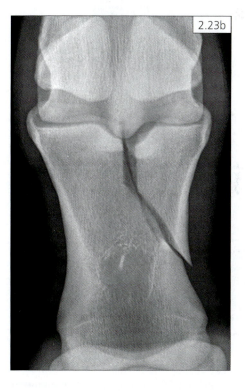

Fig. 2.23a, b Radiographs (DPl) of (a) an incomplete and (b) a complete sagittal P1 fracture with lateral propagation.

- Complete mid-sagittal fracture: fracture propagates from sagittal groove either all the way through P1 to the PIPJ or exits laterally, creating two fragments. Generally with some displacement.
- Comminuted fracture: complete fracture with multiple fragments; +/− intact strut of bone between fetlock joint and PIPJ (**Figures 2.24, 2.25**).
- Frontal fracture: fracture line in dorsal plane, propagates from articular surface and extends in dorsodistal direction. Generally incomplete and predominantly in hindlimb (**Figures 2.26–2.28**).

Cause
- High stress during full loading in sagittal groove region of proximal P1.
- Mid-sagittal fracture: generally considered an acute monotonic injury from single supraphysiological loading event. Stress fracture pathology responsible for some cases.
- Comminuted fracture: considered a severe manifestation of complete mid-sagittal fracture, although circumstances that lead to comminution poorly understood.
- Frontal fracture: stress/fatigue injury.

Risk factors
- Mid-sagittal fracture: one of the most common fetlock fractures sustained by racehorses.
- Frontal fractures: rare.
- Encountered in horses of all ages.

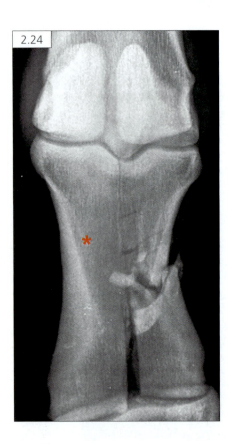

Fig. 2.24 Radiograph (DPa) of a complete/comminuted P1 fracture with extension to the pastern joint. Note the intact medial bony strut (*).

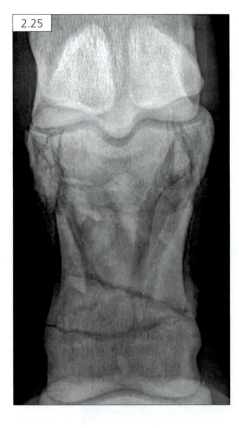

Fig. 2.25 Radiograph (DPl) of a comminuted P1 fracture.

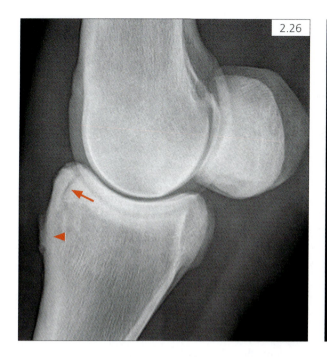

Fig. 2.26 Radiograph (LM) of a frontal P1 fracture of the forelimb fetlock. Note the linear lucency (arrow) in dorsoproximal P1, with periosteal proliferative change at the distal extent of the fracture (arrowhead).

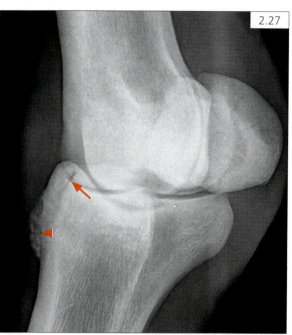

Fig. 2.27 Radiograph (DLPaMO) of a frontal P1 fracture of the forelimb fetlock. Note the linear lucency (arrow) in dorsoproximal P1, with periosteal proliferative change at the distal extent of the fracture (arrowhead).

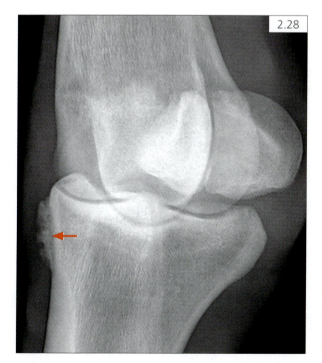

Fig. 2.28 Radiograph (DLPlMO) of a frontal P1 fracture of the hindlimb fetlock. Note the periosteal proliferative change at the distal extent of the fracture (arrow), but no evident fracture line.

- Generally during cantering/fast exercise phase of training.
- Other risk factors unknown.

History
- Mid-sagittal fracture (complete/incomplete): acute onset lameness that develops during or immediately after exercise (either on track or on return to yard).
- Comminuted fracture: severe acute lameness on track.
- Usually no history of pre-existing lameness.
- Frontal fracture: either acute lameness after exercise or mild lameness worsening with continued exercise over days/weeks. Occasionally an incidental finding without lameness.

Signs
- Lameness, presence of joint effusion and palpable pain varies with injury type/severity (*Table 2.2*).
- Typically severe lameness and obvious pain response to palpation of dorsoproximal P1; exceptions are hindlimb and some short incomplete injuries, frontal fractures.

Diagnosis
- Clinical findings strongly indicative.
- Radiography: to confirm configuration and guide management (generally unnecessary for comminuted fracture). Multiple DPa/DPl projections may be required to detect/assess fracture line (in the case of frontal plane fractures: may be best visualized on LM/slightly oblique LM projections). Repeat radiography at 7–14 days if initial screening unremarkable. Not all cases develop visible fracture line; however, development of periosteal reaction at dorsoproximal P1 strong indicator of injury (**Figures 2.29a, b**).
- Fracture configuration frequently more complicated than evident on the radiographic imaging. Consider CT assessment prior to surgical intervention.
- MRI/bone scan: may be required for radiologically silent, short incomplete fractures (rare) (**Figure 2.30**).

Table 2.2 Signs associated with P1 fractures

INJURY TYPE	LAMENESS	JOINT EFFUSION	RESPONSE TO FLEXION	PAIN ON PALPATION (DORSOPROXIMAL P1)
Mid-sagittal (forelimb)	Severe	Yes	Yes (marked)	Yes (marked)
Mid-sagittal (hindlimb)	Moderate–severe	Variable	Variable	Variable
Mid-sagittal (short incomplete)	Mild–moderate	No	No	Yes (mild)
Comminuted	Severe	Yes (+ instability/crepitus)	Not required	Not required
Frontal plane	Mild–moderate. Occasionally clinically silent	Mild (+/– palpable buttressing P1)	No	Variable

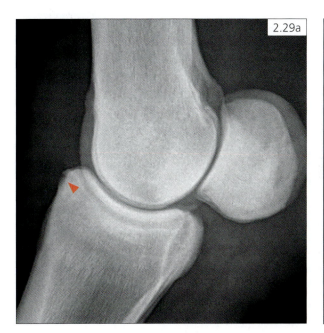
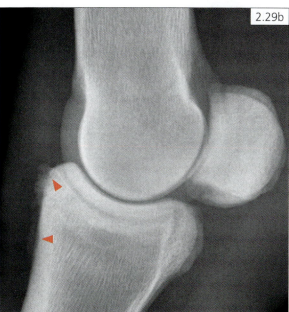

Figs. 2.29a, b Radiographs (LM) of subtle (a) and extensive (b) periosteal reaction (arrowheads) at dorsoproximal P1.

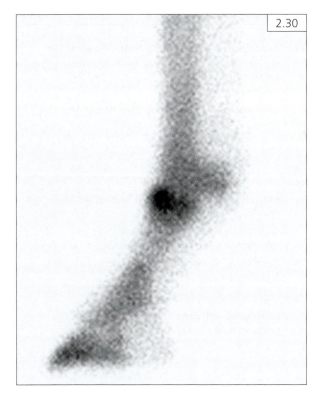

Fig. 2.30 Lateral scintigram of a radiologically silent sagittal P1 fracture.

Management
- See *Table 2.3*.
- First aid: application of immobilizing splint (Kimzey Leg Saver) or Robert Jones bandage for transport or until initial radiographic assessment.
- Clinical suspicion of P1 injury but initial radiographic screening unremarkable: stable confinement (+ immobilizing bandage) with repeat radiography at 7–14 days.

Prognosis
- See *Table 2.3*.

Condylar fracture

Condylar fracture (Mc3/Mt3) is an important injury of the racehorse fetlock. Typically develops initially as a small 'hairline' prodromal fissure originating at the articular margin of the sagittal groove and unless detected at this stage (largely clinically inapparent) may progress to more serious injury within weeks. The fracture propagates proximally into the cannon from either the lateral (most common: >80%) or the medial sagittal groove and may be incomplete or complete (**Figures 2.31a, b**). A proportion of fractures originate in the condyle rather than in the sagittal groove. The spectrum of injury varies but the majority encountered are incomplete non-displaced injuries of variable length. They are most common (80%) in the forelimb. While lateral condylar fractures usually have a simple configuration, medial injuries are frequently incomplete and spiral proximally (**Figure 2.32**) and are associated with a high risk of displacement. Comminution at the articular margin occurs in approximately 15% of cases. Concurrent fracture of P1 may occur rarely (more common in hindlimb than forelimb) (**Figure 2.33**). Concurrent axial fracture of the ipsiaxial PSB is a rare but potentially catastrophic configuration.

Table 2.3 Management of P1 fractures

INJURY TYPE	MANAGEMENT	PROGNOSIS
Mid-sagittal: Short incomplete	Conservative management: stable rest (8–12 weeks)/walking +/– immobilizing bandage in acute phase depending on initial lameness. Surgical reduction (optional).	Good prognosis (approximately 70%) for return to full use. Small proportion reinjure on return to training (unless treated surgically).
Long incomplete (non-displaced)	Surgical reduction: treatment of choice for athletic soundness. Satisfactory outcome possible with stable rest/immobilizing bandage (8–12 weeks guided by radiography); small risk of displacement in initial weeks (greater risk with hindlimb fractures: typically warrant surgery).	Good prognosis (approximately 70%) for return to full use.
Long incomplete (displaced)	Surgical reduction.	Good prognosis (approximately 70%) for return to full use.
Complete	Surgical reduction.	Complete (to lateral cortex): good prognosis (approximately 70%) for return to full use. Complete (to pastern joint): guarded prognosis (<50%) for return to racing.
Comminuted	Immediate euthanasia on humane grounds if severely comminuted/no intact strut. Surgical reduction (incorporating transfixation cast/external fixation device) under exceptional circumstances for salvage of horses with breeding value.	Hopeless prognosis for athletic use. Comminuted with intact strut: guarded–fair (>60%) prognosis for survival/paddock use with surgery.
Frontal: Dorsoproximal incomplete	Conservative management: stable rest (8–12 weeks)/walking. Rehabilitation guided by radiography.	Good/excellent prognosis for return to full use.
Mid-articular	Surgical reduction.	Guarded prognosis for athletic soundness.

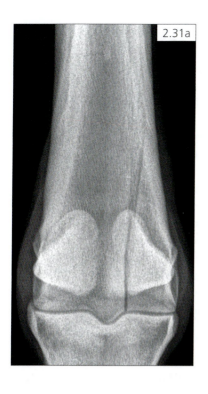 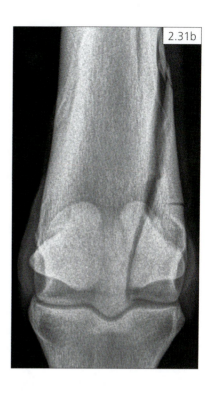

Figs. 2.31a, b Radiographs (DPa) of lateral condylar fractures (forelimb) showing fracture lines propagating (a) and exiting (with proximal comminution) (b) laterally.

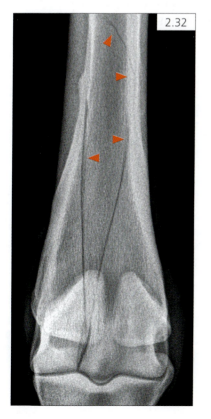

Fig. 2.32 Radiograph (DPl) of a medial condylar fracture (hindlimb) showing spiralling proximal propagation of the fracture line (arrowheads).

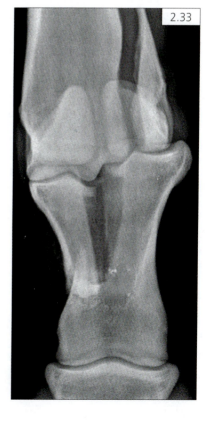

Fig. 2.33 Radiograph (DPl) of a concurrent lateral condylar and P1 fracture.

Cause
- Joint loading is primarily through the condyles.
- Adaptation to training results in greatly increased density of subchondral bone of the condyles relative to that of adjacent sagittal groove.
- Cumulative damage in response to loading may also cause site-specific microcracks in the sagittal groove; failure of bone repair to keep pace with resorption may lead to coalescence into cortical fracture.
- Combination of shear strain differential at condyle/sagittal groove interface and microcracking can result in clinical fracture when cannon subjected to high loading at faster paces.

Risk factors
- Lateral condylar fracture is one of the most common causes of racetrack catastrophic distal limb injury and the most common hurdling/steeplechase fatal injury.
- Encountered in horses of all ages.
- Generally during fast exercise/racing phase of training.
- Fast ground increases likelihood of injury.
- Catastrophic lateral condylar fracture (racing): greater risk for horses that have done no fast work during training; also for those that start racing as 3 or 4 YOs.

History
- Frequently display subtle to mild pre-existing lameness (prodromal injury/'fissure' stage) in days/weeks prior to fracture.
- Incomplete/complete fracture presents as acute-onset severe lameness; usually develops during or immediately after exercise (either on track or on return to yard).

Signs
- Prodromal injury ('fissure' fracture):
  - Subtle–mild unilateral lameness.
  - May only be apparent when ridden.
  - Usually no fetlock joint effusion or localizing signs.
- Incomplete fracture:
  - Moderate–marked lameness.
  - Mild–moderate fetlock joint effusion.
- Complete fracture:
  - Severe lameness.
  - Marked fetlock joint effusion +/– oedematous thickening over affected side of lower cannon.
  - Marked resentment to fetlock flexion.
  - Catastrophic fractures may be open/comminuted with discontinuity of bone column in mid-cannon.

Diagnosis
- Prodromal injury: diagnostic blocking, radiography +/– MRI may be required to localize injury. Not always radiologically visible and if so, can only be detected on flexed dorsopalmar/plantar radiographic projection; multiple good-quality projections may be required (**Figures 2.34a–f**).

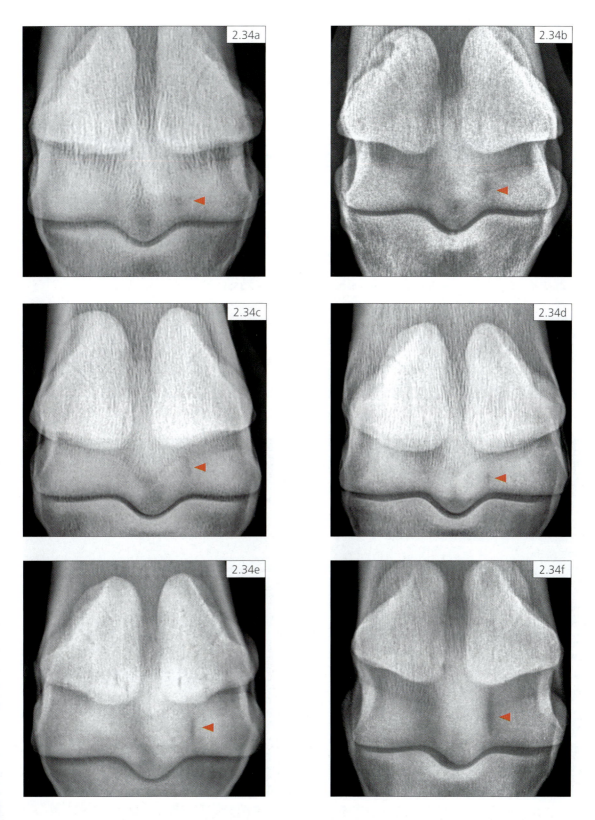

Figs. 2.34a–f Radiographs (flexed DPa) of prodromal 'fissure' fractures. These are examples of short condylar fissures (arrowheads) that were confirmed with MRI; some are radiologically indistinct.

- MRI (standing low-field): required for radiologically silent prodromal injuries; also useful to determine activity/risk of propagation of condylar fissures detected with radiographic screening (*Table 2.4*).

- Incomplete/complete fracture: clinical findings strongly indicative, confirm with radiography. Multiple oblique projections to determine extent of injury in cases with spiral configuration.

Table 2.4 Condylar fissures: MRI grading of severity and risk of fracture propagation

MR FINDINGS	RISK
Cortical fissure visible within the subchondral bone, no/minimal increased density and no STIR hyperintensity in surrounding bone (**Figure 2.35a**).	Low risk of immediate fracture if remains in full training.
Cortical fracture extending minimally into the cancellous bone with very mild, STIR/T2* hyperintensity in the cancellous bone immediately surrounding the fracture.	Moderate immediate risk of fracture if remains in full training.
Cortical fracture extending minimally into the cancellous bone with moderate/marked STIR/T2* hyperintensity diffusely within the cancellous bone of the affected condyle (**Figure 2.35b**).	High immediate risk of fracture if remains in full training.
Cortical fracture extending a variable depth into the cancellous bone with marked generalized STIR/T2* hyperintensity in one or both metacarpal/tarsal condyles (visible radiographically as short incomplete parasagittal condylar fracture).	High risk of complete fracture if horse remains in full training.

STIR, short tau inversion recovery; S. Powell (unpublished data).

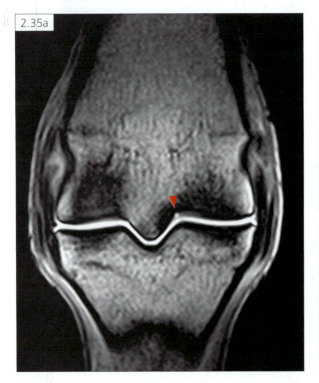
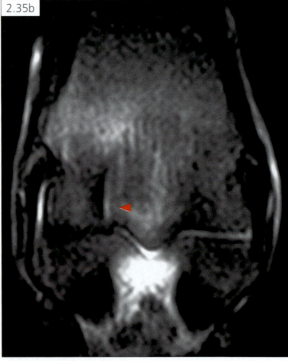

Figs. 2.35a, b MR images of a 'low-risk (a) and a 'high-risk' (b) prodromal 'fissure' fracture (arrowheads).

Management

- See *Table 2.5*.
- Injuries detected at prodromal ('fissure') stage with mild lameness require shorter rehabilitation periods and conservative management (removal from ridden exercise) is sufficient for healing in most cases; surgical placement of a single lag screw (**Figure 2.36**) may reduce risk of reinjury on return to faster paces.
- Failure to detect injury at prodromal stage will typically result in progression to incomplete/complete fracture during high intensity exercise.
- Field management of incomplete/complete fracture: application of immobilizing splint (Kimzey Leg Saver) or Robert Jones bandage for transport to surgical facility or until initial radiographic assessment.

Prognosis

- If not catastrophic, the majority of horses return to racing regardless of fracture configuration.
- Ongoing lameness (on return to training) in small proportion of cases following surgical repair: response to intra-articular medication is variable; however, risk of fracture propagation is low.

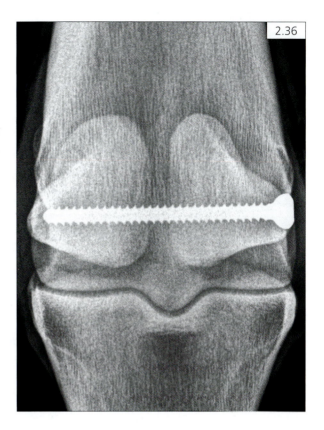

Fig. 2.36 Lag screw placement for a condylar 'fissure' fracture.

Table 2.5 Management of condylar fractures

INJURY TYPE	MANAGEMENT	PROGNOSIS
Prodromal injury ('fissure' fracture)	Removal from ridden exercise (may walk) for 4–8 weeks (determined by severity). Immobilizing bandage not required. MRI to assess healing/guide management if early return to cantering desired. Surgical placement of single lag screw (**Figure 2.36**) (may be performed as standing procedure) may lower risk of reinjury and can give confidence on return to full work.	May progress to incomplete/complete fracture if not removed from fast exercise. Conservative: good/excellent prognosis for return to full use; small proportion may reinjure. Surgery: good/excellent prognosis for return to full use.
Short incomplete (non-displaced)	Conservative management: stable rest (8–12 weeks)/walking +/− immobilizing bandage in acute phase. Rehabilitation guided by radiography. Surgical reduction for best athletic outcome.	Excellent (>80%) prognosis for return to full use with conservative management or surgery.

(continued overleaf)

Table 2.5 (continued)

INJURY TYPE	MANAGEMENT	PROGNOSIS
Long incomplete (non-displaced)	Surgical reduction is treatment of choice for athletic soundness. Satisfactory outcome possible with stable rest/immobilizing bandage; small risk of displacement in initial weeks and OA long term.	Good–excellent prognosis for return to full use with conservative management or surgery.
Complete (displaced/non-displaced)	Surgical reduction.	Good (approximately 80%) prognosis for return to full use, although less likely to race than horses with incomplete fracture. Guarded (>50%) prognosis for racing following surgery for horses with articular comminution.
Complete with concurrent axial fracture of proximal sesamoid bone	Surgical arthrodesis if paddock future desired; otherwise euthanasia on humane grounds.	Poor/hopeless prognosis for athletic soundness. Paddock salvage possible with surgery.
Open/comminuted	Usually warrants immediate euthanasia on humane grounds. Surgical reduction under exceptional circumstances for salvage of horses with breeding value.	Can be salvaged with surgery but guarded prognosis for life (>40% non-healing due to infection).

Transverse fracture

Non-articular fracture of the lower cannon (third metacarpus, Mc3); almost invariably involves the forelimb. Fracture occurs in a transverse or obliquely transverse plane in the distal metacarpal diaphysis; predilection site is above the growth plate. Injury may involve the palmar (most common) or dorsal cortices. Most commonly unilateral but bilateral injuries also occur. Severity of injury (stress/incomplete/complete) at time of initial diagnosis varies.

Cause
- Underlying mechanism unknown but currently considered to be a stress or insufficiency injury arising from dorsopalmar bending forces on the cannon.

Risk factors
- Rare condition.
- Risk factors poorly understood.
- Unraced horses appear at greater risk.
- Generally encountered in horses in trotting/early cantering phase of training.

History
- Acute- or chronic-onset forelimb lameness.
- +/– thickening around/above affected fetlock in days prior to detection of injury.

Signs
- Initial lameness variable: mild–marked.
- +/– fetlock joint effusion.
- Palpable abnormalities (if present) include soft-tissue/bony thickening on palmaromedial/lateral aspect of lower cannon +/– pain response to firm palpation.

Diagnosis
- Radiography: some cases display radiological abnormalities at initial examination (LM and oblique projections most useful) but many require repeat radiography.
- Periosteal callus on palmaro/dorso medial/lateral cannon (above level of physis); +/– palmar endocortical thickening (**Figure 2.37a**).
- Callus (sometimes profound) +/– horizontal fracture line (or radiopacity) may develop 7–14 days after injury (**Figure 2.37b**).
- MRI: rarely required for diagnosis.

Management
- Risk of complete fracture determined from initial severity of lameness/imaging findings.
- Initial radiographic screening unremarkable: stable confinement (+/– immobilizing bandage depending on severity) and repeat radiography at 7–14 days.
- Mild initial clinical and radiological signs: conservative management; stable rest/walking for 8–12 weeks.
- Moderate–marked initial lameness: stable rest with immobilizing bandage for initial 3–4 weeks; rehabilitation guided by radiographic monitoring.
- Surgical fixation considered for injuries at risk of catastrophic deterioration.

Prognosis
- Stress or incomplete fracture: good prognosis for return to full use.
- Severe initial lameness: risk of catastrophic failure with conservative or inappropriate management.

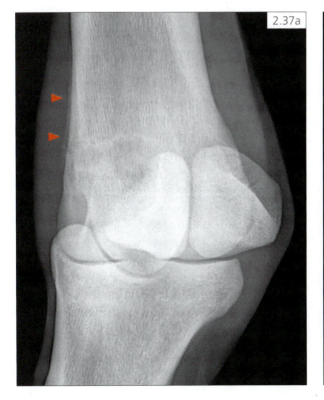
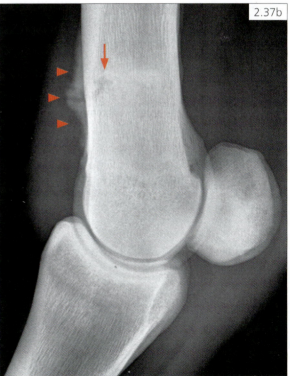

Figs. 2.37a, b Radiographs (DMPaLO/LM) of a transverse metacarpal fracture. (a) Horizontal linear radiopacity (arrow) with early periosteal proliferative change (arrowheads) extending along the dorsal aspect of the cannon. (b) Horizontal linear radiopacity (arrow) with abundant periosteal proliferative change (arrowheads).

Palmar/plantar condylar osteochondral disease (POD/'condylar stress reaction')

POD is a chronic and frequently progressive syndrome of subchondral bone +/– cartilage damage affecting load-bearing sites at the back of the fetlock, with associated loss of action or lameness. The condition does not always necessitate veterinary attention and can remain undetected throughout a racing career, but in some individuals it is performance limiting.

Most frequently occurs in hind fetlocks and is bilateral, but may occur in any limb. Affected joints typically have biaxial lesions (hindlimb pathology greatest in lateral condyle; forelimb distributed between medial and lateral condyles). Spectrum of pathology encountered can range from increased density (osteosclerosis) of condylar bone to crescentic/ovoid-shaped regions of subchondral bone collapse +/– subsequent cartilage damage in advanced cases. Associated subchondral lesions may also develop on the opposing articular face of the PSB.

Cause
- Maladaptive condition brought on by repetitive high compressive loading of subchondral bone at back of the fetlock.

Risk factors
- Common condition (prevalence unknown).
- Incidence appears to increase with age (however, 2 YOs may also be affected).
- Direct association with intensity of training/cumulative racing exposure.

History
- Insidious onset of poor action (if bilateral) or lameness, typically developing over period of months.
- Non-specific signs: trainer may report that horse 'doesn't trot' (but usually satisfied with faster paces); may display unwillingness to jump off at start of canter.
- Action typically worsens as horse approaches fast work/racing phase of training.
- +/– secondary thoracolumbar back pain/epaxial muscle spasm; many affected horses may have received treatment for a sore back.
- Lameness may sometimes be most pronounced in initial weeks of training following a long rest period.

Signs
- Hindlimb pathology: characteristic bilateral action at trot: short-striding/'rolling' of quarters/close or plaiting gait.
- Unilateral lameness (if present) can be of mild–moderate severity.
- Severely affected: may display multilimb lameness and attempt to break directly from walk to canter.
- Lameness often improves ('warms up') rapidly with exercise.
- Fetlock joints typically free from palpable abnormality.

Diagnosis
- Clinical presentation strongly indicative but non-specific.
- Diagnostic blocking: lameness improves in most cases to intra-articular blocking of fetlock joint/s (low 4- or 6-point nerve block may be required for complete abolition). Hindlimb cases may improve/switch following lateral plantar metatarsal nerve block.
- Radiography: relatively insensitive modality for detection/assessment of condition but useful for initial screening. Findings (if present) include increased/irregular radiodensity of the condyle/s (**Figure 2.38a**) (flexed DPa/PlD and LM projections) and, rarely, focal mid-condylar lucency (flexed DPa/DPl and elevated oblique projections) (**Figures 2.38b, c**). Osteoarthritic change is not typical.

Regional Musculoskeletal Conditions

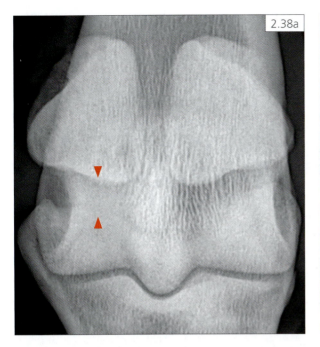

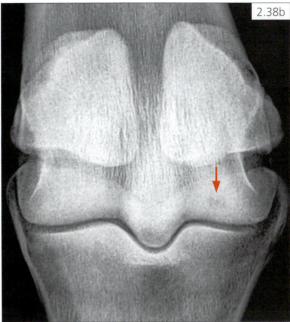

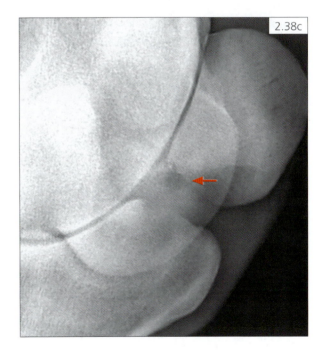

Figs. 2.38a–c Radiographs of plantar osteochondral disease. (a) Marked increase in radiodensity (arrowheads) of hindlimb lateral condyle on flexed PlD radiographic projection. Note the focal radiolucency (arrows) in the lateral metatarsal condyle on flexed DPl (b) and D45°PrL-PlDiO (c) radiographic views.

- Bone scan: characteristic pattern of IRU through affected condyles (**Figures 2.39a, b**), although not always specific or correlated to lameness; IRU usually greatest in lamest limb. Useful for diagnosis (to rule out other injuries) but not prognosis.

- MRI: diagnostic modality of choice to stage lesion (**Figure 2.40**) and differentiate from prodromal condylar fracture (p. 62).

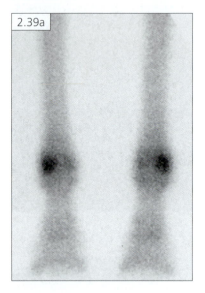

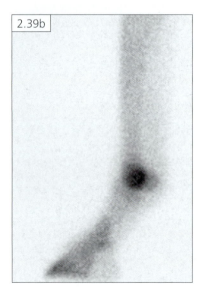

Figs. 2.39a, b Scintigrams of plantar osteochondral disease. Note the typical lateral condylar IRU; plantar (a), lateral (b) views.

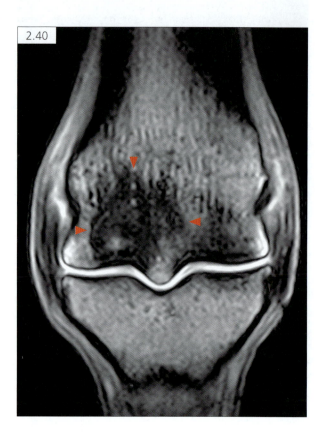

Fig. 2.40 Plantar osteochondral disease: MR T1 dorsal image through the plantar aspect of the condyles of the fetlock joint. Lateral is to the left of the image. There is extensive bone mineral densification of the lateral condyle (arrowheads) with focal T1 hyperintensity within the subchondral bone.

Management
- Some cases require initial risk assessment for other pathology (condylar fracture); necessity determined by history/clinical findings such as rapid deterioration of action.
- Many cases safely managed empirically without diagnostic imaging.
- Osteochondral changes at time of diagnosis are frequently irreversible and therefore rest is not curative.
- Treatment options are limited; mainstay is intra-articular medication (Chapter 1, p. 17): many horses respond favourably; however, quality and duration of effect varies widely.
- Modification of training regime (reduced work on uphill or synthetic tracks), use of treadmill/swimming exercise and concurrent therapies such as systemic chondroprotective medications (Chapter 1, p. 19), bisphosphonate medication (tiludronate), ESWT and altered shoeing (bar shoes/lowered heels) may be incorporated into management; efficacy undetermined and individual clinical effect likely to be limited.
- Short periods of rest (<2 months) currently considered to be of little benefit to healing of lesions and in some cases may actually lead to deterioration (subchondral bone collapse) if training resumes during resorptive phase of bone repair.

Prognosis
- Unpredictable condition: most horses remain static or display slowly deteriorating signs over one or more seasons; however, clinical improvement may also occur.
- Continued training in medium to long term usually possible aided by periodic intra-articular medication.
- Is not associated with increased risk of developing condylar fracture.
- Horses with marked pathology may have shorter/less successful careers (performance limiting); however, this is not universal and many horses (including elite performers) train satisfactorily for several seasons after diagnosis.

Synovitis
Primary synovitis (without overt underlying orthopaedic injury) is a sporadic finding and may affect one or more fetlocks. Most common in the forelimb. Joint effusion is of variable severity and usually self-limiting, although some remain palpably abnormal throughout future training.

Cause
- Undetermined in most cases.
- Acute or repetitive overextension/overloading may cause inflammation of joint capsule or support structures.

Risk factors
- Common condition.
- Any age/stage of training but most commonly in 2 YOs in cantering exercise.
- Risk factors poorly understood but possible influence of conformation/BWT/maturity relative to workload.

History
- Acute or chronic (days/weeks) onset of joint filling.

Signs
- Distension of dorsal and palmar joint pouches +/− periarticular oedema in acute phase.
- Variable response to forced flexion of joint: painful in some cases.
- +/− pain on deep palpation of joint capsule margins: may require care to differentiate from SLB desmopathy (p. 86).
- Lameness is rare and if present, is usually subtle–mild.
- Rarely, lameness of moderate severity and marked joint effusion.

Diagnosis
- Clinical findings usually sufficient.
- Imaging rarely required but warranted if lame (to rule out orthopaedic injury), or if synovitis severe or non-responsive to anti-inflammatory measures.
- Radiography/ultrasonography/MRI as dictated by clinical requirement/perceived fracture risk.

Management
- Topical anti-inflammatory therapy: osmotic dressing/cold therapy.
- No lameness: continued training, although short period of reduced exercise (walk/trot) during acute phase may be beneficial.
- Poor response to initial anti-inflammatory measures (and if orthopaedic injury not suspected): intra-articular medication +/− continuation of training.

Prognosis
- Primary fetlock synovitis rarely causes significant interruption to training.
- Articular fragmentation may occur in small proportion of cases but prognosis for continued training is good.

Dorsal osteochondral fragmentation ('chip' fracture)

Osteochondral fragments or 'chips' in the fetlock typically arise from the dorsomedial or dorsolateral aspects of the joint margin of P1. They vary in size, are usually solitary and may be displaced/non-displaced. Typically associated with other overextension pathology (soft tissue +/− subchondral bone) in joint. Predominantly in forelimb; unilateral or bilateral.

Cause
- Results from acute or repetitive overextension of fetlock and dorsal impact of P1 on lower cannon.
- Frequently part of an overloading syndrome that may include palmar or dorsal osteochondral disease (p. 66)/chronic proliferative synovitis (p. 69)/SLB desmopathy (p. 86).

Risk factors
- May occur at any age.
- Usually during cantering/fast work phase of training.
- Risk factors poorly understood: possible influence of conformation/BWT.

History
- Frequently a clinically silent incidental finding at routine imaging.
- May present with acute joint effusion +/− lameness.

Signs
- Acute phase: transient joint effusion (synovitis) +/− pain response to joint flexion +/− mild–moderate lameness; subsides over days/weeks.
- Fragmentation can also occur with little/no evidence of joint inflammation.

Diagnosis
- Clinical findings alone do not permit differentiation from primary synovitis (p. 69) but relatively mild lameness distinguishes from proximal phalangeal fracture (p. 52).
- Radiography: modelling of dorsal articular margin +/− displaced/non-displaced fragment/s (DLPaMO, LM and DPa projections most useful) (**Figures 2.41a–d**).
- Ultrasonography: rarely employed but good sensitivity for detection of fragments.

Management
- Different management options available; dictated by clinical severity and training objectives.
- Radiological severity useful as a guide but is not prescriptive.
- Conservative management: period of reduced exercise (walking/trotting for 1–4 weeks) in acute phase +/− systemic/topical/intra-articular anti-inflammatory medication to control synovitis.
- When rest period undesirable: topical and/or intra-articular anti-inflammatory therapy may permit continuation of training. Response should guide management; training in face of lameness/synovitis may lead to long-term osteoarthritic change.
- Surgical removal may be treatment of choice for some large chips or for cases that respond poorly to rest/medication.
- Long-standing fragments are generally not clinically active but may be markers of other overextension pathology in fetlock region.

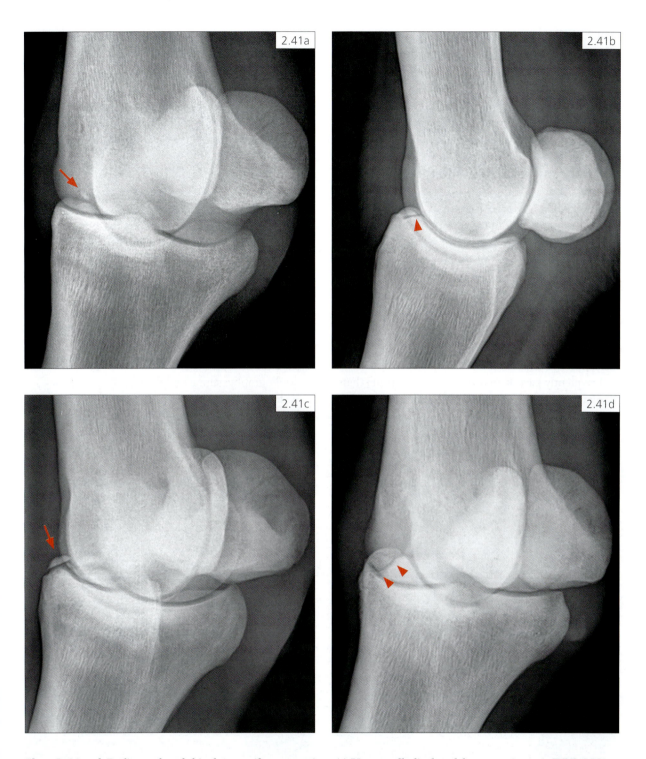

Figs. 2.41a–d Radiographs of chip fracture/fragmentation. (a) Very small, displaced fragment (arrow) (DLPaMO). (b) Moderate sized non-displaced chip fracture (arrowhead) (LM). (c) Recently displaced chip (arrow) from articular margin of P1 (DLPaMO). (d) Large osteochondral fragment (arrowheads) (DLPaMO)

Prognosis
- Good: generally results in little interruption to training.
- Surgical removal not always necessary but carries excellent prognosis for return to racing (>80%); mean time to return to full training following surgery approximately 12 weeks.

Chronic proliferative ('villonodular') synovitis
Chronic inflammatory condition of dorsal soft tissues of forelimb fetlock joint. Synovial pad within dorsal pouch of fetlock normally protects front of lower cannon but may become inflamed/thickened with repetitive trauma. Most commonly unilateral but may be bilateral.

Cause
- Repetitive overextension of fetlock causes 'pinching' of synovial pad by top of pastern.
- Frequently part of an overloading syndrome that may include dorsal osteochondral fragmentation (p. 70)/palmar or dorsal osteochondral disease (p. 66)/SLB desmopathy (p. 86).

Risk factors
- Most commonly in horses ≥3 YO.
- Risk factors poorly understood.

History
- Chronic condition with insidious onset and progression; develops over long period (months/years).
- Typically exacerbated by fast exercise.

Signs
- Visual prominence of dorsal pouch of front fetlock joint/s.
- +/– joint effusion.
- Lameness an inconsistent feature and if present, is typically mild.
- Flexion of joint resented.

Diagnosis
- Clinical findings usually definitive.
- Radiography: supracondylar lysis ('cutting back') of lower dorsal cannon, just above the condyles on LM projection. Frequently with bony proliferation immediately above the depression, at proximal attachment of joint capsule (**Figures 2.42a, b**).

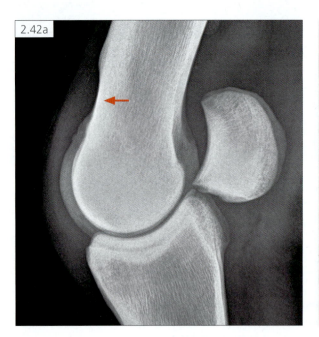
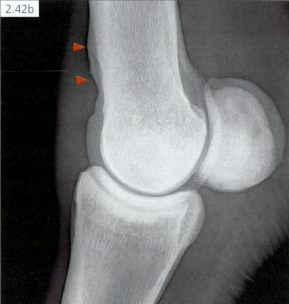

Figs. 2.42a, b Radiographs (LM) of chronic proliferative synovitis. Supracondylar lysis (arrow) (a) and periosteal proliferative change (b) (arrowheads) of forelimb fetlocks.

- Ultrasonography: employed infrequently. Mean thickness of synovial pad in affected joints 9–11 mm.

Management
- Intervention/rest not always necessary, but usually some treatment indicated by the time the condition is clinically obvious.
- Intra-articular medication +/− cold therapy may alleviate inflammation sufficiently to permit continued training.
- Surgical excision is treatment of choice for cases that do not respond favourably to medical management.

Prognosis
- Although medical/conservative management is symptomatic and not curative, many cases are manageable and continue to train/race with little interruption.
- Surgery: good prognosis for return to racing (approximately 80%). Recurrence rare.

Dorsal osteochondral disease (Mc3/Mt3)

Overextension injury of fetlock joint that can cause unilateral lameness; affects dorsal aspect of lower cannon bone. Predominantly an injury of the forelimb. Spectrum of pathology from increased density (osteosclerosis) of bone at dorsal sagittal ridge (most common location) or metacarpal condyles, to regions of subchondral bone collapse and associated cartilage damage. Osteochondral damage involves the extra-articular fibrocartilage of the dorsal recess of the joint +/− dorsal synovial pad. Often in association with adaptive change at dorsoproximal margin of P1.

Cause
- Presumed to result from repetitive overextension of fetlock and dorsal impact of P1 on lower cannon.
- May be seen in association with other fetlock overload/overextension pathologies including dorsal osteochondral fragmentation/POD/chronic proliferative synovitis.

Risk factors
- Uncommon condition.
- All ages/stages of training but typically during cantering/fast exercise phase.
- Risk factors poorly understood.

History
- Chronic- or acute-onset forelimb lameness.
- Temporary improvement with rest but recurs on return to cantering.

Signs
- Unilateral lameness of mild–moderate severity.
- +/− joint effusion.

Diagnosis
- Clinical findings non-specific.
- Diagnostic blocking: lameness improves in most cases with intra-articular blocking of fetlock joint; low 4-point nerve block may be required for complete abolition of lameness.
- Radiography: relatively insensitive: increased radiodensity on LM and/or flexed DPa projections.
- Bone scan: IRU in affected distal cannon but pattern not specific.
- Ultrasonography: most sensitive modality to detect cartilaginous damage at dorsal aspect of joint.

- MRI: diagnostic modality of choice (**Figure 2.43**) for subchondral/cancellous bone injury in this region.

Management
- Clinical/imaging severity determines necessity for rest period.
- Continued training aided by intra-articular medication possible; however, quality and duration of response varies (often poor).
- Modification of training regime (treadmill/swimming) may be beneficial.
- Stable rest/walking for 6–10 weeks +/− intra-articular medication often sufficient for resolution.

Prognosis
- Good prognosis for continued training.
- Progression to stress fracture generally considered unlikely.

Osteochondrosis: osteochondritis dissecans

Developmental defect of cartilage/subchondral bone. The fetlock is frequently the site of osteochondritis dissecans (OCD) lesions in the horse; these most commonly involve the middle or dorsal third of the sagittal ridge (any limb) and are characterized by flattening or osteochondral fragmentation. Severity varies. Less common are fragments of various sizes at the back of the joint in association with the medial (typically) or

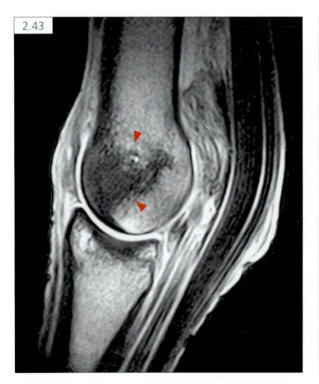

Fig. 2.43 Dorsal osteochondral disease. MR T1 sagittal image of the fetlock joint. The T1 signal abnormality (arrowheads) is biased towards the dorsal aspect of the joint in this case; the palmar aspect is relatively spared.

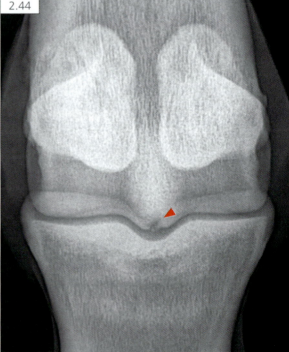

Fig. 2.44 Radiograph (DPa) of fetlock OCD. Note the sagittal ridge radiolucency (arrowhead).

lateral palmar/plantar process. These may also occur in any limb and are not always distinguishable from ununited palmar/plantar processes or overextension injuries sustained early in life. Regardless of origin most of these lesions are clinically insignificant. Occasionally, significance is attributed to axial (articular) plantar process fragments based on appearance and clinical presentation. Unilateral or bilateral.

Cause
- See Osteochondrosis (Other musculoskeletal conditions, p. 192).

Risk factors
- Sagittal ridge lesions common: prevalence in sales yearlings approximately 20–40%.
- Palmar/plantar process fragments: prevalence in sales yearlings approximately 5–7%.

History
- Typically an incidental finding at routine yearling sales radiography (subclinical at time of detection).

Signs
- +/− joint effusion (most common with sagittal ridge OCD).
- Plantar/palmar fragments typically clinically inapparent.
- Lameness is not typical of the condition.

Diagnosis
- Radiography: sagittal ridge OCD may be detectable on DPa projection (**Figure 2.44**) but is best assessed with flexed LM (**Figure 2.45**). Dorsal lesions visible on standing LM projection (**Figure 2.46**). Palmar/plantar process

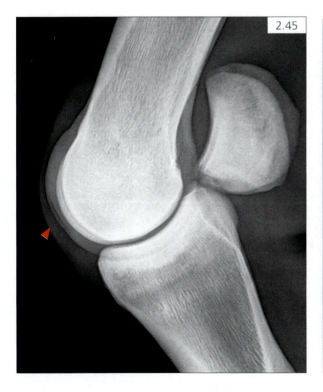

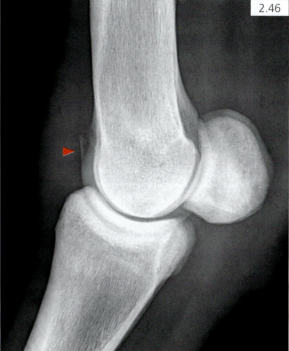

Fig. 2.45 Radiograph (flexed LM) of fetlock OCD. Note osteochondral fragment (arrowhead) of the mid-sagittal ridge.

Fig. 2.46 Radiograph (LM) of fetlock OCD. Note dorsal osteochondral fragment of the sagittal ridge (arrowhead).

lesions are detected on oblique or LM projections (**Figures 2.47a–c**).

Management
- Very rarely clinically active and treatment is generally unnecessary.
- Plantar/palmar osteochondral fragments sometimes claimed to affect action at faster paces but no evidence base to support this.
- If significant joint effusion/inflammation (rare) in early training: modified exercise +/or intra-articular medication.
- Surgical debridement occasionally warranted in clinical cases non-responsive to medical/conservative management (rare).

Prognosis
- Excellent; rarely interfere with training.

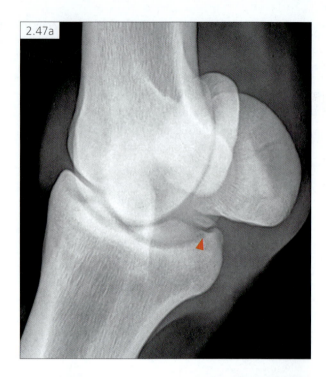
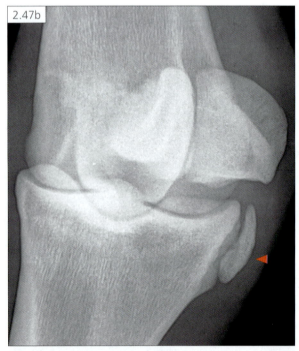
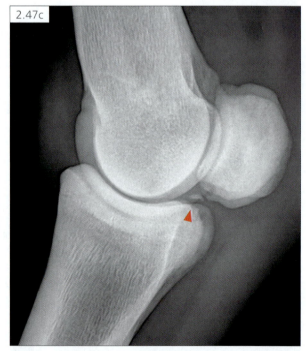

Figs. 2.47a–c Examples of plantar process fragments (hindlimb fetlocks) (arrowheads).

Osteochondrosis: subchondral bone cyst

Developmental defect of cartilage/subchondral bone. Subchondral bone cysts are encountered sporadically in association with the fetlock and PIPJ (pastern joint). Bilateral lesions are seen in about 10% of cases.

Fetlock joint cysts are usually found in the forelimb and typically in the medial condyle of the cannon bone (**Figure 2.48**), although lesions also occur in proximal P1 and dorsal sagittal ridge. In the PIPJ, midline radiolucencies in the distal articular margin of P1 are common and have generally been considered a normal variant (**Figure 2.49a**), while cysts in medial or lateral locations of either distal P1 or proximal P2 are potentially more relevant (**Figures 2.49b, c**). PIPJ cysts are most common in the hindlimb.

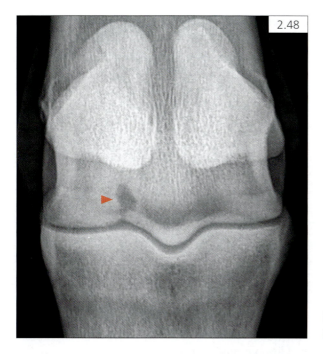

Fig. 2.48 Radiograph (DPa) of a subchondral bone cyst in the medial distal metacarpus (arrow).

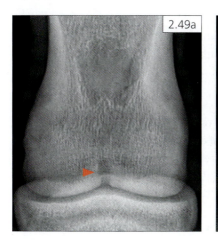 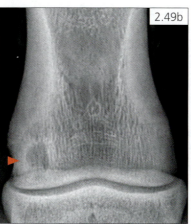 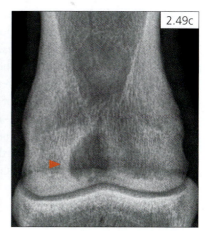

Figs. 2.49a–c Radiographs (Dpa/DPl) of subchondral radiolucencies of the PIPJ. (a) Central distal; (b) medial distal; (c) large central distal (arrowheads).

Cause
- See Osteochondrosis (Other musculoskeletal conditions, p. 192).

Risk factors
- Rare condition. Prevalence in sales yearlings: <1% for fetlock joint, <2.5% for PIPJ.

History
- Typically an incidental finding at routine yearling sales radiography (subclinical at time of diagnosis).
- May become clinically active when training commences: acute or intermittent lameness in early cantering phase.

Signs
- Most cases display no clinical signs.
- If clinically active: mild–moderate unilateral lameness +/− joint effusion.
- Fetlock: lameness often exacerbated by flexion.

Diagnosis
- Radiography: oval-shaped or irregular radiolucency +/− surrounding sclerosis; rarely, affected joints may also display evidence of arthritis.
- MRI: some PIPJ lesions are radiologically silent and MRI required for diagnosis.

Management
- Clinically silent: no treatment necessary and continue training.
- Clinically active: goal of treatment is to resolve lameness and return to full function.
- Clinically active fetlock joint cysts: intra-articular medication (corticosteroid) may be useful for short-term soundness; however, surgical debridement offers best chance of return to use.
- Clinically active PIPJ cysts: intra-articular medication (corticosteroid) may be useful for short-term soundness; surgical arthrodesis offers best chance of return to use but should be viewed as salvage procedure.

Prognosis
- Most do not cause lameness; however, unpredictable behaviour and can be career-threatening if become clinically active.
- Clinically active fetlock joint cysts: guarded prognosis with conservative management; prognosis for return to full use is good (approximately 80%) with surgery.
- Clinically active PIPJ cysts: poor prognosis for soundness with conservative management; prognosis for return to full use is improved but guarded with surgical arthrodesis (better prognosis for hindlimb).

Pastern joint (PIPJ) osteoarthritis

OA of the PIPJ (pastern joint) is rare and when encountered usually affects a single limb (forelimb or hindlimb). It may occur in association with osteochondrosis (subchondral bone cyst) or as a primary condition.

Cause
- Frequently undetermined.
- May result from acute/chronic PIPJ instability/subluxation.
- May occur secondary to a subchondral bone cyst (p. 77).

Risk factors
- Any age/stage of training.
- Risk factors unknown.

History
- Chronic-onset lameness.

Signs
- Mild–severe unilateral lameness.
- Firm non-painful thickening/altered profile of affected PIPJ.

Diagnosis
- Radiography: osteoarthritic change including dorsoproximal osteophyte/s P2, narrowing of joint space +/− altered subchondral density (**Figure 2.50a, b**).

Management
- Determined by clinical severity, chronicity and stage of training.
- Early disease best managed by rest (stable rest/walking for 8–12 weeks) +/− anti-inflammatory medication.

- Mild/chronic disease: intra-articular medication +/− continued training may be possible.
- Remedial shoeing (raised heels/improved breakover) may assist management.
- Severe disease/poor response to conservative management: consider surgical arthrodesis

Prognosis
- Guarded–poor prognosis for athletic soundness with rest/medication.
- Improved (but guarded) prognosis for return to full use with surgical arthrodesis.

Sesamoiditis

Widely used but ambiguous term describing a spectrum of radiological changes of the PSBs that can be found in young (yearling/2 YO) racehorses. Condition is defined radiologically (see below) and as described here does not include those milder radiological changes that are considered variants of normality. Characterized by areas of demineralization +/− entheseous new bone deposition predominantly on abaxial margin of sesamoid. Results in greater relative prominence of vascular channels or enlargement/change in the contour of the sesamoid on radiography. May be seen uniaxially or biaxially in forelimb and hindlimb sesamoid bones.

Cause
- Underlying cause is not 'inflammation' of the sesamoid bone as such, but rather maladaptive change to stresses primarily acting at interface with SLB.
- Likely association with SLB desmopathy in some cases.
- Proximal abaxial border of sesamoid bone is site of attachment of the SLB as well as entry point for blood supply.

Risk factors
- Approximately 2–3% of yearlings affected by marked sesamoiditis (one or more sesamoids).
- Risk factors poorly understood but nutrition and loading/conditioning early in life (foal) may be of importance.

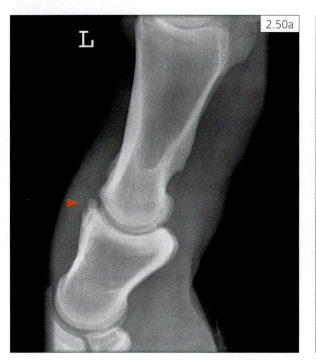
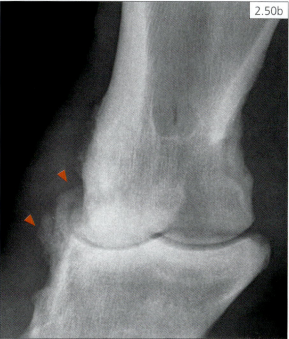

Fig. 2.50a, b Radiographs [LM (a) and DLPlMO (b)] of PIPJ osteoarthritis. Note the abundant articular and periarticular modelling (arrowheads) of the dorsomedial joint margin.

History
- Usually a 'radiological diagnosis': first detected at routine sales radiography.

Signs
- Frequently no palpable/visible abnormality of sesamoid bone or fetlock.
- Firm, non-painful prominence/enlargement of affected sesamoid/s may accompany more severe radiographic change.
- Lameness is not a feature but may be present with concurrent, active SLB desmopathy (p. 86).

Diagnosis
- Radiography: features that characterize condition include entheseous bone on the proximal abaxial or basilar margins (at SLB and distal sesamoidean ligament attachments respectively); ≥3 enlarged (>2 mm width) or irregularly-shaped vascular channels in abaxial margin; large poorly defined irregularities in bone density involving body of sesamoid bone; abnormal abaxial profile (**Figures 2.51a–c, 2.52a–c**).

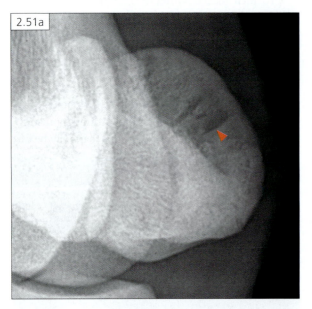

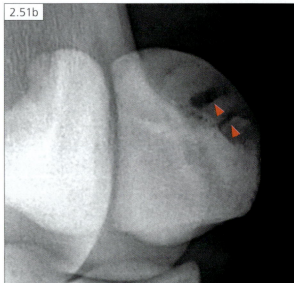

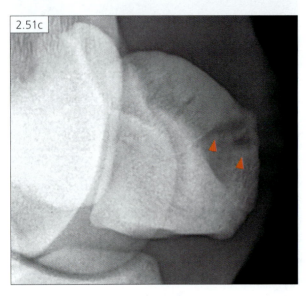

Figs. 2.51a–c Radiographs (DLPaMO/DMPaLO) of sesamoiditis. Note the enlarged vascular channels (arrowheads).

- Ultrasonography: assessment of associated SLB important in cases of moderate–marked radiological abnormality or if palpable abnormality (thickening/pain) at SLB/sesamoid interface.

Management
- If clinically silent and detected as incidental finding: no treatment required but may serve to guide management.
- Marked radiological changes: patient approach to training (to permit gradual strengthening/maturation of ligament/bone junction) generally advocated to limit risk of injury.

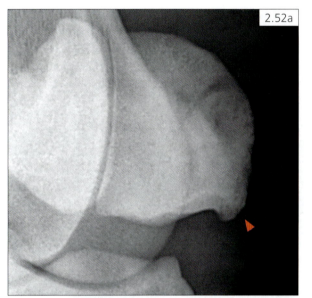
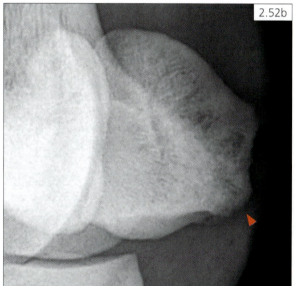
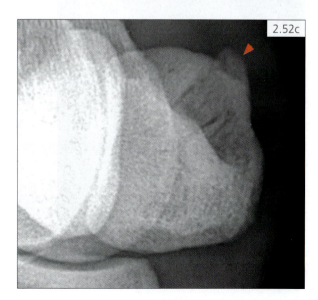

Figs. 2.52a–c Radiographs (DLPaMO/DMPaLO) of sesamoiditis. Note the altered abaxial contour/entheseous proliferation (arrowheads).

- Concurrent SLB desmopathy (p. 86) may have greater impact on trainability and should be monitored/managed appropriately.
- Medical (acetylsalicylic acid/isoxuprine) or physical (ESWT) therapy sometimes advocated but no evidence of efficacy.

Prognosis
- Most cases of mild–moderate sesamoid bone changes detected at routine radiography do not interfere with training.
- Does not predispose to sesamoid bone fracture.
- Yearlings with moderate to severe radiological changes have fewer race starts at 2 and 3 YO, but direct association with sesamoid injury is unlikely.
- Horses with significant radiological changes and concurrent SLB desmopathy are at greater risk of interruption to training as 2 YO if injury becomes clinically active (can be career-threatening in rare cases).
- No effect of forelimb/hindlimb on prognosis.

Proximal sesamoid bone fracture
PSB fracture may occur during training or can be encountered as long-standing radiological lesions from previous foal injury. Several configurations of fracture occur; fracture type, severity and location of affected sesamoid (forelimb/hindlimb, medial/lateral) can determine management and outcome of injury:
- **Apical fractures**: most common configuration (**Figures 2.53a, b**). Associated with partial disruption of SLB. Occur more frequently in hindlimb.
- **Mid-body fractures**: when uniaxial usually affects forelimb medial sesamoid (**Figure 2.54**). Biaxial (mid-body medial + apical/oblique lateral PSB) fractures are potentially catastrophic due to loss of suspensory support of fetlock (**Figure 2.55**). May be comminuted and usually associated with distraction of fragments.

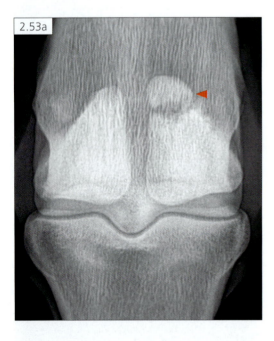
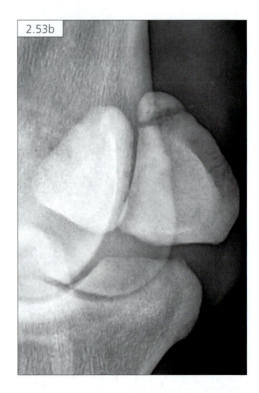

Figs. 2.53a, b Radiographs (DPl/DLPaMO) of a long-standing apical (arrowhead) proximal sesamoid bone fracture.

- **Abaxial fractures**: true avulsion fracture with moderate–severe disruption of SLB (**Figure 2.56**). Predominantly in forelimb and medial sesamoid. May be articular or non-articular.

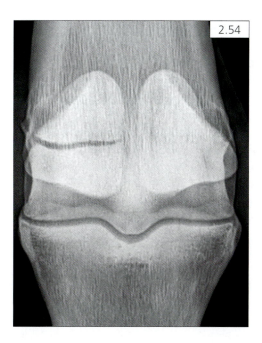

Fig. 2.54 Radiograph (DPa) of a mid-body proximal sesamoid bone fracture.

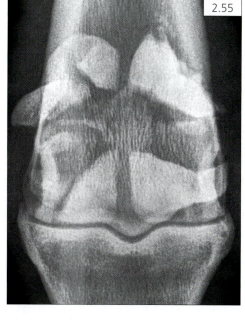

Fig. 2.55 Radiograph (DPa) of a comminuted biaxial proximal sesamoid bone fracture (forelimb).

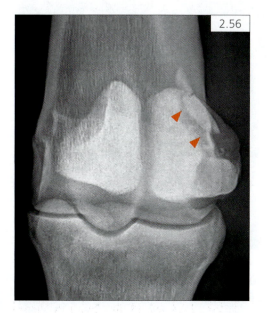

Fig. 2.56 Radiograph (DLPaMO) of an abaxial/avulsion fracture of a lateral proximal sesamoid bone. Note the distraction of the fragment (arrowheads).

- **Basilar fractures**: fragment of variable size from base of sesamoid (**Figure 2.57a**); partial displacement typical. Predominantly affects forelimb medial sesamoid.
- **Axial fractures**: predominantly in forelimb. Invariably associated with a concurrent (displaced) condylar fracture of the cannon bone (**Figure 2.57b**) (p. 58).

Cause
- Many are acute monotonic overloading injuries but proportion are predisposed by cumulative microdamage/modelling of sesamoid.
- Sesamoid bone and suspensory ligament strengthen at different rates during conditioning.
- SLBs more likely to injure early in training and sesamoid bones later in training (if overloaded).
- Training induces changes in bone density that make zone just below apex of sesamoid structurally the weakest point.
- Sesamoid subject to high tensile strains on palmar/plantar aspect from suspensory attachments and compressive force from condyle of cannon bone dorsally.
- Mid-body fractures propagate from flexor to articular surface and may be preceded by microfractures.

Risk factors
- Biaxial mid-body fractures are an important cause of catastrophic racetrack injury (particularly on dirt and synthetic tracks): typically in older horses and more likely in horses that have been campaigned intensively during season of injury.
- Risk factors for other configurations poorly understood.
- Sesamoiditis is not associated with greater risk of fracture.

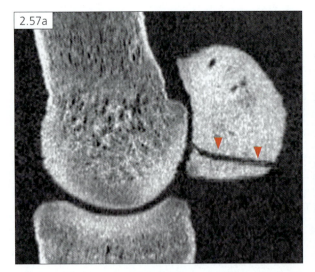
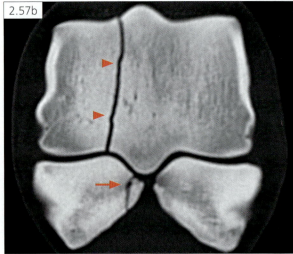

Fig. 2.57a, b (a) CT image (bone algorithm/sagittal) of a forelimb basilar proximal sesamoid bone fracture (arrowheads). (b) CT image (volume rendered) of an axial fracture of forelimb proximal sesamoid bone (arrow) with concurrent lateral condylar fracture (arrowheads).

Regional Musculoskeletal Conditions

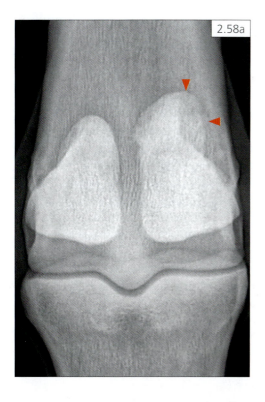

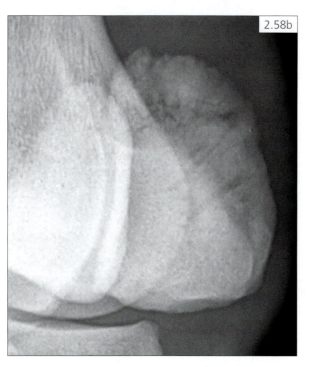

History
- Acute-onset lameness during or after racing/fast work.
- Long-standing (settled) injuries may be detected at routine radiography (**Figures 2.58a, b**).

Signs
- Clinical findings vary with fracture configuration and severity.
- Mild–marked unilateral lameness.
- Focal swelling and pain on palpation of affected sesamoid.
- +/– fetlock joint effusion.
- Biaxial fractures: severe lameness and dropping (hyperextension) of fetlock due to complete disruption of suspensory apparatus.
- Subfracture threshold (or prodromal) injuries can occur (rarely): moderate–marked unilateral lameness with reluctance to place heel of affected limb to ground and typically no clinical abnormality of fetlock region.

Figs. 2.58a, b Enlarged proximal sesamoid bone (arrowheads) resulting from a juvenile sesamoid fracture.

Diagnosis:
- Radiography: fractures usually well-defined on standard and elevated oblique projections.
- Ultrasonography: assessment of suspensory/distal sesamoidean ligament attachments not essential but may assist management.
- Bone scan: not necessary for overt fracture but may permit detection of prodromal fracture (**Figure 2.59**).
- MRI: may be of some use in differentiating the causes of increased scintigraphic activity but sensitivity and specificity currently undetermined.

Management/prognosis
- See *Table 2.6*.

Suspensory ligament branch desmopathy

Injuries to the SLB typically take the form of a focal palmar/plantar insertional tear at the interface with the PSB (+/− enlargement of branch). More generalized/extensive damage (sometimes to the level of suspensory ligament bifurcation) is far less common and usually represents chronic injury. Clinical injury most frequently affects a single SLB but subclinical defects may be present at other sites. Medial branches are overrepresented and injury is more common in the forelimbs. Injuries involving the dorsal face of the SLB may communicate with the fetlock joint.

Cause
- Likely that some injuries arise from acute overextension or asymmetrical loading of the fetlock and others from repetitive strain injury of ligament/sesamoid bone interface.
- Clinical and subclinical lesions occur frequently in untrained yearlings (+/− sesamoiditis, p. 79) and may predispose to clinical injury when exposed to increased loading in early training.

Risk factors
- Clinical injury usually first encountered in 2 YOs during early cantering phase of training; likely to be preceded by pre-existing subclinical injuries (from yearling/foal stage) in many cases.
- Clinical injuries are less common in older horses; may be seen in association with other fetlock overextension pathology.
- Clinical injury also seen in yearlings prior to/during sales preparation (occasionally foals).
- Risk factors poorly understood but loading/conditioning early in life (foal) may be of importance.
- Increased risk with some poor conformation types (toe in: lateral branch; toe out: medial branch).
- Mediolateral imbalance of hoof frequently cited as risk factor but rarely observed in clinical cases.

History
- Subclinical lesions may be detected during pre-purchase imaging (yearlings and horses-in-training).
- Clinical injury: usually insidious onset with mild signs in early stages contributing to delayed detection in many cases.

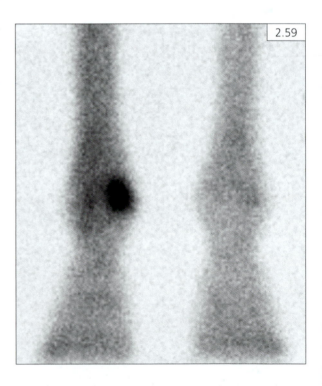

Fig. 2.59 Plantar scintigram of marked focal IRU in the medial sesamoid bone. This injury was radiologically silent.

Table 2.6 **Management and prognosis for proximal sesamoid bone fractures**

FRACTURE TYPE	MANAGEMENT	PROGNOSIS
Apical	Surgical removal of fragment gives best chance of return to racing.	Size/geometry of apical fragment does not influence prognosis but location does.
	Conservative management is acceptable alternative: stable rest/walking for 8–12 weeks.	Conservative management: generally a good prognosis for racing.
		Surgery: excellent prognosis for hindlimb or lateral forelimb fractures.
		Medial forelimb sesamoid: guarded prognosis for return to racing (<50%) regardless of management.
Mid-body	Uniaxial fractures: consider surgical fixation if athletic future desired. Lengthy rehabilitation (up to 1 year) regardless of management.	Uniaxial: fair prognosis (60–70%) for return to some athletic use following surgical fixation; guarded prognosis for racing.
	Biaxial fractures: may justify euthanasia; salvage for paddock use possible with surgery (fetlock arthrodesis) or long-term splinting.	Biaxial fractures are a career-ending/life-threatening injury.
Abaxial	Surgical removal of fragment gives best chance of return to racing.	Surgery: good prognosis (>70%) for return to racing. Fractures involving both apical and abaxial margins have less favourable outcome.
	Conservative management acceptable alternative with lower success rate.	
Basilar	Surgical removal of fragment gives best chance of return to racing (when fragment does not involve entire base of bone).	Surgery: good prognosis (>70%) for return to racing.
	Conservative management acceptable alternative with lower success rate.	Conservative management: guarded prognosis (<50%) for racing
		Factors with negative influence on outcome include large fragment size (full dorsopalmar width), displacement (>3 mm) and comminution.
Axial	Not usually treated (concurrent condylar fracture may be repaired by surgical arthrodesis for paddock salvage only).	Prognosis for athletic use poor/hopeless.
Prodromal fracture	Continued training without rest period carries risk of sesamoid bone fracture.	Excellent prognosis for return to full use.
	Conservative management: stable rest/walking for 6–10 weeks +/− anti-inflammatory medication.	

Signs

- Prominence/enlargement of affected branch or sesamoid region, +/− overlying oedematous thickening.
- +/− focal pain response to deep palpation, particularly at level of SLB/sesamoid interface.
- +/− palpable enlargement/loss of border definition of branch with limb in flexion.
- +/− fetlock joint effusion.
- Lameness is uncommon and frequently may only be observed when ridden on deep track; likely that loading 'stretch' pain (on extension of fetlock) is responsible in these cases.
- Lameness (if present) is mild–moderate.

Diagnosis
- Clinical findings alone are strongly indicative.
- Ultrasonography: required to characterize location and severity of injury. Focal hypoechogenic lesion/enlargement/loss of border definition/periligamentous thickening/irregular sesamoid bone interface (**Figures 2.60a–d, 2.61a, b**). Ultrasound does not always permit determination of articular component to injury.
- Radiography: not necessary for diagnosis but may assist management by determining health of associated sesamoid bone. Single or multiple enlarged vascular channels +/– entheseous modelling (**Figure 2.62**) are typical but not universal.

Management
- Management dictated by clinical severity, stage of training and career goals.
- Subclinical or subtle lesions (no lameness): no alteration in training required; however, vigilance for clinical deterioration.
- Clinical injuries early in training: consider conservative management to improve likelihood of long-term soundness (stable rest/walking for 8–12 weeks +/– ultrasonographic monitoring +/– ESWT). Ultrasonographic resolution is typically slow and should not dictate management.

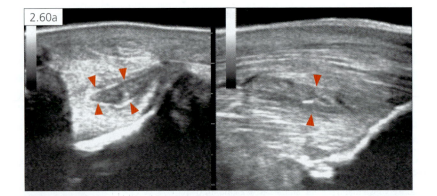

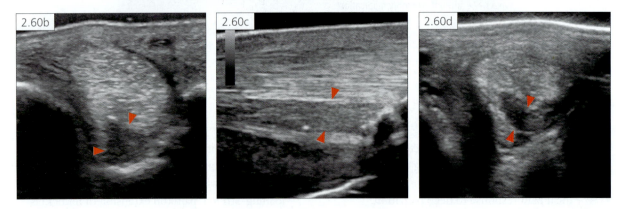

Figs. 2.60a–d Ultrasonograms (transverse, longitudinal) of SLB desmopathy. Note the insertional tear at the palmar (arrowheads) (a) and axial (arrowheads) (b–d) margins of the branch.

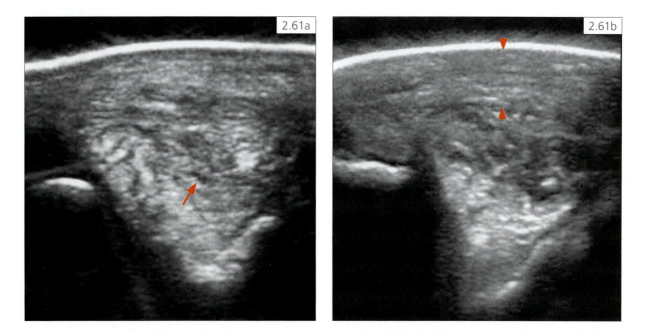

Figs. 2.61a, b Ultrasonograms (transverse) of SLB desmopathy. Examples of diffuse irregularity of fibre pattern (arrow) and periligamentous thickening (arrowheads).

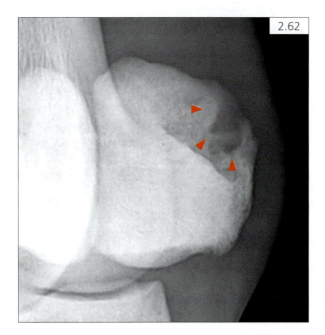

Fig. 2.62 Radiograph (DMPaLO) of sesamoid bone radiological changes (arrowheads) associated with SLB desmopathy.

- Clinical injuries later in training or when removal from training is difficult to justify: continued training may be possible aided by short period (2–6 weeks) of reduced exercise and aggressive anti-inflammatory therapy (topical/cold therapy/ intra-articular medication). Satisfactory progress judged by maintenance of soundness (clinical +/or ultrasonographic appearance of SLB may deteriorate slightly). With appropriate management there is no risk of serious breakdown.
- Extensive injuries (including those to suspensory ligament bifurcation): may require lengthy rehabilitation.
- Shoeing: balancing foot and remedial shoeing (caudal support) may be beneficial.
- Ultrasound-guided intralesional medication (biological regenerative products): currently little evidence of efficacy but may be justifiable.
- Arthroscopic surgery: consider for recurrent/ troublesome injuries with articular component.
- Treadmill-assisted rehabilitation and training may be beneficial to control loading at SLB/sesamoid interface.
- Treatments used in human sports medicine for insertional Achilles tendinitis, such as sclerotherapy/prolotherapy, may offer some promise for recurrent/chronic injuries but currently investigational in racehorses.

Prognosis
- Prediction of outcome difficult and not directly related to ultrasonographic severity.
- Most injuries settle with a period of rest but some interruption to training can often be expected in short term.
- Presence/absence of lameness and severity of palpable abnormality at initial diagnosis often a reasonable guide to likelihood of training on without deterioration/interruption.
- Long-term persistence of ultrasonographic irregularity can be expected.
- Recurrent lameness and early retirement in small proportion of cases; likely that underlying overextension of fetlock in these cases contributes to poor outcome.
- Injuries with articular involvement: more likely to recur or cause ongoing lameness if treated conservatively; prognosis for return to full use following surgery is good (>70%).

Distal sesamoidean ligament desmopathy
Injury to the distal sesamoidean ligament/s (DSL) below the back of the fetlock most commonly involves a single structure; concurrent damage to both the straight and oblique DSL is rare. May be seen in association with other fetlock overextension pathologies, such as condylar or SLB injuries.

Injuries of the straight DSL occur in the forelimb or hindlimb and may be bilateral in a small number of horses. Injuries of the oblique DSL are more common in the forelimb; the medial branch is most frequently involved but may be biaxial. Avulsion injuries (sesamoid) occur but are rare.

Cause
- Overextension injury of fetlock.
- Not known whether acute overload or cumulative fatigue is responsible.

Risk factors
- Rare condition.
- Usually encountered in horses in fast work/racing stage of training.
- More common in older horses.
- Risk factors poorly understood but long/slack pastern conformation may predispose.

History
- Typically acute onset; lameness/swelling may first be noted in days following fast work/racing.
- May initially be mistaken for infection.

Signs
- Unilateral lameness of mild–moderate severity, usually worse when ridden.
- Diffuse thickening and loss of definition of back of pastern in some (not all) cases.
- Pain response to deep palpation of affected ligament.
- Very rarely, complete biaxial rupture results in luxation of PIPJ.

Diagnosis

- Ultrasonography: loss of border definition/enlargement/disrupted fibre pattern of affected ligament. Injuries to straight DSL may appear as core lesions (**Figure 2.63a**) or generalized hypoechogenicity; periligamentous thickening is common. Entheseous change (**Figure 2.63b**) may occur at the base of sesamoid
- Radiography warranted if concern over possible sesamoid involvement.

Management

- Conservative management: stable rest, supportive bandaging and anti-inflammatory medication in acute phase, followed by controlled exercise (+/− ultrasonographic monitoring).
- A 6-month rehabilitation period is typical.

Prognosis

- Mild–moderate lesions: good (>70%) prognosis for return to full use.
- Severe lesions: often recur and carry guarded prognosis for continued soundness.
- Presence of other pathology related to fetlock overextension may affect likelihood of return to racing.

Superficial digital flexor tendinitis (insertional branch)

Injury to the SDFT may occur at the level of its insertion in the mid-pastern region. Generally involves only the insertional portion of the tendon (avulsion fractures are rare). Usually a core lesion; diffuse injury less typical. Most common in forelimb. Lateral branch is most commonly involved, with both branches being affected in small proportion of cases. Unilateral or bilateral.

Cause

- Overextension injury of fetlock.
- Not known whether acute overload or cumulative fatigue is responsible.
- Appears distinct from the more typical SDFT tendinitis in the metacarpal region.

Risk factors

- Rare condition.
- Usually encountered in horses in fast work/racing stage of training.
- Risk factors poorly understood but long/slack pastern conformation may predispose.

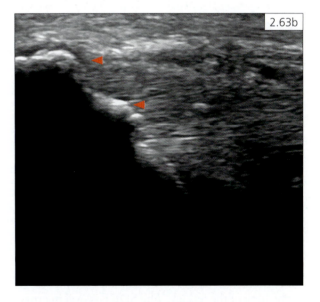

Figs. 2.63a, b Ultrasonograms of DSL desmopathy. (a) Transverse image of a straight DSL core lesion (arrowheads). (b) Longitudinal image of entheseous irregularity at the oblique DSL–sesamoid interface (arrowheads).

History
- Lameness at exercise/local thickening may develop over several days.

Signs
- Focal thickening at back of mid-pastern.
- Pain response to palpation.
- +/− mild–moderate lameness.
- +/− dorsal subluxation of PIPJ during stance phase.

Diagnosis
- Ultrasonography: enlargement/disrupted fibre pattern/reduced echogenicity of affected branch.

Management
- Rehabilitation as for metacarpal SDFT injuries (see below); controlled exercise guided by ultrasonographic monitoring.

Prognosis
- Fair–good prognosis for return to full use.
- Long-term thickening of branch plus irregular fibre pattern on ultrasonography can be expected.
- Reinjury is rare.

THE METACARPUS/METATARSUS ('CANNON')

Applied anatomy

The anatomy of the metacarpal/metatarsal ('cannon') region is similar in the forelimb and hindlimb, with some minor differences in relative size and position of soft-tissue structures (**Figure 2.64**). The cannon (Mc3/Mt3) bone extends from the carpus/tarsus to the fetlock and aside from the flexor tendon/ligament bundle at the back of the leg is little protected by soft tissue. The small splint bones (Mc/Mt2 and Mc/Mt4) adhere to the medial and lateral aspects of the cannon, respectively, by interosseous ligaments and articulate with the carpus/tarsus at their head. The thin distal portion of each splint bone is only loosely affiliated with the cannon.

A flexor tendon bundle comprising the SDFT and the DDFT descends from the level of the carpus/tarsus to the back of the fetlock. The SDFT is oval in cross-section in the high cannon and becomes progressively flattened as it approaches the fetlock. Deep to the DDFT in the upper half of the cannon is the accessory ligament of the DDFT (AL-DDFT/'inferior check ligament'), which arises from the palmar carpal ligament and back of C3/C4 and merges with the DDFT mid-cannon. Deep to all these structures and lying immediately adjacent the back of the cannon is the suspensory ligament. The suspensory ligament arises largely from the top of the palmar/plantar cannon but also, in part, from the lower row of carpal/tarsal bones, and in its proximal portion consists of muscle and connective tissue as well as ligament. It is tightly confined on three sides in the upper cannon by the cannon and splint bones but emerges as a distinct ligamentous body. Just below the mid-cannon it splits into two SLBs, each diverging to attach to its respective PSB. In the forelimb, interposed between the tendon bundle and the AL-DDFT down to nearly mid-cannon, is the potential space of the carpal synovial sheath, which is only palpable when effused; the tarsal sheath is the corresponding structure in the hindlimb.

Examination

Change in profile (bowing) of the tendon bundle may be noted on visual appraisal; palpation of both limbs weight bearing will also permit subjective assessment of any difference in heat between the legs. Assessment of individual tendons and ligaments is best performed with the leg raised; thickening/rounding and focal soreness of the SDFT are detectable with light palpation of the tendon edges and should be distinguished from thickening of the skin/subcutaneous structures. Responses should be compared with the opposite limb. The medial and lateral edges of the proximal suspensory ligament are not palpable as they are bordered by the splint bones; however, pressure on the ligament against the back of the cannon may elicit a pain response. The shin and splint bones are also best palpated with the leg raised; care should be taken not to apply pressure simultaneously to other sites that may confound the diagnosis.

Superficial digital flexor tendon disease ('tendinitis')

The SDFT is the main load-bearing tendon in the forelimb. Its elasticity (stretches by 10–16% at maximum loading during high speed exercise) has 'shock absorbing' and energy storing roles in locomotion. The structure of the SDFT matures by around 2 YO, with little/no adaptation or strengthening possible after maturity.

Acute or degenerative 'strain' of the SDFT in the forelimb is a potentially career-ending injury. Lesions typically occur in the cannon region, with injuries at or above the level of the carpus or in the fetlock/pastern region being rare. Disruption of tendon fibres frequently manifests as a central 'core lesion'; however, generalized inflammation and focal tears of tendon margins are also encountered. Most commonly unilateral but bilateral injuries can occur.

Cause
- During fast work, peak strains within the SDFT are close to their physiological limit: tendon is on a biomechanical 'knife edge'.
- Factors that lead to higher SDFT strains can result in clinical injury.
- Weight-bearing load is dampened by action of forearm muscles; muscle fatigue at closing stages of fast work can therefore lead to greater SDFT peak strains.
- Force on limb is proportional to speed: greater risk of SDFT injury on fast ground.
- Ageing causes some structural weakening in tendon over time; cumulative high-intensity exercise accelerates this process.
- Possible role of 'overheating' of tendon matrix in centre of tendon during exercise.
- Damage from direct trauma or 'bandage bind'/'bow' is far less common than overload injury.

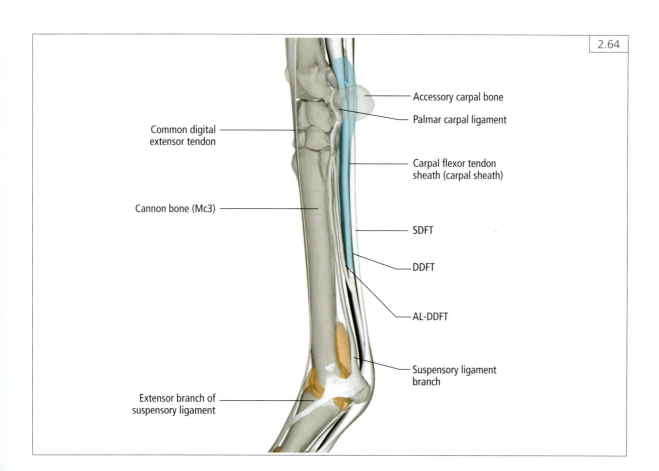

Fig. 2.64 Major structures of the forelimb cannon (lateral view, splint bone removed).

Risk factors
- Incidence rate in flat racing/training is approximately 3%/year.
- Risk of SDFT strain during racing approximately 0.5–0.6/1,000 starts in flat races in the UK and USA.
- Primarily affects horses ≥3 YO and risk increases considerably with age.
- Racehorses in jump racing disciplines at greater risk than flat racehorses.

History
- Acute or chronic in onset depending on severity and location of injury.
- Heat/swelling usually first noted within 24 hours of fast work/racing, but can also develop at slower cantering paces.
- Routine use of cold therapy/bandaging may mask early warning signs.

Signs
- Heat and/or thickening of tendon bundle.
- +/− pain response to palpation.
- Limb examined both weight bearing (for change in profile) and in flexion (for focal thickening/rounding of edge/pain). Opposite limb palpated for comparison.
- Location and extent of injury determines appearance: ranges from subtle to marked 'bowing' in profile.
- Lameness not a consistent feature: typically no lameness with mid-cannon lesions of mild–moderate severity.
- Lameness more likely when injury runs into the confined spaces of carpal canal or digital tendon sheath.

Diagnosis
- Clinical signs sufficient for diagnosis in cases of marked ('bowed') injury.
- Ultrasonography: to confirm and quantify extent of injury; best assessed approximately 1 week after injury.
- Cross-sectional area of normal tendon in range of 0.9–1.2 cm^2 and should be similar at same level in opposite limb.
- Injury associated with generalized or focal enlargement of tendon plus reduced echogenicity and fibrillar disruption, which may vary in severity (**Figures 2.65–2.68**).

Management
- See Rehabilitation (Chapter 1, p. 24).
- Tendon injuries repair with tissue that is strong but inelastic.
- Goal of treatment is to modify the acute inflammatory response and assist healing so that mechanical properties of the healed tendon are optimized.
- Range of management options available; all involve lengthy recuperation with graded return to loading (up to 12 months for return to racing).
- Rarely, continued training without a rest period may be possible in some horses with minor injuries providing the tendon and lesion remain static clinically and on ultrasound. Some horses with focal marginal lesions can continue in full exercise without significant deterioration in the appearance of the tendon.

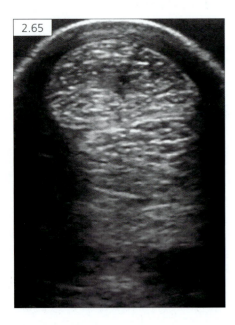

Fig. 2.65 Ultrasonogram (transverse) of a SDFT lesion of mild severity (upper cannon). Note the irregular echogenicity.

Prognosis
- Return to fast work/racing is possible for most mild–moderate injuries.
- Following return to training: guarded prognosis for continued racing soundness (approximately 50% of horses complete three starts and few horses race ≥5 times without reinjury).
- Better prognosis with controlled exercise than uncontrolled pasture rest.
- Increasing severity of injury is associated with lower likelihood of return to racing, shortened racing career and drop in racing class.
- Bilateral tendinitis associated with poor prognosis (25% complete three starts) for racing.

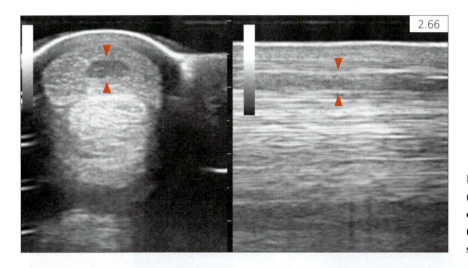

Fig. 2.66 Ultrasonograms (transverse and longitudinal) of a SDFT core lesion (arrowheads) of medium severity.

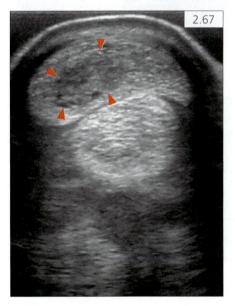

Fig. 2.67 Ultrasonogram (transverse) of a SDFT core lesion of marked severity. Note the large zone of reduced echogenicity (arrowheads).

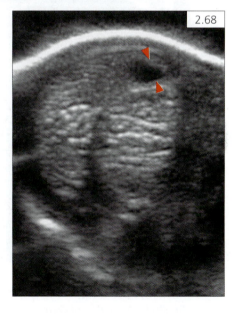

Fig. 2.68 Ultrasonogram of a SDFT showing a lateral margin injury (arrowheads).

- Carpal/proximal cannon SDFT lesions: poor prognosis for racing and frequently display ongoing lameness.
- Regardless of severity most injuries can sustain paddock or non-racing athletic careers.

'Juvenile' tendinitis

Uniform enlargement without fibre disruption of the forelimb SDFT through the cannon or carpal regions in the young horse appears to be a distinct condition from SDFT disease (p. 92).

Condition usually affects one limb but is bilateral in approximately one-third of cases. Generally develops at yearling/early 2 YO stage, with affected tendons typically remaining enlarged long term.

Cause
- Considered to be an adaptive (or maladaptive) response to conditioning exercise in some individuals.

Risk factors
- Occurs predominantly in yearlings/2 YOs.
- Occurs during early (yearling preparation or light cantering) phase of training.
- Risk factors not known.

History
- Typically chronic onset (weeks/months) of tendon thickening.
- Often first noted during pre-purchase examinations.

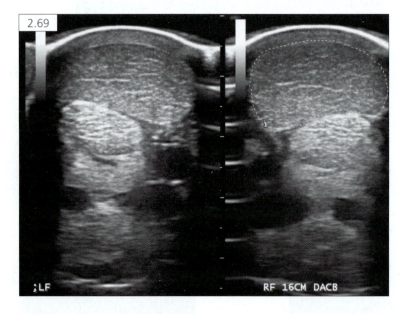

Fig. 2.69 Ultrasonograms (transverse) of 'juvenile' tendinitis (forelimb). Note the marked enlargement of both tendons.

Signs
- Uniform non-painful thickening of one or both forelimb SDFTs.
- Can usually be differentiated from SDFT disease by history and clinical findings (absence of heat/pain on palpation/lameness/focal enlargement).
- Frequently associated with distension of distal recess of carpal synovial sheath.

Diagnosis
- Clinical findings strongly indicative.
- Ultrasonography: undertaken if differentiation from true SDFT injury desired. Affected tendons have homogeneous appearance with normal/reduced echogenicity and parallel fibrillar pattern (**Figure 2.69**); enlargement (>1.7 cm^2) in cross-sectional area (CSA) is sometimes profound (up to 2.5× normal CSA: 2.8 cm^2).

Management
- Interruption to training programme rarely necessary.
- Risk of progression to clinical SDFT injury is considered low but should be determined on individual basis.
- Where enlargement is profound/rapid in onset/associated with peritendinous inflammation: rest or modified exercise (removal from cantering) recommended. Duration determined by severity and career goals; walking/trotting for 6–10 weeks frequently sufficient.
- +/– medical therapy (systemic steroidal/non-steroidal anti-inflammatories).
- Reduction in size of tendon should not generally be expected.

Prognosis
- Good prognosis for continued training as likely to race at 2, 3 and 4 YO as unaffected horses.
- Tendon usually remains thickened long term and may affect resale.

Suspensory ligament desmopathy: forelimb

The suspensory ligament acts along with the flexor tendons to limit overextension of the fetlock joint. Injury to the suspensory ligament can be manifested by fibre disruption, generalized enlargement or maladaptive change at the bone/ligament interface in the proximal cannon. Along with palmar cortical stress injury/fracture (p. 105), it is an important cause of subcarpal lameness. Injury usually occurs at site of origin of the ligament in the proximal third of the cannon; injuries to the body of the ligament are rare. Unilateral (most common) or bilateral. SLB injuries are considered elsewhere (p. 86).

Cause
- Likely to result from cumulative damage incurred by repetitive strain/overload of suspensory apparatus during exercise.

Risk factors
- Incidence rate approximately 3–5%/year.
- Typically in 2 YOs during early–mid cantering phase of training but may occur at all ages.
- Injuries in horses ≥3 YO are more likely to be chronic and involve the ligament/bone interface.
- Mid-body injuries are rare and almost invariably occur in older horses.
- Risk factors for development of injury (track surface/conformation/training regime) poorly understood.

History
- Unilateral forelimb lameness that develops acutely or over several days.
- Lameness often transient; horse may be sound within several hours of initial reporting.

Signs
- Mild–moderate unilateral lameness.
- Lameness usually worse when ridden +/– on soft surface +/– with affected leg on outside of circle.
- Many cases have no associated palpable abnormality of limb.
- Enlargement of suspensory ligament +/– pain response to deep palpation in some horses (should be compared with opposite limb).

Diagnosis
- Lameness arising from subcarpal/lower carpal region is a diagnostic challenge due to non-specificity of regional nerve blocks and conventional imaging.

- Diagnostic blocking: frequently does not permit differentiation of subcarpal from middle carpal joint lameness. Lameness may be exacerbated by nerve blocking of foot.
- Ultrasonography: interpretation difficult due to frequently irregular appearance of normal suspensory ligament (presence of muscle and fat tissue) and variability between individuals; also poor correlation with pathology. Size/echogenicity of forelimb ligaments should be symmetrical: signs of injury include enlargement, loss of dorsal border definition and focal or diffuse reduced echogenicity relative to opposite limb (**Figures 2.70a–c**).
- Radiography: to assess proximal cannon/carpal regions (**Figures 2.71a–c**).
- Practical diagnosis is typically one of elimination of other pathology (i.e. distal limb and carpus) using combination of ultrasonography and radiography.
- MRI is superior imaging modality but not widely used.

Management
- Uncomplicated proximal suspensory desmopathy in 2 YOs: conservative management (stable rest/walking for 6–8 weeks) usually sufficient.

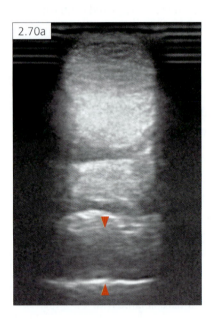
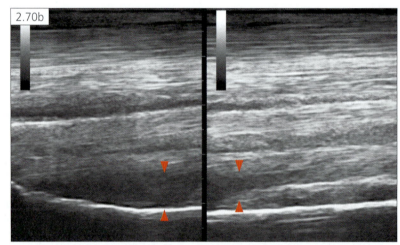
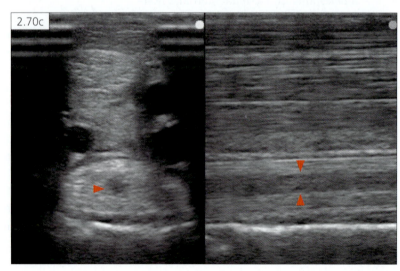

Figs. 2.70a–c Ultrasonograms of suspensory ligament desmopathy. Hypoechoic dorsal margin (arrowheads) of proximal suspensory ligament on transverse (a) and longitudinal (b) images. (c) Injury to mid-body of forelimb suspensory ligament: core lesion (arrowheads) and enlargement.

- Proximal suspensory desmopathy with concurrent disease of bone interface: requires more conservative approach (stable rest/walking for 8–12 weeks) +/− ultrasonographic monitoring +/− ESWT.
- Persistence/recurrence of lameness following rest period (with other pathology ruled out): periligamentous infiltration of corticosteroid may permit continued training.
- Continued training in acute phase aided by corticosteroid medication +/− ESWT of subcarpal region (or in the face of deteriorating action) risks development of more severe pathology with consequent poorer prognosis for recovery.

Prognosis
- Proximal suspensory desmopathy in juvenile: excellent prognosis for return to soundness; recurrence rare.
- Proximal suspensory desmopathy in older horse with concurrent bone disease: guarded; may recur.
- Suspensory body desmopathy: guarded–fair prognosis for return to full soundness.

Suspensory ligament desmopathy: hindlimb

Less common than the forelimb equivalent. Injury usually occurs in proximal third of the cannon; injuries to body of ligament are rare. Proximal suspensory ligament of the hindlimb differs from the forelimb by being constrained on three sides by bone borders (cannon and both splints) and on its plantar face by a strong fascial band: enlargement of the ligament may result in a compartment syndrome with compression/inflammation of the plantar metatarsal nerves and ongoing lameness. Pathology usually bilateral with lameness manifesting in a single limb. Suspensory ligament branch injuries are considered elsewhere (p. 86).

Cause
- Likely to result from cumulative damage incurred by repetitive strain/overload of suspensory apparatus during exercise.
- Subsequent enlargement of ligament/compartment syndrome may cause ongoing lameness.

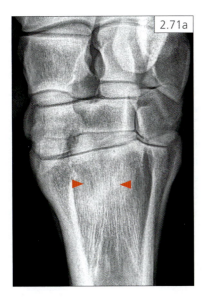 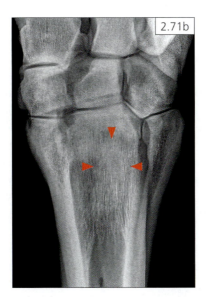 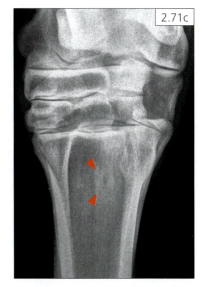

Figs. 2.71a–c Radiographs of the proximal cannon. Note the mild and markedly irregular radiodensity at the suspensory ligament origin (arrowheads) of the proximal metacarpus (a, b, respectively, DPa) and the proximal metatarsus (c, DPl).

Risk factors
- Rare condition.
- Occurs in horses in cantering/fast work phase of training.
- Typically in horses ≥3 YO.
- Straight-through-the-hock conformation may predispose to injury.

History
- Onset of lameness may be acute or chronic.
- May display reluctance to break from stalls gate.

Signs
- Mild–moderate unilateral lameness, typically with shortened cranial phase and toe catch.
- Lameness usually worse when ridden.
- Positive response to limb flexion is common.
- Large head of lateral splint and deep location of proximal suspensory ligament limits access for palpation.

Diagnosis
- Diagnostic blocking: may not permit differentiation of subtarsal from distal hock joint lameness.
- Ultrasonography: moderate sensitivity; signs of injury include enlargement, loss of dorsal border definition and focal or diffuse reduced echogenicity relative to opposite limb.
- Radiography: of limited use; changes include increased densification of proximal metatarsus (**Figure 2.71c**) and endosteal reaction (LM projection).
- Bone scan: often unremarkable but IRU in some cases.
- Practical diagnosis is typically one of elimination of other pathology (i.e. distal limb and lower hock).

Management
- Acute lameness: conservative management generally recommended; stable rest/ walking for 6–12 weeks.
- Low-grade or more chronic lameness (with acceptable ultrasonographic appearance): periligamentous infiltration of corticosteroid +/− ESWT may permit continued training. Poor or short-lived response necessitates further imaging or rest period.

Prognosis
- Most horses are manageable with rest +/or medication.
- Acute-onset lameness is associated with better long-term outcome than chronic lameness.
- Recurrence of lameness due to persistent compartment syndrome may occur in some horses: guarded prognosis for racing.
- Releasing fasciotomy plus neurectomy (deep branch of lateral plantar nerve) carries good prognosis for return to soundness in horses with satisfactory conformation; racing following neurectomy is prohibited in most jurisdictions.

Avulsion fracture of proximal suspensory ligament origin

Small avulsion fracture with focal associated damage to proximal suspensory ligament; predominantly occurs in forelimb. May represent 'end stage' of proximal suspensory ligament desmopathy in some horses.

Cause
- Avulsion fracture of suspensory ligament attachment.
- Often preceded by stress remodelling at bone/ligament interface.

Risk factors
- Rare condition.
- Occurs in horses in cantering/fast exercise phase of training.
- Risk factors poorly understood.
- Horses trained on in face of developing subcarpal lameness (aided by systemic/local anti-inflammatory medication) may be at greater risk.

History
- Typically acute-onset lameness noted after cooling-off from exercise.

Signs
- Moderate–severe unilateral lameness.
- Palpable heat/thickening in proximal cannon region.

- Marked pain response to palpation of suspensory ligament origin.

Diagnosis
- Radiography: crescent-shaped lucency in proximal cannon (DPa projection) (**Figures 2.72a, b**).
- Ultrasonography: fracture fragment and associated torn suspensory ligament readily detected on longitudinal and transverse images.
- Bone scan: rarely required for diagnosis. Intense focal IRU at site of injury.

Management
- Conservative management: requires longer rehabilitation period than for simple proximal suspensory ligament desmopathy; stable rest/walking for 12–18 weeks with ultrasonographic monitoring.
- +/– ESWT.

Prognosis
- Good prognosis for return to full use with appropriate rehabilitation.

Accessory ligament of the deep digital flexor tendon ('inferior check' ligament) injury

The AL-DDFT prevents overloading of the DDFT by sharing the load during the late stance phase. Injuries occur only sporadically in flat racehorses and predominantly in the forelimb (hindlimb AL-DDFT is small/vestigial structure). Usually unilateral. Typically affects the ligament near its junction with the DDFT in the mid-cannon region, and disruption at site of injury is often extensive.

Cause
- Strength and elasticity of ligament decreases with age.

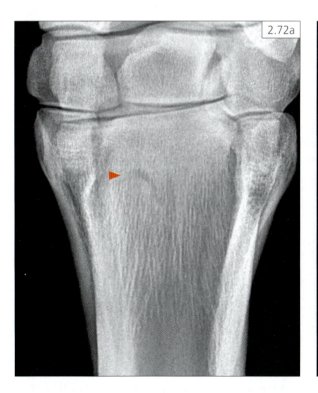 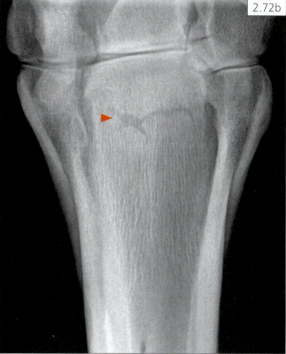

Figs. 2.72a, b Radiographs (DPa) showing radiolucency (arrowheads) of the proximal Mc3, indicating an avulsion fracture.

- Likely to result from acute overload during high-intensity exercise, although role of chronic degeneration poorly defined.

Risk factors
- Rare condition.
- Usually an injury of older horses.

History
- Acute-onset soft-tissue thickening (cannon) +/− lameness.

Signs
- Soft-tissue thickening at junction of the mid and upper third of the cannon, immediately forward of the flexor tendon bundle.
- Mild pain response to palpation.
- +/− mild–moderate lameness.

Diagnosis
- Clinical findings strongly indicative.
- Ultrasonography: obvious enlargement/loss of echogenicity/loss of border definition of ligament (**Figure 2.73**).

Management
- Conservative management: stable rest/walking for 8–12 weeks (shorter rehabilitation period possible for mild injuries).
- Systemic and topical (cold therapy) anti-inflammatory measures in initial phase.
- Adhesions to DDFT or SDFT may occur during healing; may cause transient inflammation/thickening on return to faster exercise. Of no concern unless lame.
- Rarely, chronic or recurrent lameness on return to training: surgery (desmotomy) considered for these cases.

Prognosis
- Good (>70%) prognosis for return to full use.
- Risk of recurrence low but affected horses may be at greater risk of other soft-tissue overload injuries (suspensory ligament/SDFT) on return to fast exercise.
- Permanent thickening at site of injury can be expected; cosmetic blemish only.
- Affected horses appear predisposed to AL-DDFT injury in opposite limb during subsequent training; may imply degenerative cause.

Dorsal metacarpal disease ('sore/bucked shins')

Soreness and palpable thickening of front of cannon/s of variable severity. Predominantly affects forelimbs; unilateral or bilateral. Pain/inflammation associated with acute phase can interrupt training; permanent bony thickening of affected part of cannon may result in some cases.

Cause
- Maladaptive modelling response of cannon bone to training-imposed stresses: at slower paces, dorsopalmar bending of cannon occurs and tensile ('stretching') forces act on the front of the shin; at faster paces, the predominant force is compression.
- Tension stimulates deposition of new bone at front of cannon bone, causing dorsomedial thickening.

Risk factors
- Common in 2 YOs during cantering/fast exercise phase of training.
- Horses in their first training cycle (regardless of age) at greater risk.

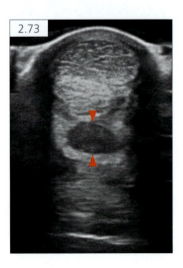

Fig. 2.73 Ultrasonogram (transverse) showing disruption to the AL-DDFT (arrowheads) in the mid–upper metacarpus.

- Prevalence varies widely with training programme/geographical location; can be as high as 20–40%.
- Greater risk on harder/faster tracks due to higher strains on forelimb.

History
- Initial palpable heat/soreness/thickening of cannon/s frequently noted in day/s after fast exercise.
- Some horses display reluctance to train freely at speed.

Signs
- Palpation: tenderness/heat to front of cannon; usually affects dorsomedial aspect of upper half of cannon. May be focal or diffuse.
- +/− swelling/thickening of contour of cannon at same site.
- Severity varies between individuals.
- +/− shortening of forelimb action (bilateral).
- Unilateral lameness is rare and more typically associated with progression to cortical stress fracture.

Diagnosis
- Clinical findings are definitive.
- Radiography only required if lame and cortical stress fracture suspected.

Management
- Determined by severity and horse/trainer factors.
- Mild pain with minimal 'bucking': often requires no alteration in training, although intermittent exacerbation with fast exercise/racing may necessitate short periods of reduced exercise +/− anti-inflammatory medication.
- Moderate–marked pain ('grunting' response to palpation): treat symptomatically with reduced exercise until pain diminishes. 2–4 weeks without cantering generally sufficient; may walk/trot/swim.
- Acute phase: topical anti-inflammatory measures (cold therapy/clay) useful.
- Continued training without rest may result in permanent change in profile of cannon (cosmetic blemish only). Small associated risk of development of dorsal cortical stress fracture (p. 107).
- Chronic/recurrent cases non-responsive to rest: counter-irritation including periosteal scarification (Chapter 1, p. 30)/ESWT/bisphosphonate medication associated anecdotally with successful resolution in some troublesome cases.

Prevention
- Exposure to faster speeds (and therefore more 'compression' force on cannon) stimulates better adaptive modelling of bone.
- Introduction of fast work at earlier stage in training programme, providing distances trained at speed are restricted (initially ≤200 metres), may be useful.
- Intentionally 'bucking' shins not recommended.

Prognosis
- Excellent prognosis for return to full use.
- Interruption to training uncommon and rarely more than a few weeks.
- Very few horses develop stress fractures.

Splints (metacarpal/metatarsal exostosis)
Inflammation and enlargement of the small metacarpal or metatarsal (splint) bones. Severity varies considerably between individuals. Most frequently affects the medial splint of the forelimb; only rarely in hindlimb (when it is usually lateral). Bilateral lesions are common. Splint fractures sometimes arise as a more severe manifestation of the condition or secondary to direct trauma or fetlock overextension.

Both 'true' splints and splint fractures go through a period of active inflammation before 'setting' as a non-painful permanent bony thickening.

Cause
- Medial splint bone of forelimb bears considerable load (along with cannon); splint enlargement may represent maladaptive response to these loads.
- Shear forces acting on interosseous ligament between splint bone and cannon are the cause of many 'splints'.
- Direct trauma (typically interference injuries) can also cause periosteal reaction/fracture.

- Fracture of the distal ends ('buttons') of splints: fatigue injury caused by physical deviation following SLB desmopathy (p. 86) or secondary to overextension of fetlock (fibrous attachment to PSBs).

Risk factors
- Any age/stage of training but most common in 2 YOs in early cantering phase.
- Offset carpal conformation predisposes to injury (greater load bearing through medial splint rather than cannon).

History
- Chronic- (most common) or acute-onset lameness +/− swelling; typically develops over days/weeks.

Signs
- Initially: pain on palpation +/− oedema/soft-tissue thickening at affected site.
- Followed within days by palpable thickening of underlying splint bone.
- Splint enlargement: lameness a variable feature (absent–moderate).
- Splint fracture (proximal and mid-body): moderate–severe lameness +/− overlying wound in cases of direct trauma.
- Splint fracture (distal): mild lameness plus poorly defined thickening of the inside of the lower cannon/fetlock.
- Severity of lameness and palpable pain response corresponds broadly to degree of resulting splint enlargement.

Diagnosis
- Clinical findings sufficient in most cases and imaging rarely necessary.
- Radiography: warranted if splint fracture suspected (**Figures 2.74a, b**); multiple lesion-oriented oblique projections may be required to detect fracture line.

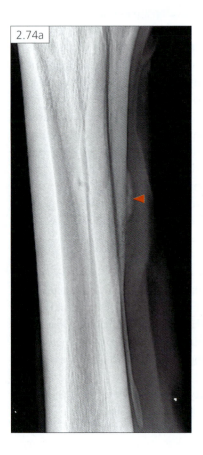
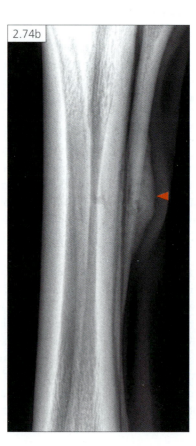

Figs. 2.74a, b Radiographs (DMPaLO) of splint enlargement. (a) Acute phase with active periosteal proliferative change. (b) Settled splint enlargement (arrowheads).

Management
- Clinical severity and lameness guide management.
- Acute phase: anti-inflammatory therapy (topical DMSO/corticosteroid, cold therapy).
- No lameness: interruption to training programme not necessary; however, short period (1–2 weeks) of walking/trotting beneficial to allow splint to settle.
- Lame: reduce level of exercise (to walking/trotting) until splint 'sets' (palpable pain and lameness subsides).
- Recurrent/problematic despite rest: counter-irritation measures (Chapter 1, p. 30) may be considered.
- Lateral splints: frequently slow-setting; low-grade ridden exercise +/− counter-irritation may be preferable to complete rest.
- Fractures require considerably longer rehabilitation period than splint enlargement.
- Open/comminuted splint fractures: surgical intervention may be warranted.
- Distal splint fractures (**Figure 2.75**): most resolve with conservative management (painless non-union). Surgery sometimes warranted.

Prognosis
- All carry good prognosis for return to full use.
- Initial severity of lameness/palpable pain is a good predictor of length of interruption to training required.
- Medial splints: generally minimal interruption to training; 1–4 weeks out of cantering is typical.
- Lateral splints: more likely to cause significant interruption to training and may remain lame for many weeks/months.
- Splint fractures: may require rehabilitation period of 8–12 weeks.

Palmar cortical stress reaction/fracture
Bone fatigue injury of upper cannon, predominantly in forelimb. Along with proximal suspensory ligament desmopathy (p. 97), is an important cause of subcarpal lameness in young racehorses. Primarily affects palmar cortex/medulla in region of attachment of medial lobe of suspensory ligament, sometimes with associated inflammation of medial splint bone and interosseous ligament. Spectrum of injury ranges from stress reaction to incomplete cortical fracture. Usually unilateral.

Cause
- Stress/fatigue injury.
- Distraction forces from suspensory +/− interosseous ligaments may contribute to strains on palmar cortex of Mc3.

Risk factors
- Common condition.
- Typically in 2 YOs during trotting/early cantering phase of training.
- Risk factors not known.

History
- Acute-onset lameness.

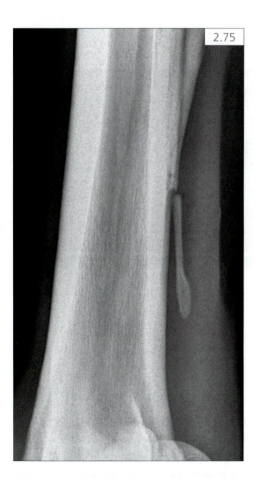

Fig. 2.75 Radiograph (DMPaLO) of a distal splint fracture.

Signs
- Moderate–marked unilateral forelimb lameness.
- Frequently no localizing signs.
- +/– pain response to palpation of subcarpal region.

Diagnosis
- Confirming diagnosis can be difficult as conventional imaging (radiography/ultrasonography) frequently unremarkable.
- Diagnostic blocking: may not permit differentiation of subcarpal from middle carpal joint lameness.
- Radiography: radiological changes not present in all cases (up to 30% without abnormality) at time of injury but may develop over subsequent months. Increased densification +/– vertical/oblique linear lucency in medial proximal cannon (DPa projection) (**Figure 2.76a**); endosteal reaction (LM projection).
- Ultrasonography: suspensory ligament usually unremarkable; +/– periosteal irregularity proximal cannon.
- Bone scan: intense focal IRU.
- MRI: the gold standard imaging modality due to inconsistent radiographic/ultrasonographic features of condition. Bone marrow oedema-type pattern +/– cortical fissure (**Figure 2.76b**).

Management
- Conservative management: stable rest/walking for 6–8 weeks depending on severity.

Prognosis
- Good prognosis for return to full athletic use.
- Some horses subsequently develop low-grade middle carpal joint lameness later in career; may represent ongoing maladaptive response to loading of limb.

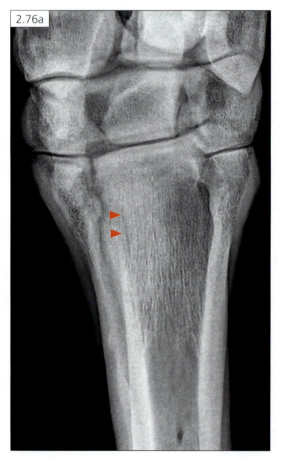

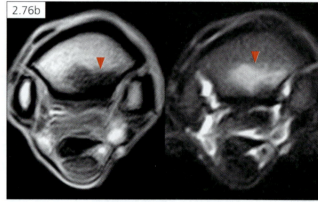

Figs. 2.76a, b Proximal metacarpal fatigue injury. (a) Radiograph (DPa): note the indistinct radiolucency (arrowheads). (b) MR T1 (left) and STIR (right) transverse images of right proximal Mc3 at level of suspensory ligament origin; medial is to the right in both images. T1 hypointensity and STIR hyperintensity in palmaromedial aspect.

Dorsal cortical stress fracture

Incomplete fracture of the dorsal cortex of the cannon bone. Predominantly in forelimb. Can develop in upper, mid- or lower cannon and usually located dorsolaterally. Short oblique fracture line.

Cause
- Stress/fatigue injury.
- May develop as progression of bucked shins (p. 102) that have received insufficient rest.

Risk factors
- Rare condition.
- Most common in 3 YOs.
- Risk factors unknown.

History
- Typically chronic-onset lameness (worsening over days/weeks), although may arise acutely following fast exercise/racing.

Signs
- Small (≤1 cm) focal bony thickening of front of forelimb cannon.
- Considerable focal pain on palpation.
- Mild–moderate unilateral lameness.

Diagnosis
- Clinical findings strongly indicative.
- Radiography: oblique fracture line in dorsal cortex (LM/DPa projections) +/− periosteal/endosteal reaction depending on chronicity of injury (**Figures 2.77a, b**).

Management
- Continued training without rest may result in complete diaphyseal fracture (catastrophic).
- Conservative management: stable rest/walking for 6–10 weeks.
- Surgery (cortical drilling/screw placement): sometimes advocated for non-healing chronic injuries.

Prognosis
- Fair to good prognosis for return to full use with conservative management.
- Good prognosis with surgery.

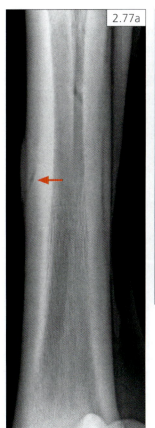
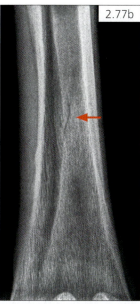

Figs. 2.77a, b Radiographs (LM, DPa) of dorsal Mc3 fatigue fractures. (a) Linear radiolucency (arrow) and associated dorsal cortical thickening. (b) Small linear radiolucency (arrow).

THE CARPUS

Applied anatomy

The carpus ('knee') is a compound articulation between the forearm and cannon and comprises three joints and two rows of carpal bones (**Figures 2.78a, b**). The primary movement of the carpus is flexion/extension in the sagittal plane. At faster paces full extension occurs just prior to the foot landing; when the carpal joints close the tight-packed configuration of the small bones keeps the carpus fixed and the leg rigid as the body passes over it during stance.

The lowermost (carpometacarpal) carpal joint does not 'open' and is rarely associated with problems. This joint is separated from the middle carpal joint by the distal row of carpal bones (C2, 3, 4). The two high-motion (middle carpal and antebrachiocarpal) joints are separated by the proximal row of carpal bones (radial, intermediate and ulnar carpal bones). The accessory carpal bone sits prominently at the back of the proximal row, articulating with the ulnar carpal bone and lower radius. It forms part of the outer border of the carpal canal, through which the flexor tendons course.

The carpal joints are palpable at the front of the carpus between the constraining extensor tendons. All of the joints also have outpouchings at the back of the leg. The palmar pouch of the middle carpal joint is just below the accessory carpal bone and that of the antebrachiocarpal joint is on the outside of the lower forearm, between the back of the radius and the tendon of the ulnaris lateralis muscle.

The carpal bones are held together by several intercarpal and collateral ligaments; these provide stability and prevent overextension. Two large extensor tendons (the extensor carpi radialis and common digital extensor) run over the front of the carpus. The retinaculum that restrains the extensor tendons at the front of the carpus also forms the thick medial and palmar borders of the carpal canal. The carpal canal contains the carpal synovial sheath, which encloses the SDFT and DDFT and extends above the carpus for 8–10 cm and below the carpus to the mid-cannon (with the distal recess terminating at the junction of the DDFT and the AL-DDFT). At the back of the carpal bones the dense palmar carpal ligament is the foundation of the AL-DDFT ('inferior check' ligament), which runs down into the cannon to its union with the DDFT. The AL-SDFT ('superior check' ligament) is a fan-shaped band that arises from the caudomedial radius and joins the SDFT at the back of the carpus.

The growth plate of the lower radius (immediately above the carpus) has traditionally been used to assess skeletal maturity. Bone turnover at this growth plate starts to subside rapidly at around 20 months of age, and radiological 'closure' occurs at 24–30 months.

Load-bearing compression forces act primarily through the 'dorsal load path' at the front of the limb, and training stimulates increased density of the struts of cancellous bone (trabeculae) that are oriented proximodistally. While training adaptations allow for greater load bearing, increased bone density also causes increased bone stiffness. The majority of training-related pathology occurs within the middle carpal joint. The largest and most important bone in the distal row is the third carpal bone, which has two main load-bearing facets corresponding to the opposing bones in the proximal row. The radial facet (opposite the radial carpal bone) is the largest, is subject to the greatest forces and consequently is most frequently affected by training-related maladaptive changes. Together with the opposing articular margin of the radial carpal bone, these sites form the regions of the carpus most likely to sustain injury.

Synovial spaces
- Carpometacarpal and middle carpal joints: always communicate.
- Middle carpal and antebrachiocarpal joints: rarely communicate.

Examination

The conformation of the carpus (particularly offset knees) may influence the risk of injury and assessment may direct the lameness investigation. Evidence of middle carpal or radiocarpal joint effusion may be subtle and is best discerned by palpation of the front of the knee with the limb weight bearing. Joint effusion can be differentiated from subcutaneous bursae (arising from direct trauma) by observing the communication between the dorsal and palmar synovial pouches. With the limb raised, firm palpation of the bone borders most prone to injury (dorsodistal radial carpal bone/dorsoproximal third carpal bone/dorsodistal radius) may elicit a pain response and indicate fracture/

Regional Musculoskeletal Conditions

Figs. 2.78a, b Major structures of the carpus: (a) dorsal and (b) flexed lateral views.

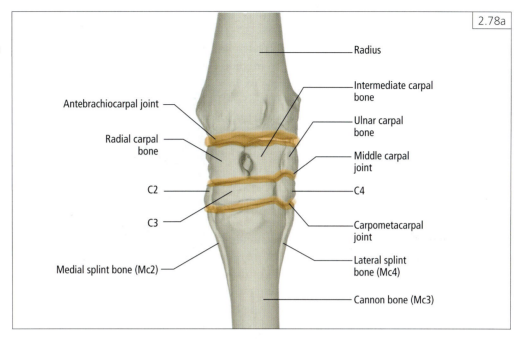

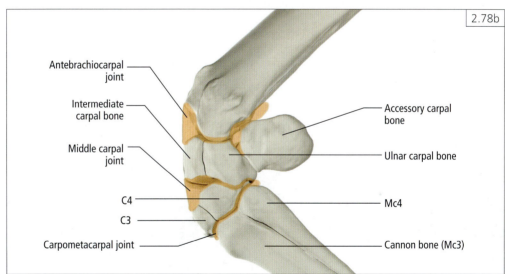

framentation. Forced full flexion of the knee should never be painful and, if so, often indicates marked joint effusion and likely injury.

Carpal lameness

Carpal ('knee') lameness is common in all age groups and can be associated with a spectrum of pathology from subchondral bone injury to OA or fracture. Progression is unpredictable and considerable individual variation in presenting signs, radiological changes and outcome occurs.

Pathology or lameness frequently affects both limbs. The middle carpal joint is the site most frequently involved in carpal lameness; pathology primarily affects the axial portions of the radial and third carpal bones, which face each other across the joint space. Antebrachiocarpal joint lameness is less common; pathology most commonly affects the distal radius or proximal row of carpal bones (predominantly radial carpal bone; less commonly intermediate carpal bone).

Most carpal lameness is associated with relatively mild radiological findings; these typically include increased densification or mild modelling of the third +/or radial carpal bones. Correlation between radiological severity and arthroscopic evidence of OA is poor. Increased density of the third carpal bone is manifested by thickening or loss of trabeculation +/or corticomedullary definition on the DPr-DDiO ('skyline') radiographic projection. There is variation between individuals in the area of the bone affected and its severity (mild/moderate/severe); it is also common for one limb to be affected to a greater degree. Osteochondral fragmentation ('chip' fracture) of the articular margin of the radial carpal (**Figures 2.79, 2.80a, b**) and/or third carpal bone is usually a progression of degenerative modelling (**Figure 2.81**); fragmentation involving the antebrachiocarpal joint (**Figures 2.82a–c**) may also arise from degenerative change or may be acute with no obvious pre-existing pathology.

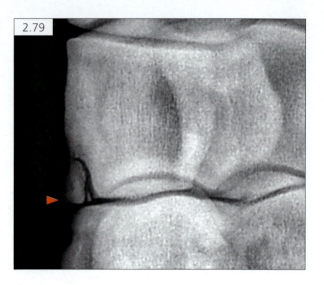

Fig. 2.79 Radiograph (DLPaMO) of a moderate-sized, displaced chip fracture (arrowhead) of the radial carpal bone.

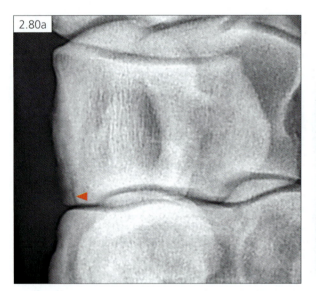

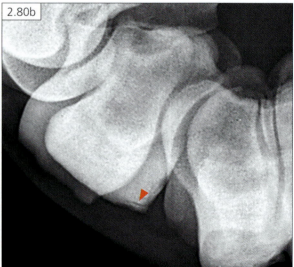

Figs. 2.80a, b Radiographs of non-displaced chip fractures (arrowheads) of the radial carpal bone: DLPaMO (a) and flexed LM (b) projections.

Regional Musculoskeletal Conditions

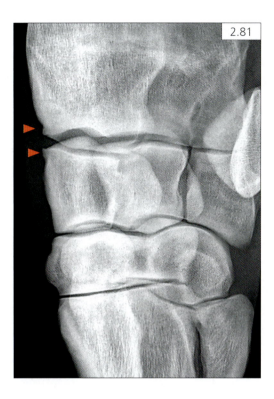

Fig. 2.81 Radiograph (DLPaMO) of mild antebrachiocarpal joint modelling (arrowheads).

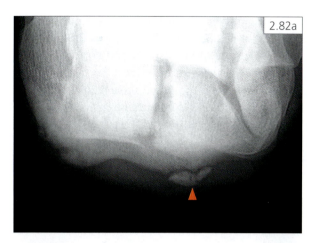

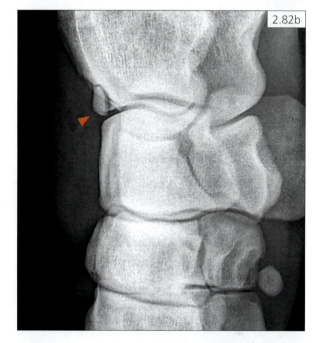

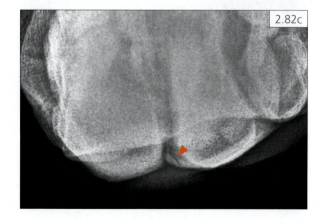

Figs. 2.82a–c Radiographs of antebrachiocarpal joint fragmentation. Note the distal radial chip fracture (arrowheads) on the skyline (a) and DMPaLO (b) projections; note the proximal intermediate carpal bone chip fracture (arrowhead) on the skyline (c) projection.

Configurations of third carpal bone injury include chip (**Figures 2.83a, b**), slab (**Figures 2.84a–c**) and sagittal (**Figure 2.85**) fractures and cortical fissures (**Figure 2.86**); these occur almost invariably in the portion of third carpal bone subject to the greatest load (radial facet). Chip fracture/fragmentation affects the proximal articular border of the radial facet, while slab fracture commonly occurs in the frontal plane and extends full thickness between the proximal and distal articular margins. Cortical fissures occur in the proximal weight-bearing face of the bone.

Modelling and fragmentation of the distal intermediate carpal bone is rare and not always clinically relevant.

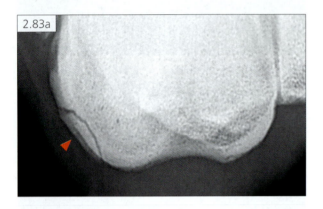

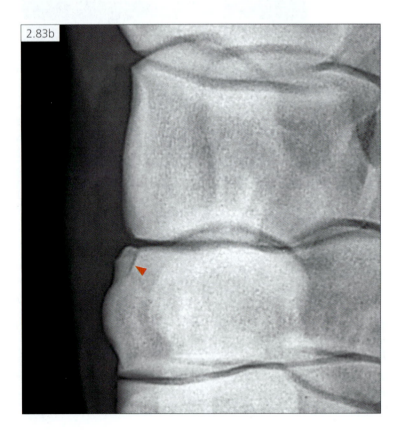

Figs. 2.83a, b Radiographs of a third carpal bone chip fracture (arrowheads): flexed D35°PrDDiO (a) and DLPaMO (b) projections.

Regional Musculoskeletal Conditions

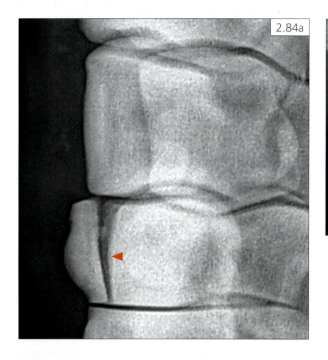

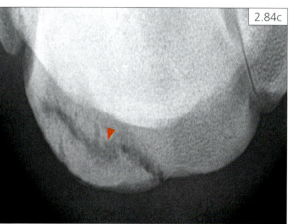

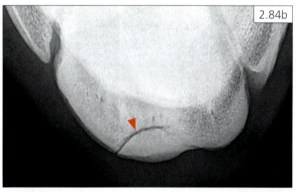

Figs. 2.84a–c Radiographs of a third carpal bone slab fracture (arrowheads): DLPaMO (a) and flexed D35°PrDDiO (b, c) projections.

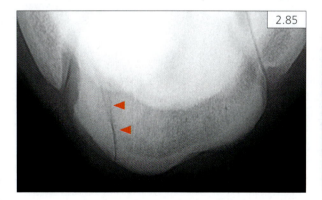

Fig. 2.85 Radiograph (flexed D35°PrDDiO) of a third carpal bone sagittal fracture (arrowheads).

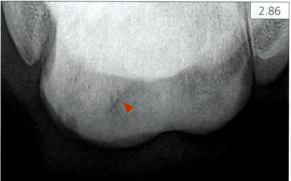

Fig. 2.86 Radiograph (flexed D35°PrDDiO) of a third carpal bone 'fissure' fracture (arrowhead) with surrounding increased radiodensity.

Palmar carpal fracture/fragmentation is encountered only rarely. When discrete and involving the ulnar carpal bone it represents an avulsion injury of the lateral palmar intercarpal ligament. Fracture of the palmar border of the radial carpal bone (+/− ulnar or intermediate carpal bones) is usually a traumatic injury sustained during anaesthetic recovery (**Figure 2.87**).

Cause
- Middle and antebrachiocarpal joints are high motion.
- Dorsal margins of the third carpal bone and radial carpal bone are subjected to considerable compressive forces during weight bearing at faster paces.
- Loading forces are greatest through axial portion of knee and proximal cannon.
- Training causes adaptive change; in some individuals becomes maladaptive, leading to subchondral bone injury.
- Increased density of subchondral bone/associated cartilage damage can lead to reduced compliance and greater susceptibility to fracture (chip/fragmentation/slab fracture). However, fractures frequently occur in non-sclerotic third carpal bones and the relationship is not linear.

Risk factors
- Any age/stage of training.
- Poor carpal conformation: depending on severity, 'offset' (middle carpal joint lameness) and 'back-at-knee' (antebrachiocarpal joint lameness) conformation may increase risk.
- Body type/condition (heavy), maturity, training regime and track surface may be risk factors

History
- Many affected horses conform to following general features:
  - Low-grade lameness that typically warms up with exercise.
  - Pathology often bilateral and may present as wide-based forelimb action rather than overt lameness.
  - Insidious progression over weeks/months.
  - More severe, acute lameness seen with fractures or with some subchondral bone collapse/necrosis or stress injuries.
  - Slab fracture (third carpal bone): acute moderate–marked lameness, usually following fast work.

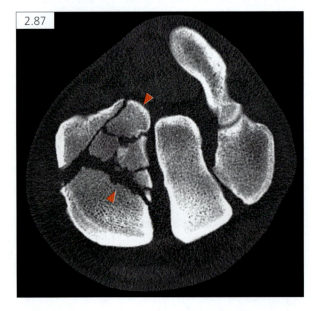

Fig. 2.87 CT image (bone algorithm/transverse) of a palmar carpal fracture. Note the comminution of the radial carpal bone (arrowheads).

Signs
- Unilateral or bilateral lameness.
- Variable severity: subtle to severe (with slab fracture).
- +/− palpable joint effusion.
- Unless acute fracture, typically no pain/restriction to carpal flexion.
- Chip fracture/fragmentation: frequently a pain response to deep palpation of affected site (with limb flexed).
- Slab fracture (third carpal bone): marked effusion of middle carpal joint/pain on flexion of carpus.
- Cortical fissure (third carpal bone): typically no joint effusion.

Diagnosis
- History and clinical findings often strongly indicative; confirmation with diagnostic blocking +/− imaging.
- Adaptive radiological changes are present in many 'normal' horses; interpret imaging findings with caution.
- Not always possible to distinguish middle carpal joint lameness from subcarpal/suspensory pain by diagnostic blocking/conventional imaging.
- Radiography (middle carpal joint): assessment of distal articular margin of radial carpal bone (DLPaMO/flexed LM projections) and third carpal bone (flexed D35°PrDDiO/'distal row skyline' projection) of both forelimbs is important. Increased density/loss of trabecular definition of the radial facet (less commonly intermediate facet) of the third carpal bone (**Figures 2.88a–d**);

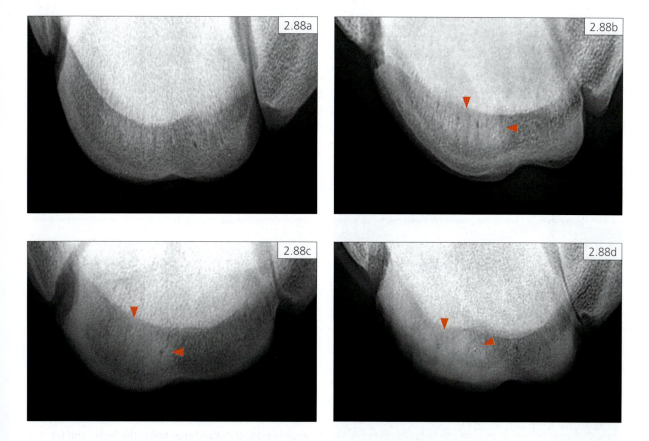

Figs. 2.88a–d Radiographs (flexed D35°PrDDiO) of the third carpal bone. Normal trabeculation (a). Mild (b), moderate (c) and marked (d) increase in densification of the radial facet (arrowheads).

increased density/focal lysis/spurring distal radial carpal bone (**Figures 2.89a–c**). Activity at both sites is also encountered (**Figure 2.90**). Bone modelling over the dorsal margin of the radial carpal bone is an indicator of prior joint activity/distension (**Figure 2.91**).

- Radiography (antebrachiocarpal joint): distal radial pathology best assessed on DMPaLO and skyline distal radius/proximal row projections; modelling/spurring/fragmentation of articular margins.
- Bone scan/MRI: useful in investigation of moderate/severe carpal lameness if radiography unrewarding (**Figure 2.92**).

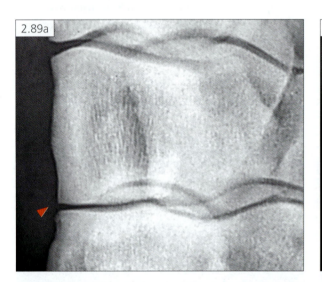
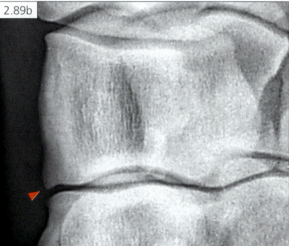
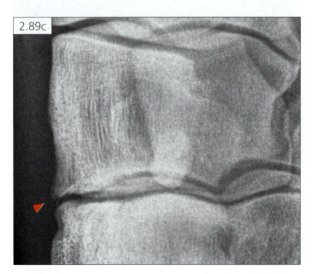

Figs. 2.89a–c Radiographs (DLPaMO) of modelling of the dorsodistal margin of the radial carpal bone (arrowheads). (a) subtle angularity, (b) 'beak' and (c) lytic/active modelling.

Regional Musculoskeletal Conditions

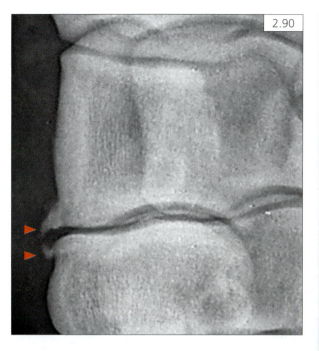

Fig. 2.90 Radiograph (DLPaMO) of active modelling of the facing dorsal margins of the radial and third carpal bones (arrowheads).

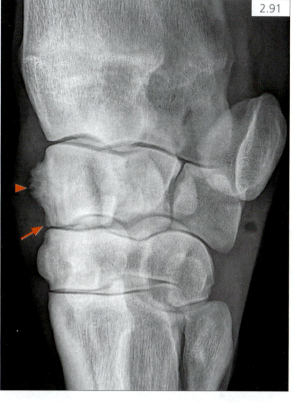

Fig. 2.91 Radiograph (DLPaMO) of modelling of the dorsal radial carpal bone (arrowhead) indicative of previous joint effusion. Note also the active modelling of the distal articular margin of the radial carpal bone (arrow).

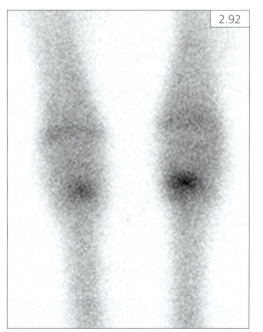

Fig. 2.92 Scintigram (dorsal) showing intense third carpal bone IRU (radiography unremarkable).

Management

- See *Table 2.7*.
- Management dependent on clinical and radiological severity, stage of training and career targets. For most carpal lameness there is no direct relationship between clinical and radiological severity, and radiology findings are not prescriptive. In general:
  - Insidious-onset, low-grade lameness: continued training (+/– intra-articular medication).
  - Acute-onset, moderate lameness: assess risk of further injury through imaging and determine whether rest period necessary.
  - Radiography does not necessarily permit accurate assessment of fracture risk (with continued training) unless prodromal fracture (linear radiolucency) already visible.
- Significant lameness in young horse: consider exercise modification or rest to minimize risk of long-term unsoundness.
- Continued training aided by intra-articular medication: management guided by quality/duration of response; if short-lived (<4–5 weeks) or poor response, period of rest should be considered.
- Antebrachiocarpal joint generally more forgiving than middle carpal joint with respect to lameness/trainability.
- Continued training/racing in the face of mild–moderate lameness is possible but may result in radiological deterioration: implications for resale.

Table 2.7 Management and prognosis for carpal injuries

INJURY TYPE	MANAGEMENT	PROGNOSIS
Middle carpal joint (radial carpal bone fragmentation/fracture)	Dependent on clinical and radiological severity/stage of training/career targets. Continued training aided by intra-articular medication frequently possible: short initial period (1–4 weeks) of reduced exercise may be beneficial. Surgery sometimes warranted to optimize longer-term soundness: determined by chip size/configuration/displacement.	(Ongoing carpal lameness can be expected on return to full work and may require management: intra-articular medication/chondroprotective agents.) Good prognosis for continued training with appropriate management. Once carpal arthritis established, will always be evident radiologically regardless of surgical intervention.
Middle carpal joint (third carpal bone fracture):		(Ongoing carpal lameness can be expected on return to full work and may require management: intra-articular medication/chondroprotective agents.)
Chip fracture/fragmentation	Surgery optimizes athletic outcome.	Guarded to fair prognosis for racing soundness.
Displaced slab fracture	Surgical reduction.	Conservative management: poor prognosis for paddock/racing soundness. Surgery: fair prognosis for return to racing.
Non-displaced slab fracture	Surgical reduction optimizes athletic outcome. Conservative management for non-racing use.	Surgery: fair prognosis for racing soundness. Conservative management: guarded prognosis for racing soundness.
Sagittal slab/cortical fissure	Conservative management: duration of rest dependent on initial severity of lameness/risk of fracture propagation: typically stable rest/walking for 8–10 weeks. Surgical reduction may be considered for some sagittal slab fractures.	Short fissures: good prognosis for return to full use. Sagittal slab fracture: guarded prognosis for return to full soundness (conservative or surgery.)
Catastrophic, comminuted fracture of proximal or distal row of carpal bones	Euthanasia in most cases. Surgery (pancarpal arthrodesis) may permit salvage for paddock use, but considered heroic.	Surgery: guarded prognosis for paddock use.

Table 2.7 (continued)

INJURY TYPE	MANAGEMENT	PROGNOSIS
Carpometacarpal joint (articular fracture of dorsoproximal Mc3) (**Figure 2.93**)	Conservative management: dependent on initial severity of lameness but typically require <4 weeks out of ridden exercise +/− intra-articular medication.	Good prognosis for return to full use.
Antebrachiocarpal joint fracture/fragmentation	Dependent on clinical and radiological severity/stage of training/career targets. Continued training aided by intra-articular medication frequently possible: short initial period (1–4 weeks) of reduced exercise may be beneficial. Poor or short-lived response to medication: rest/surgery. Large chip fractures associated with significant, acute lameness: surgical removal optimizes longer-term soundness.	Good prognosis for athletic soundness with appropriate management.
Palmar carpal fracture/fragmentation:		
Ulnar carpal bone–lateral palmar intercarpal ligament avulsion	Surgical debridement is treatment of choice for athletic use.	Ulnar carpal bone (with surgery): excellent (approximately 90%) prognosis for return to full use.
Multiple/radial carpal bone fragmentation post trauma	Severe injuries: euthanasia or surgery for paddock salvage.	Multiple palmar carpal fragments: guarded prognosis for return to full use (approximately 50%). Severe injuries (sustained during falls/anaesthetic recovery) frequently have a poor prognosis for soundness/survival.

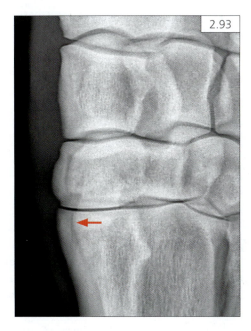

Fig. 2.93 Radiograph (DLPaMO) showing non-displaced radiolucency (arrow) of the dorsoproximal Mc3 with carpometacarpal joint involvement.

Prognosis
- Most cases respond favourably to intra-articular medication or exercise modification.
- Small proportion progress to further carpal injury with continued training.
- Small proportion remain troublesome regardless of management (rest/medication/surgery).

Distal radial subchondral bone injury
Poorly defined injury of lower forearm encountered occasionally in horses in full work. Appears to be separate condition from antebrachiocarpal arthritis, involving primarily the distolateral radius, although some cases have an articular component.

Cause
- Unknown.

Risk factors
- Rare condition.
- Usually encountered in horses in fast work.
- Risk factors unknown.

History
- Acute unilateral lameness.

Signs
- Moderate–marked forelimb lameness.
- Typically without palpable abnormality of limb.
- Occasionally, antebrachiocarpal joint effusion.

Diagnosis
- Diagnostic blocking: variable response to blocking of antebrachiocarpal joint.
- Radiography: usually unremarkable.
- Bone scan: marked diffuse IRU in distolateral weight-bearing aspect of radial epiphysis (**Figures 2.94a, b**).
- MRI/CT: may permit detection of focal radiologically silent lesion.

Management
- Conservative management: stable rest/walking for 6–10 weeks.
- Rationale for use of bisphosphonate therapy (although no current evidence base of efficacy).

Prognosis
- Good prognosis for return to racing.

Carpal sheath tenosynovitis
Effusion of the carpal synovial sheath may have several causes and most are benign with respect to training. Mild synovial effusion encountered in early training may be a response to loading of the limb and is often self-limiting. More severe carpal sheath effusion can also be found with injury to soft-tissue structures within or adjacent to the carpal canal (AL-SDFT, SDFT or radial head of DDFT) and may be synovial or haemorrhagic.

Cause
- Most mild/bilateral cases arise from simple synovitis with no significant underlying pathology.
- Injuries may be primary or may arise from direct trauma caused by bone irregularities of the canal borders: includes bony growths of lower forearm (distal radial osteochondromata; physeal spurring/exostosis) and accessory carpal bone fracture.
- Osteochondroma: cartilage-capped bone growth formed by a displaced 'island' of growth plate tissue. Found in lower third of radius, proximal to growth plate; growth ceases with skeletal maturity.

Risk factors
- Mild/bilateral (and clinically insignificant) effusion commonly seen in 2 YOs as response to early training.

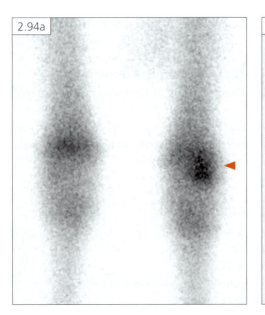
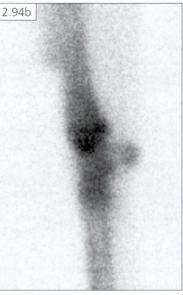

Figs. 2.94a, b Scintigrams (dorsal/lateral) of a distal radial subchondral bone injury. Note the marked IRU (arrowhead), which should be differentiated from normal physeal activity.

- More severe pathology is rare and can occur at any age/stage of training.
- Risk factors unknown.

History
- Mild synovitis in young horses: usually insidious onset; may be mistaken for thickening of upper metacarpal flexor tendon bundles.
- Effusion arising from true injury is usually acute in onset and may follow any exercise pace.
- Osteochondroma: carpal sheath effusion and recurrent lameness.

Signs
- Clinical findings variable.
- Mild effusion: usually only distal pouch (top half of cannon) filled; non-painful thickening around upper flexor tendon bundle.
- Moderate/marked effusion: prominence of proximal pouch (lateral aspect of lower forearm).
- If lameness present, often direct relationship with severity of distension: marked acute effusion may be associated with severe lameness and resentment of carpal flexion.
- +/− pain on palpation of palmar soft-tissue (musculotendinous) structures above carpus.

Diagnosis
- Imaging generally only necessary if lame or marked effusion.
- Ultrasonography: used to determine presence of lesions involving the principal soft-tissue structures.
- Radiography: LM projection for detection of physeal exostosis ('spur') (**Figure 2.95**) or osteochondroma (**Figure 2.96**) of caudal margin of lower radius.

Management
- Mild effusion/no lameness: no treatment or modification of training required.
- If marked/progressive/lameness, diagnostic imaging to rule out obvious pathology.

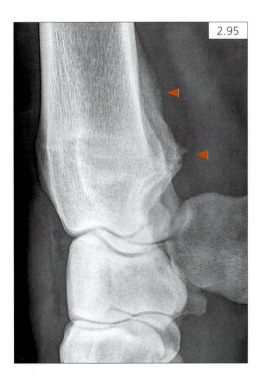

Fig. 2.95 Radiograph (LM) of active modelling of the distal radius (arrowheads).

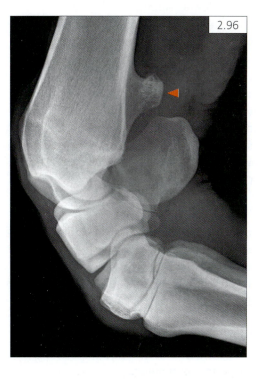

Fig. 2.96 Radiograph (flexed LM) of a radial osteochondroma (arrowhead).

- If no significant pathology detected, intra-thecal medication (corticosteroid).
- Poor/short-lived response to medication should prompt further imaging or rest according to the diagnosis.
- Osteochondroma or physeal spur (if causing impingement): surgical removal along with debridement of torn DDFT tissue (if present).
- Tearing of radial head of DDFT: surgical debridement (tenoscopy).

Prognosis
- 'Adaptive', non-painful distension in young racehorses: self-limiting and rarely interferes with training.
- Tearing of radial head of DDFT: excellent prognosis following surgery.
- AL-SDFT desmopathy (p. 134): good–excellent prognosis for return to full use with conservative management (stable rest/walking for 6–10 weeks).
- Radial osteochondroma: excellent prognosis following surgery.
- Exostosis of caudal radial physis: excellent prognosis following surgery.

Accessory carpal bone fracture

Fracture of the accessory carpal bone at the back of the carpus typically results from trauma. Most common configuration is a frontal slab fracture (**Figure 2.97**); there is invariably displacement of the major fragments and comminution may occur. Involvement of the carpal synovial sheath may result from disruption of the carpal canal border; concurrent laceration of the DDFT is common.

Cause
- Traumatic hyperextension injury of carpus caused by racing/training fall.
- Results from distraction forces on accessory carpal bone by muscular attachments (flexor carpi ulnaris and ulnaris lateralis).

Risk factors
- Rare condition.
- Any age or stage of training.

History
- Acute-onset lameness, usually following a fall.
- Occasionally encountered as incidental finding in clinically normal horse during radiographic imaging: presumed in these cases to be long-standing and of no future concern.

Signs
- Moderate–marked unilateral forelimb lameness.
- Generalized (often marked) thickening of soft tissues around back of carpus.
- Carpal synovial sheath effusion usually present but may not be evident until acute swelling dissipates.
- Flexion of carpus resented.
- +/– instability/crepitus/pain on palpation of accessory carpal bone with limb in partial flexion.

Diagnosis
- Clinical findings strongly indicative.
- Radiography: required for diagnosis. Several projections to determine fracture configuration/comminution.

Management
- Conservative management: 8–12 weeks stable rest with immobilizing bandage (full-limb Robert-Jones bandage; leg in extension) for initial few weeks.
- Radiographic union does not occur but functional union sufficient for return to athletic use including racing.
- Surgical fixation rarely undertaken; tenoscopy of the carpal synovial sheath may be warranted in some cases of fracture comminution.

Prognosis
- Fair prognosis for return to racing soundness.
- Long-term chronic distension of carpal synovial sheath may occur; can be managed medically.

Radial physitis

Inflammation of the growth plate (physis) at the lower extremity of the radius is occasionally encountered in yearlings entering training. Subsequent inhibited bone lengthening on affected side of limb can result in further deviation of carpal conformation.

Cause
- Excessive or asymmetrical loading (lunging/walker exercise) of immature limb during early training.
- Compressive forces from excessive loading stimulate inflammation of growth plate.

Risk factors
- Usually occurs in yearlings during sales preparation.
- Poor carpal conformation, rapid growth, nutrition and excessive loading of limb are risk factors.

History
- Prominence of lower forearm noted in pre- or early training.

Signs
- Prominence of medial aspect of one or both lower forearms, immediately above carpus.
- Heat/pain response to palpation when active.
- +/– mild lameness.

Diagnosis
- Clinical findings definitive.
- Radiography: DPa projection to confirm/assess severity and activity; thinning of physeal cartilage and adjacent proliferative bone reaction (**Figure 2.98**).

Management
- Conservative management: restricted exercise (stable rest/walking) until affected site free from pain.
- NSAID medication +/– polysulphated glycoaminoglycans in initial phase.
- Feed restriction to slow growth rate/reduce BWT may be beneficial: reduce calorific intake by 25% + low-quality roughage for approximately 6 weeks. Ensure correct calcium:phosphorus ratio in diet.

Prognosis
- Prognosis good for athletic soundness.
- Training in the face of active physitis may result in permanent angular limb deformity (consequences for soundness in training).

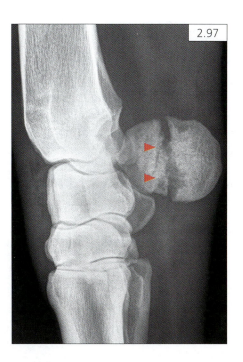

Fig. 2.97 Radiograph (LM) of an accessory carpal bone fracture. Note the frontal fracture configuration (arrowheads) and lytic change at the fracture site indicative of a healing injury.

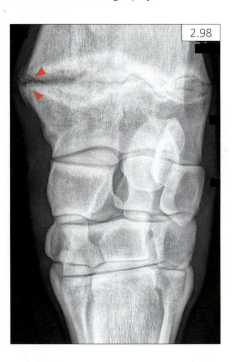

Fig. 2.98 Radiograph (DPa) of radial physitis: flaring of medial physis (arrowheads).

THE UPPER FORELIMB

Applied anatomy

The upper forelimb (**Figure 2.99**) functions primarily as a 'shock absorber' (propulsion being the role of the hindlimb). There is no bony articulation between the forelimb and the axial skeleton; rather, the upper forelimb is attached to the trunk by the muscles and ligaments of the shoulder girdle. This is composed largely of the latissimus dorsi and serratus ventralis muscles, which connect the thoracolumbar fascia and caudal cervical vertebrae to the inside of the humerus and scapula, respectively. The pectoral muscles, running from the sternum to the inner aspect of the humerus, serve to stabilize the limb just before and during the stance phase.

The scapula articulates with the humerus at the shoulder joint. The shoulder joint is notable for having no collateral ligaments and it is stabilized by the large muscle bellies that surround it; consequently, the joint capsule is not directly palpable. At the point

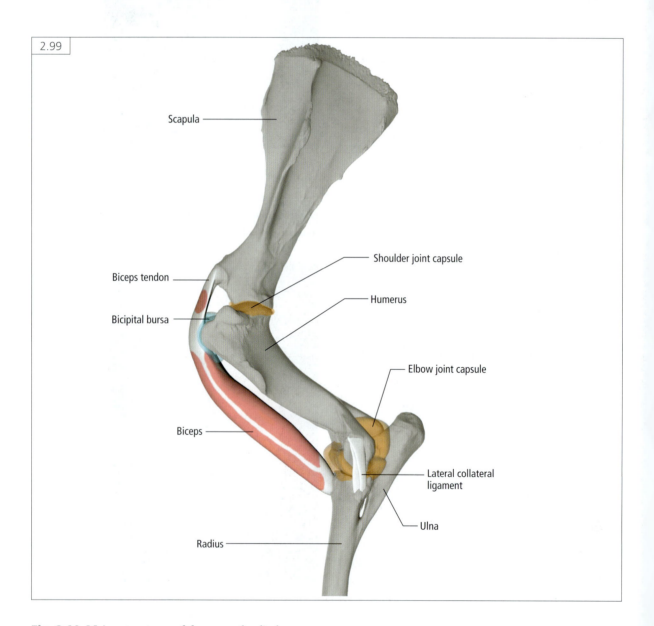

Fig. 2.99 Major structures of the upper forelimb.

of the shoulder the strong and bilobed biceps tendon passes over the front of the joint from its origin on the supraglenoid tuberosity of the scapula. After running through the bicipital synovial bursa over the intertuberal groove of the humerus it descends to attach to the top of the radius (below the elbow joint). The biceps brachii muscle acts to extend the shoulder and flex the elbow, and its action is opposed by the triceps brachii muscle, which attaches to the point of the elbow.

As with the shoulder, the elbow joint acts primarily as a hinge with movements restricted to flexion/extension. The humeral condyles articulate with the proximal radius and partly with the prominent olecranon process of the ulna, which forms the point of the elbow. The joint has cranial and caudal compartments, with muscles surrounding the cranial and medial aspects. Although the elbow joint has little soft tissue overlying it laterally, distension of the joint is not readily apparent due partly to the lateral collateral ligament, which limits rotational movement.

Synovial communications
- Shoulder joint and bicipital bursa: communication in approximately 20% of limbs.

Examination
With the horse weight bearing, the upper forelimb, forearm and pectoral regions should be observed for muscular symmetry. Muscle atrophy may be manifested by greater prominence of some of the bony features of the upper limb such as the scapular spine. Effusion of the shoulder and elbow joints is rarely detectable clinically, although marked distension or inflammation of the bicipital bursa is usually apparent. Flexion and extension of the limb or deep palpation of the point of the shoulder may elicit a pain response and allow localization to the shoulder/bicipital bursa region. The biceps brachii muscle both limits and links elbow joint extension to shoulder joint flexion; drawing the limb caudally such that overextension of the elbow is achieved with shoulder flexion indicates an injury to the biceps tendon/muscle unit.

Humeral stress fracture
Despite being a bone of robust dimensions, the humerus may sustain stress injury in response to repetitive loading. The spectrum of injury encountered ranges from subclinical/mild to catastrophic (oblique or spiralling diaphyseal fracture, **Figure 2.100**). If complete fracture occurs, contraction of the shoulder muscles causes overriding of fragments and shortening of the limb.

The main predilection sites are the craniodistal (medial epicondylar region), caudoproximal and caudodistal humerus. Proximal lesions are more likely to be severe or propagate to complete fracture. Lameness is typically unilateral but pathology may be bilateral.

Cause
- Stress/fatigue injury.
- Tensile strains act at distomedial and cranial humerus; compressive strains at caudal humerus during stance.

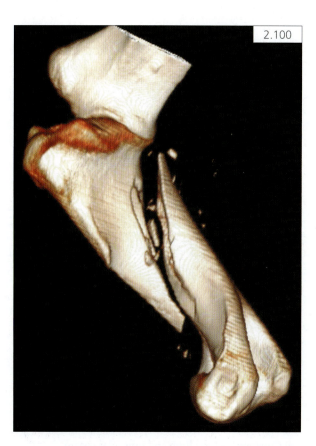

Fig. 2.100 Postmortem CT scan (volume rendered) of a comminuted humeral fracture.

Risk factors
- Any age/stage of training; however, typically encountered in horses in light exercise (trotting or cantering).
- Most common in horses that are unraced or have only run once.
- Horses that are returning from a recent rest period (for unrelated reason) at greater risk.
- Racing surface: proximal lesions more commonly encountered on dirt than on synthetic tracks.

History
- Acute-onset forelimb lameness; usually no history of preceding lameness.
- Incomplete (stress) injury: lameness usually first noted during warm-up for daily exercise.
- Complete fracture: acute severe lameness during exercise; horse may fall at time of injury. Must be examined on track as horse usually unwilling to move.

Signs
- Clinical findings dependent on severity of injury (incomplete/complete).
- Incomplete fracture: moderate–marked lameness characterized by reduced cranial phase to gait; often noticeable at walk. Limb usually palpably normal.
- Complete fracture: severe lameness, usually with marked swelling/sweating of proximal limb/shoulder and visible shortening of upper limb with muscle spasm (**Figure 2.101**). Guarding of limb +/– crepitus may be observed on manipulation. Concurrent damage to radial nerve common and associated with inability to protract limb.

Diagnosis
- Complete/displaced fracture: clinical findings usually sufficient for diagnosis; radiography sometimes needed for confirmation.

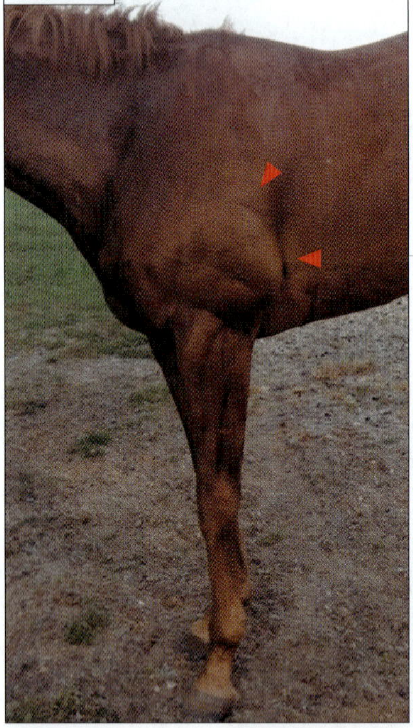

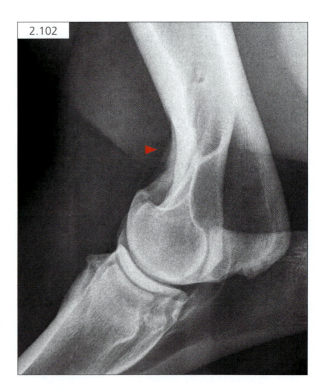

Fig. 2.101 Complete humeral stress fracture. Note the shortening of the limb and muscular spasm (arrowheads).

Fig. 2.102 Radiograph (ML) of a humeral stress fracture. Note the proliferative modelling (arrowhead) at the craniodistal humerus.

- Incomplete fracture: requires radiography +/– bone scan. Poor sensitivity of radiography due to impaired radiological definition of upper forelimb; changes evident in approximately 50% of cases and include cortical thickening, endosteal and/or periosteal proliferation at predilection sites (**Figure 2.102**).
- Incomplete fracture/stress injury: bone scan frequently needed for definitive diagnosis. Focal IRU (variable intensity) at predilection site (**Figures 2.103a, b**).

Management
- Complete fracture: immediate euthanasia usually warranted.
- Incomplete fracture: conservative management; determined by clinical/imaging severity but typically stable rest/walking for 8–10 weeks. Caution advised as displacement of humeral fractures can occur at slow paces (trotting).

Prognosis
- Incomplete (stress) fractures: excellent prognosis for return to full use. Small proportion recur.
- Complete fractures: generally catastrophic in adult horses and warrant immediate euthanasia on humane grounds. A number of cases of complete fracture have survived with conservative management (salvage for paddock use only); however, requires careful case selection and prognosis for survival is poor–guarded. Supporting limb laminitis (p. 46) is a significant risk and welfare of horse should be the primary concern.

Scapular stress fracture
Stress injury with predilection site at the lower end of the scapular spine. Rarely detected at subclinical/early clinical phase; typically encountered at time of complete/catastrophic fracture, suggesting that warning signs are subtle or masked by bilateral nature of pathology.

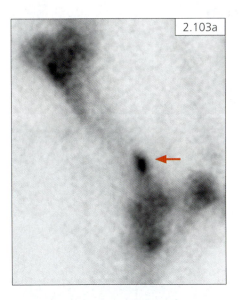
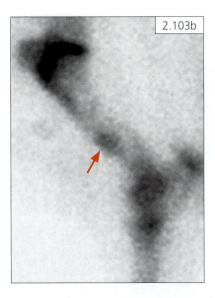

Figs. 2.103a, b Scintigrams (lateral) of humeral stress fracture. Note the focal IRU (arrows) in the caudodistal (a) and mid-humerus regions (b).

Fracture may propagate transversely across the neck of the scapula and distally to the articular surface. Complete fracture often results in severe comminution (**Figures 2.104a, b**). Pathology frequently bilateral.

Cause
- Stress/fatigue injury.
- Spine of scapula serves to limit mediolateral bending of body of scapula during load bearing; stress failure of this supporting strut can result in profound collapse of lower scapula.

Risk factors
- Rare condition (racetrack fatalities: <0.4/1,000 starters).
- Usually encountered in horses currently in fast exercise/racing phase of training.
- Complete fracture may occur at fast or slow cantering paces.
- Most common in horses ≥3 YO.

History
- Acute-onset, unilateral or bilateral forelimb lameness.
- Complete fracture: occurs during training/racing; horse may fall at time of injury and typically regains feet. Must be examined on track as horse usually unwilling to move.

Signs
- Complete fracture: severe forelimb lameness with swelling/guarding/crepitus/instability of lower shoulder blade region. Affected limb may bear weight due to support of muscular girdle but horse shows marked distress at any attempt at movement.
- Incomplete fracture: moderate–marked lameness characterized by reduced cranial phase to gait; often noticeable at walk. May elicit pain response to palpation of the scapular spine.

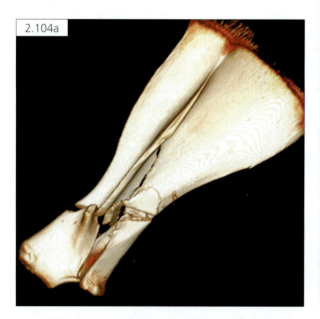 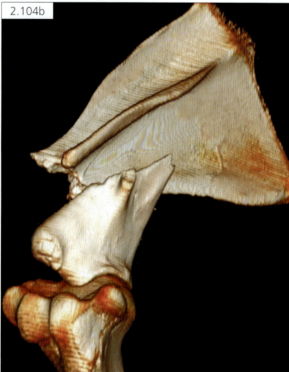

Figs. 2.104a, b Postmortem CT images (volume rendered) of a comminuted (a) and a transverse/complete (b) scapular fracture.

Diagnosis
- Clinical findings sufficient to diagnose complete/catastrophic fracture.
- Incomplete fracture: requires bone scan for definitive diagnosis: focal, often intense IRU.
- Ultrasonography: callus may be detected at lower end of scapular spine/scapular neck.

Management
- Incomplete fracture: conservative management (typically stable rest/walking for 8–10 weeks).
- Complete (catastrophic) fracture: immediate euthanasia.

Prognosis
- Incomplete fractures carry a good prognosis for return to full use.
- Complete fractures are catastrophic and carry a hopeless prognosis for survival.

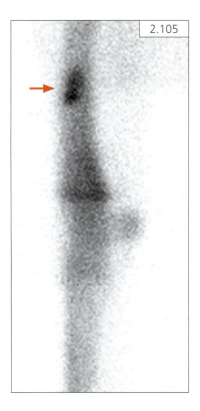

Fig. 2.105 Scintigram (lateral) of a radial stress fracture. Note the intense IRU (arrow) in the mid-radius region.

Radial stress fracture
Stress injury with predilection site in mid to lower third of the shaft of the radius. Severity at time of detection varies between individuals; however, complete fracture is rare. Unilateral or bilateral.

Cause
- Stress/fatigue injury.
- Mid to upper radius subjected predominantly to craniocaudal bending forces (cranial cortex loaded in tension, caudal cortex in compression) while lower radius undergoes largely torsional strains.

Risk factors
- Rare condition.
- Risk factors poorly understood.
- More common in young horses (2 YO).
- Usually encountered in horses in early cantering exercise.

History
- Acute-onset lameness, usually first noted during warm-up for daily exercise.

Signs
- Unilateral forelimb lameness of moderate–marked severity.
- Limb typically palpably normal.
- Occasionally, pain on deep palpation/percussion of medial mid-shaft of radius.

Diagnosis
- Strong clinical suspicion of proximal limb stress fracture (radius/humerus/scapula) may warrant radiographic imaging in the first instance.
- Radiography: findings often subtle/indistinct at initial examination; repeat radiography at 7–14 days post injury. Increased radiodensity of diaphyseal medulla/endocortical callus +/– short fracture line.
- Bone scan: may be required if radiography unrewarding; focal IRU (**Figure 2.105**).
- Diagnostic blocking: negative response to distal limb analgesia (blocking generally contraindicated if stress fracture suspected).

Management
- Conservative management: determined by clinical/imaging severity but typically stable rest/walking for 8–10 weeks.
- If risk of deterioration/displacement, consider tying up for initial weeks pending radiographic review. Measures to minimize risk of supporting limb laminitis (p. 46).
- Complete fracture (invariably with fragment displacement): euthanasia. Surgical repair possible but poor prognosis for survival.

Prognosis
- Good prognosis for return to full use in cases of incomplete fracture.

Shoulder osteochondrosis

Developmental osteochondral defects of the shoulder joint are less common than at other sites. They develop early in life and usually first cause lameness in early training. They include OCD and bone cyst lesions. Unilateral or bilateral.

OCD lesions primarily involve the caudal half of the joint: osteochondral defects of one or both articular margins. Subchondral bone cysts may be single or multiple and are typically found in the mid-distal scapular (less commonly mid-humeral) joint margin. Both forms of osteochondrosis may be associated with secondary arthritis, depending on severity and duration of pathology.

Cause
- See Osteochondrosis (Other musculoskeletal conditions, p. 192).

Risk factors
- Rare condition.
- Usually encountered in 2 YOs.

History
- Lameness usually first noted early in training (yearling or 2 YO stage).
- Intermittent in nature, responding favourably to rest in short term.

Signs
- Unilateral forelimb lameness of variable severity; intermittent or persistent.
- Limb usually palpably normal.
- +/– boxy/upright foot on affected limb in some cases.

Diagnosis
- Clinical features often suggestive of upper forelimb problem but are non-specific.
- Diagnostic blocking: total/partial response to intra-articular blocking of shoulder joint.
- Radiography: ML projection most useful. Signs often subtle. OCD lesions: irregular subchondral radiodensity or flattening/loss of congruity of joint margin. Cysts: subchondral lucencies with associated sclerotic rim. Most obvious feature of both types of lesions is often secondary arthritic change (modelling/lipping of caudoventral angle of scapula).

Management
- Conservative management (rest +/– intra-articular medication) in cases without marked clinical or radiographic findings. Rest period of 3–4 months out of ridden exercise.
- Surgery may give best chance of positive outcome for more severely affected cases, although not all lesions accessible.

Prognosis
- Prognosis for racing soundness poor to guarded regardless of management (<50% return to athletic use). Some manageable with periodic intra-articular medication.
- Prognosis worsens with severity of radiological findings at initial presentation.

Biceps bursitis/tendinitis

Injuries to the biceps tendon or the synovial (bicipital) bursa that surrounds it occur sporadically. Most frequent is septic tenosynovitis of the bursa, causing progressive and severe lameness. Less common are non-septic tenosynovitis and true tendinitis/enlargement of the biceps tendon.

Cause
- Septic tenosynovitis usually the result of a penetrating injury (commonly pitchfork) but closed/haematogenous infection can occur.
- Non-septic tenosynovitis or tendinitis may arise from traumatic stretching/flexion of shoulder during a fall or blunt trauma to point of shoulder. In some cases may arise from undefined repetitive loading factors.

Risk factors
- Septic tenosynovitis may occur at any age/stage of training.
- Tendinitis very rare and usually in 2 YOs in cantering phase of training; risk factors unknown.

History
- Septic tenosynovitis: forelimb lameness that worsens (to become severe) over several days.
- Non-septic tenosynovitis/tendinitis: acute- or chronic-onset unilateral forelimb lameness.

Signs
- Unilateral forelimb lameness of variable severity.
- Shortened cranial phase of stride.
- +/- pain response to palpation of biceps/point of shoulder region or flexion of shoulder.
- Septic tenosynovitis: severe lameness/swelling +/- pain response at point of shoulder +/- fever. External wound may not be readily apparent.

Diagnosis
- Clinical features usually indicative of upper forelimb origin but non-specific.
- Ultrasonography: assessment of biceps tendon (enlargement/irregular echogenicity/ loss of border definition), bursa and intertuberal grooves (**Figure 2.106**).
- Diagnostic blocking: elimination of lower limb lameness; response to blocking of bicipital bursa may be partial/total.
- Radiography: useful to assess irregularities of associated bone margins: intertuberal groove/ enthesious reaction at radial tuberosity/ intratendinous calcification.
- Synoviocentesis (for suspected septic tenosynovitis).

Management
- Septic tenosynovitis: requires hospitalization and emergency tenoscopy/lavage.
- Non-septic bursitis/tendinitis: conservative management (typically stable rest/walking for 8–12 weeks) +/- intrathecal medication. Rehabilitation guided by clinical/ultrasonographic monitoring.

Prognosis
- Septic tenosynovitis: fair prognosis for return to soundness with prompt surgical management. Prognosis declines with chronicity.
- Non-septic tenosynovitis/tendinitis: good prognosis for return to full soundness.

Shoulder fracture: supraglenoid tuberosity

The most common fracture involving the point of the shoulder. The supraglenoid tuberosity is the bony prominence upon which the biceps brachii tendon attaches. Fracture typically runs through the growth plate of the tuberosity, regardless of age (growth plate

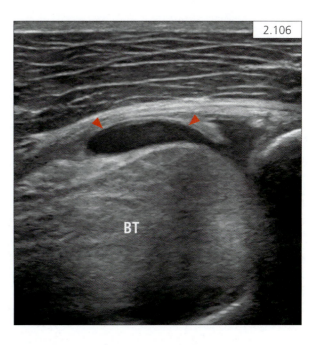

Fig. 2.106 Ultrasonogram (transverse) of a biceps bursal effusion (arrowheads). BT, biceps tendon.

closes between 1 and 2 years of age). Fracture fragment is usually distracted cranially/distally due to the pull of the biceps tendon. Injuries vary in severity (simple or comminuted) and frequently have articular (shoulder joint) involvement.

Cause
- Traumatic injury.
- Occurs either through direct trauma or following overflexion of shoulder (during a fall).

Risk factors
- Rare condition.
- Sporadic injury at any age/stage of training.

History
- Acute-onset unilateral forelimb lameness.
- Usually follows a fall or collision.

Signs
- Unilateral forelimb lameness of moderate–marked severity.
- Shortened cranial phase of stride.
- +/− pain on palpation of point of shoulder.
- Local inflammation/swelling may be minimal.
- Manipulation: concurrent flexion of shoulder and extension of elbow indicative of loss of integrity of biceps tendon/supraglenoid unit (**Figure 2.107a**).
- Atrophy of muscles of shoulderblade (supraspinatus and infraspinatus) may follow acute phase if concurrent damage to suprascapular nerve at point of shoulder.

Diagnosis
- Radiography (ML projection) is definitive (**Figure 2.107b**).

Management
- Surgery: removal (less commonly fixation) of fracture fragment offers best chance of return to soundness; full function of biceps tendon is not a necessity for athletic activity.
- Conservative management (stable rest/walking for 12–16 weeks): satisfactory for paddock use. Results in non-union and generally not considered if return to racing desired.

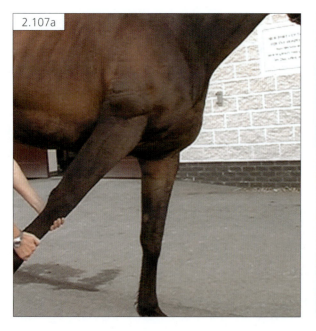
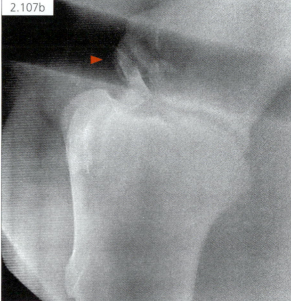

Figs. 2.107a, b Supraglenoid tuberosity fracture. (a) Concurrent extension of elbow and flexion of shoulder with caudal retraction of limb. (b) Radiograph (ML) showing a displaced fracture fragment (arrowhead).

Prognosis
- Surgery: fair to good prognosis for return to athletic use.
- Prognosis best for injuries with minimal displacement/fragmentation/articular involvement.
- Conservative management: good prognosis for survival; poor prognosis for athletic soundness.

Elbow osteochondrosis
Developmental osteochondral defects of the elbow joint include OCD and bone cyst lesions. Less common than osteochondrosis found in the lower limb. They develop early in life and usually first cause lameness in early training. OCD lesions can involve articular margin of medial condyle of humerus or proximomedial radius. Cysts most common in proximomedial radius but also occur in distal humerus. Both may be unilateral or bilateral and secondary arthritis may develop depending on severity and duration of pathology.

Cause
- See Osteochondrosis (Other musculoskeletal conditions, p. 192).

Risk factors
- Rare condition.

History
- Lameness usually first noted early in training (yearling or 2 YO stage).
- Acute or intermittent in nature, responding favourably to rest in short term.

Signs
- Unilateral forelimb lameness, generally of moderate severity.
- Limb usually palpably normal.

Diagnosis
- Diagnostic blocking: positive response to blocking of elbow joint.
- Radiography: (CrCd and ML projections most useful) changes may be subtle; secondary arthritic change may be more obvious than primary lesion. OCD: irregular subchondral radiodensity/loss of congruity or flattening of joint margins (**Figure 2.108**). Cysts: subchondral lucencies with associated sclerotic rim.

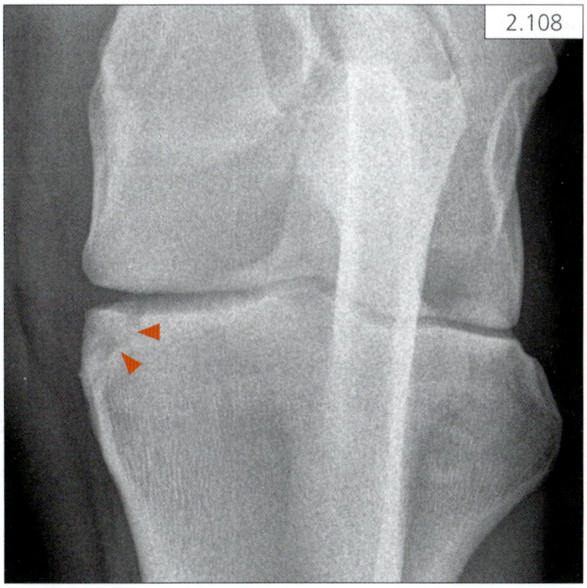

Fig. 2.108 Radiograph (CrCd) of elbow osteochondrosis. Note the indistinct focal subchondral radiolucency in the proximomedial radius (arrowheads).

Management
- OCD: conservative management (stable rest/walking +/− intra-articular medication). Rest period dependent on clinical/radiographic severity but typically 1–3 months out of ridden exercise.
- Cyst: intra-articular medication +/− continued training as initial approach; surgical access is poor and generally considered an option of last resort.

Prognosis
- OCD: fair prognosis for racing soundness with conservative management. Periodic intra-articular medication may be required to maintain soundness.
- Cyst: prognosis for return to racing soundness is guarded.

Capped elbow ('shoe boil')
Focal swelling at point of elbow caused by direct trauma. Initial inflammation typically resolves to leave semi-permanent acquired subcutaneous bursa or fibrous pad. Typically unilateral.

Cause
- Self-trauma: elbow struck by heel of same leg while horse lying down.

Risk factors
- Any age/stage of training.

History
- Acute onset.
- Not associated with exercise.

Signs
- Fluctuant, fluid-filled bursa over point of elbow (**Figure 2.109**); painful in initial phase.
- +/− superficial abrasion and local infection.
- +/− mild lameness.

Diagnosis
- Clinical findings definitive.

Management
- Systemic and topical (osmotic/non-steroidal creams) anti-inflammatory medication in acute phase.
- Do not require rest.
- Treatment may be desired for large bursae remaining after acute inflammation has subsided. Favourable response to intra-thecal medication (corticosteroid) or surgical drainage.
- Prevent recurrence by use of pastern ('donut'/'sausage') boot on affected leg (**Figure 2.110**) while stabled: blocks contact between shoe and point of elbow when lying down.

Prognosis
- Rarely interferes with training.
- May remain a minor cosmetic blemish.

Accessory ligament of the superficial digital flexor tendon ('superior check' ligament) desmopathy
The AL-SDFT assists the SDFT and suspensory ligament in preventing overextension of the forelimb during load bearing. Strain of the ligament can cause lameness +/or effusion of the carpal synovial sheath, with which it has a close association. Typically a solitary and unilateral injury.

Cause
- May sustain injury through acute overload of limb or accumulated degenerative change.
- Loading conditions predisposing to injury, and relationship to concurrent tendon/suspensory problems poorly understood; muscle fatigue may play a role.

Risk factors
- Rare condition.
- Predominantly an injury of older (≥4 YO) horses.
- May arise during slow (including trotting) or fast exercise phases of training.

History
- Acute- or chronic-onset forelimb lameness.

Signs
- Palpable thickening (+/− pain) of lesion site caudal/medial lower forearm when limb held in flexion.
- +/− unilateral forelimb lameness of mild–moderate severity; may be intermittent.
- +/− carpal synovial sheath effusion (in proximal cannon +/− lower forearm).

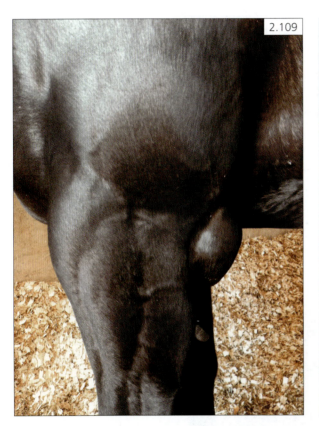

Fig. 2.109 Typical appearance of a capped elbow.

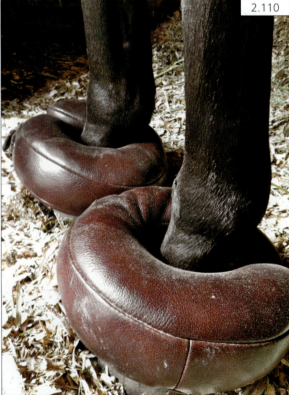

Fig. 2.110 Pastern boot used for prevention of capped elbow.

Diagnosis
- Ultrasonography: enlargement/reduced echogenicity/focal fibre disruption of affected ligament (**Figure 2.111**).

Management
- Conservative management: stable rest/walking for 8–10 weeks with ultrasonographic monitoring to guide return to ridden exercise.
- Anecdotal evidence that swimming/water treadmill during rehabilitation may delay healing.
- Intra-thecal medication unnecessary.
- Surgical debridement may be warranted in some cases.

Prognosis
- Excellent prognosis for return to racing with appropriate management (approximately 90%).
- Reinjury or subsequent injury of suspensory ligament may occur on return to training; presumed to result from altered loading of flexor tendon/suspensory apparatus.

THE TARSUS (HOCK)

Applied anatomy
The tarsus (hock), in common with the carpus, is composed of multiple bones and joints and acts as the articulation between the cannon and the upper limb (**Figure 2.112**). The lower row of tarsal bones is dominated by the third tarsal bone (T3), while the second row has the correspondingly large central tarsal bone. Along with the fused 1st and 2nd and the 4th tarsal bones these make up the distal hock joints. The largest bones in the hock are the calcaneus (part of which forms the point of the hock) and the ridged talus. The hock has three primary joint compartments relevant to the clinician: the tarsometatarsal (TMT) and distal intertarsal (DIT) are low motion joints associated with the distal tarsal bones, while the tibiotarsal joint is the large articulation between hock and tibia.

The soft-tissue structures of primary importance are found at the back of the hock. The tendons of two muscles that cover the caudal tibia merge to become the DDFT. The tendon forms just above the level of the tibiotarsal joint and courses down a groove on the medial aspect of the plantar hock to enter the cannon from a medial position. The DDFT runs through the tarsal synovial sheath, which (just as the carpal sheath does in the forelimb) extends from just above hock to the upper third of the cannon.

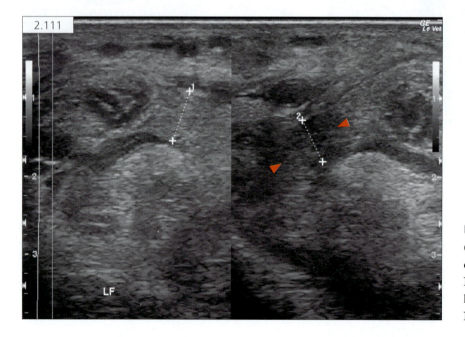

Fig. 2.111 Ultrasonogram (transverse) of AL-SDFT desmopathy (right screen). Note the disruption to the ligament (arrowheads). Normal limb in left screen.

The 'Achilles' tendon bundle associated with the point of the hock is made up of the gastrocnemius tendon and SDFT. While the gastrocnemius tendon is positioned behind the SDFT in the upper limb, as it approaches the hock it falls to the outside, then cranial to the SDFT, to insert on the point of the hock. The SDFT broadens to form a cap over the point of the hock then courses down the back of the cannon into the lower limb. These tendons have a close association with the calcaneal synovial bursae.

Flexion of the hock occurs entirely in the uppermost (tibiotarsal) joint, which is the articulation between the trochlea of the talus and the lower end of the tibia. There is minimal movement (primarily translational/rotational) at the small joints of the hock. The distal joints are loaded in compression. Because of the reciprocal apparatus in the hindlimb, flexion of the normal hock cannot occur in isolation to flexion of the fetlock, stifle and hip.

Synovial communications

- TMT and DIT joints: direct communication in approximately 25% of hocks; diffusion of drugs between these joints in majority (75–100%).
- TMT and tibiotarsal joints: communicate in small proportion (<5%) of hocks.
- Proximal intertarsal and tibiotarsal joints: communicate in all cases and have a common joint capsule.
- Subcutaneous calcaneal bursa communicates in approximately 40% of hocks with a synovial space made up of two compartments (intertendinous and gastrocnemius calcaneal bursae) that interpose between and around the tendons.

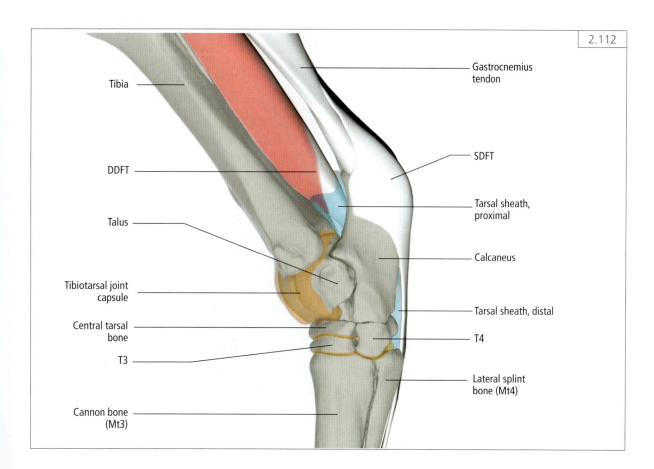

Fig. 2.112 Major structures of the hock.

Examination

Conformation of the hock/hindlimb may influence risk of injury and assessment can assist lameness investigation. 'Straight through the hock' conformation is associated with reduced energy absorption and may contribute to the development of distal hock joint OA or suspensory ligament desmopathy. 'Sickle-hock' conformation may predispose to the development of 'curb'. Palpation of the limb while weight bearing permits assessment of tibiotarsal joint or tarsal sheath effusion; however, examination of most other structures is best done with the limb raised. Firm palpation of the front of the lower hock/upper cannon may elicit a pain response in the presence of a fracture involving the lower hock bones or metatarsus.

Distal hock joint osteoarthritis ('bone spavin')

Lameness arising from OA of the lower hock (TMT/DIT) joints is less prevalent in racehorses than in disciplines that require sharp turns or jumping. The condition is largely defined by localization of lameness to the site (and elimination of other pathology) rather than imaging, as it is not consistently associated with an obvious radiological abnormality.

Cause
- Causative factors unknown.
- Loading (compression) forces are greatest on outer aspect of front of lower hock/upper cannon.

Risk factors
- Uncommon condition.
- Any age/stage of training.
- Tarsal bone collapse (foal), sickle-, straight or cow-hocked conformation may predispose.

History
- Onset of lameness usually chronic.
- Change in gait (such as reluctance to use particular lead at canter) may be noted rather than overt lameness.

Signs
- Mild unilateral or bilateral hindlimb lameness.
- Rarely, acute lameness of moderate severity.
- Reduced hock flexion, lower and shorter limb flight during swing phase of the gait when trotting.
- Toe catch and positive response to flexion test may be features but are not specific.
- Hock palpably normal.

Diagnosis
- Exclusion of other possible local causes of lameness (proximal suspensory ligament desmopathy, tarsal bone fracture).
- Diagnostic blocking: complete or partial response to intra-articular blocking of TMT and/or DIT joints.

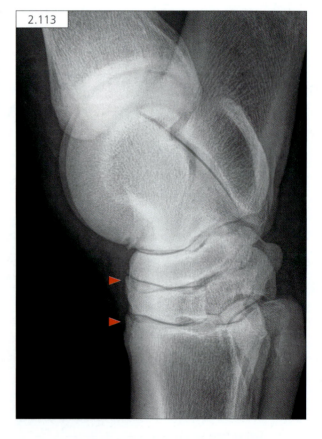

Fig. 2.113 Radiograph (LM) showing modelling (arrowheads) of TMT and DIT joints and dorsal T3.

- Radiography (and less commonly bone scan): generally reserved for cases that fail to respond to intra-articular medication or those that display uncharacteristically severe lameness.
- Little correlation between radiological changes (spurring at top of Mt3/altered density of articular margins of small hock bones/joint space narrowing, **Figure 2.113**) and lameness.
- Bone spurs in lower hock (**Figure 2.114a**) are found in up to one-third of yearlings and are generally of little importance. May arise from OA or insertional strains of dorsal ligament/tendons; radiological differentiation not usually possible.
- Marked arthritic change involving DIT joint tends to be more significant than similar change in TMT joint (**Figure 2.114b**).

- Bone scan: of limited use; variable degree of focal IRU and poor correlation between increased activity and lameness.

Management
- Rest or reduction in training intensity generally not recommended.
- Intra-articular medication (corticosteroid) as required (Chapter 1, p. 17).
- Unsatisfactorily response to joint medication should prompt review to ensure that original diagnosis was correct.
- Cases non-responsive to conventional medication: systemic bisphosphonate therapy or fusion/arthrodesis (chemical/surgical) of affected joint/joints can be considered; fusion is considered treatment of last resort and very rarely warranted in racehorses.

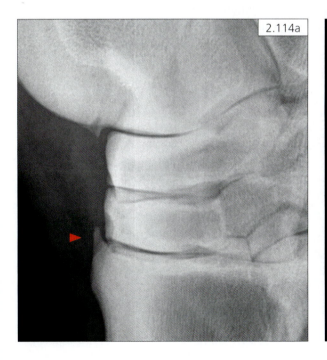

Fig. 2.114a Radiograph (LM) of a proximal Mt3 'spur' (arrowhead).

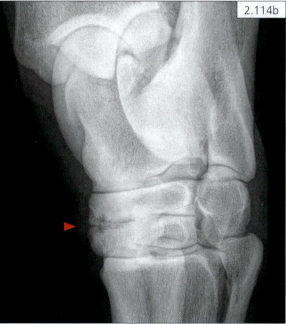

Fig. 2.114b Radiograph (DLPlMO) showing marked osteoarthritic change involving the DIT joint (arrowhead).

Prognosis
- Rarely interferes with training.
- Most cases manageable with periodic intra-articular medication.
- Deterioration of action or unsatisfactory response to medication indicates need for further investigation.

Osteochondrosis: osteochondritis dissecans

Osteochondral lesions develop in the foal. Predilection sites are the distal intermediate ridge, the medial and lateral malleoli of the tibia and the lateral trochlear ridge of the talus (within the tibiotarsal joint) (**Figure 2.115**); also 'teardrop' fragments of the distal talus. Unilateral or bilateral.

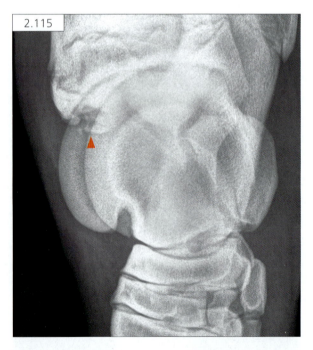

Fig. 2.115 Radiograph (DMPlLO) of tarsal osteochondrosis. Note the osteochondral fragmentation (arrowhead) and lysis of the distal intermediate ridge of the tibia.

Cause
- See Osteochondrosis (Other musculoskeletal conditions, p. 192).

Risk factors
- Tarsal osteochondrosis lesions found in approximately 4–8% of sales yearlings.

History
- Typically an incidental finding at routine or pre-purchase radiography.
- Less commonly present with joint effusion +/– lameness; onset of signs usually insidious.

Signs
- Frequently clinically silent.
- +/– effusion of uppermost (tibiotarsal) hock joint: 'bog spavin'.
- Lameness an inconsistent feature; when present is usually mild.

Diagnosis
- Radiography is imaging modality of choice.
- Ultrasonography: used less frequently but can be more sensitive than radiography for some osteochondrosis lesions.

Management
- If detected at early yearling stage: surgical removal generally advocated in view of potential to affect saleability or cause joint effusion/lameness in training.
- If detected after yearling-sale purchase or later in career: management dependent on clinical signs. In presence of lameness +/– joint effusion attributable to osteochondrosis lesion: intra-articular medication in first instance and surgery only if poor response. No treatment required if clinically silent.

Prognosis
- Rarely interrupts training.

- Good prognosis for continued (or return to) athletic soundness.
- Horses that have osteochondrosis surgery as yearlings are just as likely to race as 2 and 3 YOs as their siblings.
- Surgery resolves joint effusion in most cases.
- Size of distal intermediate ridge lesions has no effect on prognosis.

Third tarsal bone fracture

Fracture of the third tarsal bone (T3) typically occurs in the frontal plane and traverses the bone from the distal intertarsal to the tarsometatarsal joints ('slab' fracture). Usually a complete fracture, less commonly incomplete. Unilateral.

Cause
- Acute injury sustained during fast exercise.
- Results from compressive forces through portion of lower hock subject to greatest loading.

Risk factors
- Uncommon condition.
- Affects all ages; usually in horses in fast exercise phase of training.
- Wedge-shaped conformation of T3 (**Figures 2.116a, b**) may predispose to injury (risk is currently unquantified but appears to be greatest with more severely wedged/collapsed bones).

History
- Acute-onset hindlimb lameness, usually noted after cooling off following fast work.
- Lameness may diminish rapidly over initial days if rested.
- Less commonly: mild–moderate hindlimb lameness, progressively worsening over days/weeks.

Signs
- Moderate–severe unilateral hindlimb lameness.

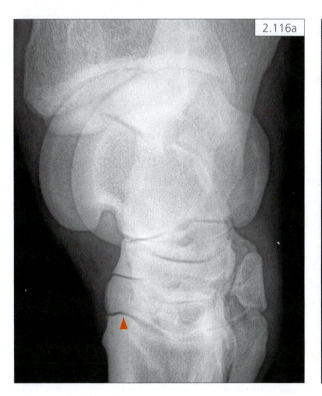 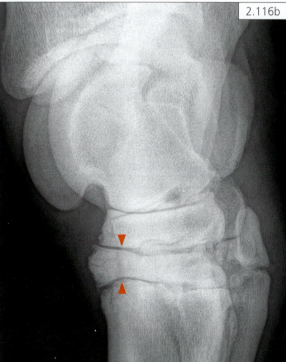

Figs. 2.116a, b Radiographs (DMPlLO) showing mild (a) and marked/collapsed (b) wedge-shaped T3s (arrowheads).

- No visible abnormality of limb.
- Consistent, mild-marked pain response to palpation of front of lower row of hock bones.
- Occasionally, subtle soft tissue thickening/heat at same site.

Diagnosis
- Radiography: fracture line usually only visible on DMPlLO projection (**Figures 2.117, 2.118**); multiple projections may be required.
- If not visible at initial examination, repeat radiography 7–14 days post injury.
- Bone scan: sometimes required if radiography inconclusive; intense focal IRU.

Management
- Most cases respond well to conservative management: stable rest (4–8 weeks)/walking (4–6 weeks).
- Surgical fixation does not greatly improve outcome and is rarely indicated, but should be considered when fracture fragment considerably displaced or for incomplete fractures.

Prognosis
- Good prognosis for return to full use.
- Frequently display mild/moderate hock lameness (may be bilateral) on return to cantering: respond favourably to intra-articular medication.
- Reinjury is rare, although fracture of T3 in opposite hock may occasionally occur.

Central tarsal bone fracture
Fracture of the central tarsal bone occurs in the frontal plane and may be complete or incomplete. Unilateral.

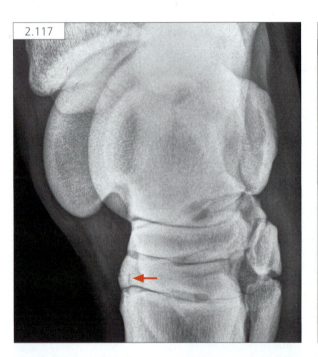

Fig. 2.117 Radiograph (DMPlLO) of an incomplete T3 slab fracture. Note the short radiolucent fracture line (arrow).

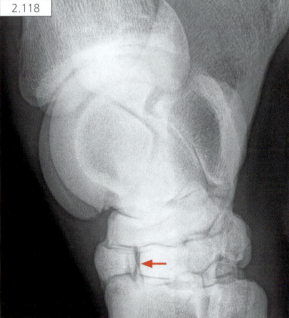

Fig. 2.118 Radiograph (DMPlLO) of a complete T3 slab fracture. Note the fracture line (arrow) extending between the TMT and DIT joints, with slight displacement of the fracture fragment.

Cause
- Presumed to result from compressive forces during loading as for T3 fracture.

Risk factors
- Rare condition.
- Affects all ages; usually in horses in fast exercise phase of training.
- Risk factors unknown.

History
- Acute-onset hindlimb lameness, usually noted after cooling off following fast work.

Signs
- Moderate–severe unilateral lameness.
- No visible abnormality of limb.
- Consistent, mild–marked pain response to palpation of front of hock.
- +/− tibiotarsal joint effusion.

Diagnosis
- Radiography: fracture line best visualized on DPl/DPl oblique or LM projections (**Figure 2.119**).
- If not visible at initial examination, repeat radiography at 7–14 days post injury.
- Bone scan: sometimes required if radiography inconclusive; intense focal IRU.

Management
- Surgical fixation offers best chance of return to racing soundness.
- Conservative management: stable rest (6–8 weeks)/walking (4–6 weeks) an acceptable but less successful option.

Prognosis
- Surgery: good prognosis for return to racing (approximately 70%).
- Conservative management: guarded–poor prognosis for return to full use (approximately 30%).

Dorsoproximal articular stress fracture of the third metacarpal bone

Stress fracture of the dorsoproximal Mt3 (cannon) is a sporadic injury. Fracture configuration is typically oblique and in the frontal plane with articular (TMT joint) involvement. Usually incomplete, although minimally displaced complete fractures can occur. Unilateral or bilateral.

Cause
- Stress injury.
- Peroneus tertius/cranial tibial tendon insertions at top of cannon may contribute to cyclical loading at site.

Risk factors
- Rare condition.
- Typically in horses in cantering/fast exercise phase of training.
- Risk factors unknown.

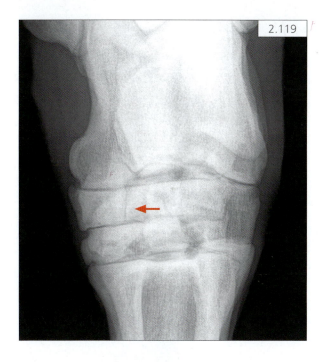

Fig. 2.119 Radiograph (DPl) of a central tarsal bone fracture. Note the linear radiolucency (arrow) through the central tarsal bone.

History
- Acute-onset hindlimb lameness is most typical, but chronic/low-grade poor action may also occur.

Signs
- Typically a unilateral, moderate–marked lameness.
- Less commonly: bilateral hindlimb lameness/poor action that may resemble that associated with other pathology (e.g. tibial stress fracture).
- +/– pain response to palpation of front of high cannon/low hock region.
- +/– prominence of soft tissue/bone at site.

Diagnosis
- Radiography is definitive: oblique fracture line propagating from TMT joint to dorsolateral cortical margin of upper cannon bone +/– periosteal reactivity in region of distal end of fracture (**Figures 2.120a, b**).

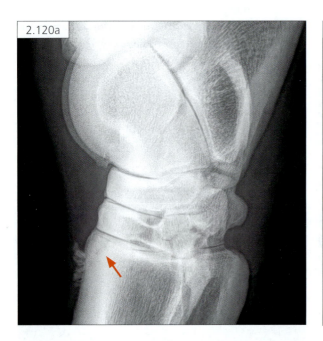

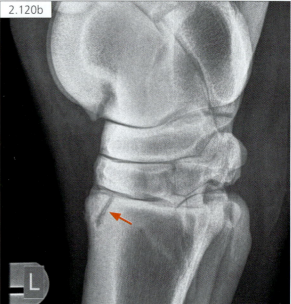

Figs. 2.120a, b Radiographs (LM) of a dorsoproximal articular stress fracture of Mt3. Note the faint (a) and clear (b) oblique fracture line (arrows) and associated periosteal proliferative change in the proximal Mt3.

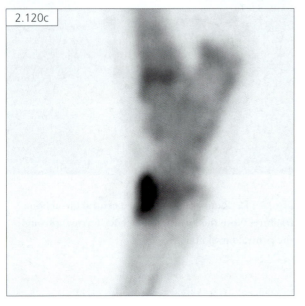

Fig. 2.120c Scintigram (lateral) showing marked IRU at dorsoproximal Mt3.

- Bone scan sometimes undertaken as initial imaging modality in horses with bilateral lameness: marked focal IRU at affected site/s (**Figure 2.120c**).

Management
- Conservative management: stable rest (4–6 weeks)/walking (4–6 weeks).

Prognosis
- Excellent prognosis for return to full use.

Lateral malleolar fracture

The lateral malleolus forms the lower outer aspect of the tibia and serves as an attachment point for the long and short collateral ligaments of the hock. Fracture typically results in a displaced articular (tibiotarsal joint) fragment. Unilateral.

Cause
- Acute traumatic injury.
- Collateral attachments and origin as a separate centre of ossification (fuses with tibia in 1st year) may predispose it to avulsion fracture.

Risk factors
- Rare condition.
- More common in jumping disciplines (hurdling/steeplechasing) than in flat racing.

History
- Acute-onset lameness: usually sustained during a fall, while being cast or from direct trauma such as a kick.

Signs
- Unilateral hindlimb lameness generally of moderate severity.
- Typically some effusion of tibiotarsal joint.
- +/– painful soft-tissue thickening over outside of hock in acute phase.

Diagnosis
- Clinical findings are non-specific.
- Radiography: definitive. Best observed on a DPl or D5°MPlLO projection (**Figure 2.121**).
- Ultrasonography: lateral malleolar fracture always involves some disruption to the short +/– long collateral ligaments. Ultrasound assessment not essential but may assist surgical planning.

Management
- Surgery (arthroscopic removal) is treatment of choice.
- May also respond favourably to conservative management: stable rest (4–6 weeks)/walking (4–6 weeks).

Prognosis
- Surgery: good–excellent prognosis for return to full use.
- Conservative management: fair–good prognosis for return to full use.

Capped hock

Distension of acquired bursa over point of hock resulting from non-septic inflammation. Variable severity; unilateral or bilateral.

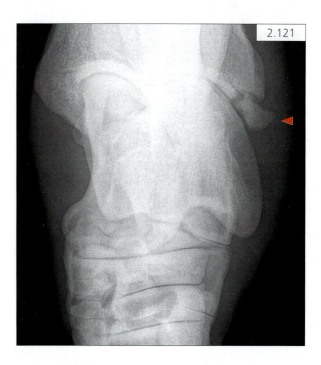

Fig. 2.121 Radiograph (D5°MPlLO) of a lateral malleolar fracture. Note the recently displaced fragment (arrowhead) from the lateral malleolus of the tibia.

Cause
- Cause generally remains unknown but frequently arises from direct trauma (e.g. kicking walls).
- Can be exercise induced.

Risk factors
- All ages/stages of training but most common in horses in early training (yearling/2 YO).
- Risk factors not known.

History
- Acute or chronic in onset.
- When acute, typically follows incident such as being cast in stable.

Signs
- Unilateral or bilateral subcutaneous enlargement over point of hock (**Figure 2.122**).
- Severity varies from mild to marked distension.
- Lameness is usually not a feature, even with marked distension.
- Usually no pain on palpation.

Diagnosis
- Clinical findings definitive.

Management
- Treatment generally not required.
- If lame with marked distension/palpable pain: further investigation (imaging/synoviocentesis) to rule out bursal infection or tendon injury.
- Short period of rest +/− topical anti-inflammatory therapy may be beneficial.
- Medication of bursa with corticosteroid warranted in some circumstances if cosmetic improvement desired.

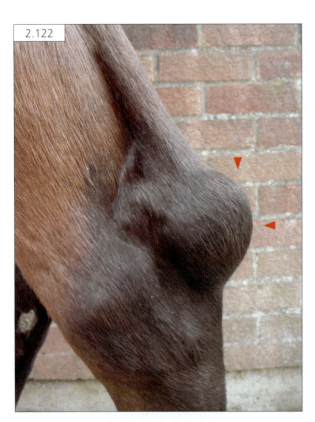

Fig. 2.122 Subcutaneous bursa (arrowheads) characteristic of capped hock.

Prognosis
- Rarely interferes with training; cosmetic blemish only.

Thoroughpin

'Thoroughpin' is a general term used to describe non-septic effusion of the tarsal synovial sheath. Unilateral or bilateral.

Cause
- As with effusion of the carpal synovial sheath, thoroughpin can arise from a number of causes including synovitis or injury to either the lining of the sheath or the structures (DDFT) that run through it.
- Simple synovitis (without overt injury) is most common.

Risk factors
- Rare condition.
- Any age/stage of training.
- Risk factors unknown.

History
- Typically chronic onset (over days/weeks).

Signs
- Well-defined fluid-filled swelling above hock, between Achilles tendon bundle and back of tibia (usually most prominent on outside of leg) +/− distension of sheath immediately below hock around flexor tendon bundle.
- Distinguish from other fluid swellings that can occur in same region: 'bog spavin'/false thoroughpin/calcaneal bursa.
- Not usually associated with lameness.
- Presence of lameness may indicate injury to either the associated bones of hock or DDFT (or infection) and should prompt further investigation.

Diagnosis
- Clinical findings usually definitive.
- Investigation only warranted if lame (rare).
- Radiography: DMPlLO and skyline projection of calcaneus useful to determine presence of bone involvement.
- Ultrasonography: may be useful to assess synovial lining, DDFT and bone margins of tarsal sheath.
- Synoviocentesis if infection suspected.

Management
- In the absence of lameness: no treatment or rest usually required.
- Short phase of reduced exercise/topical/systemic anti-inflammatory therapy may be beneficial to overall cosmetic outcome if thoroughpin has developed acutely.
- Marked effusion: intra-thecal medication (corticosteroid).
- Injury to structures within the sheath (DDFT, tarsal bones) is rare: surgery (tenoscopy) and rest offer best chance of resolution.

Prognosis
- Generally excellent: rarely interferes with training.
- May resolve spontaneously.
- Chronic distension of sheath may persist for medium term; usually considered cosmetic blemish only.

False thoroughpin

Discrete, fluid-filled swelling between Achilles tendon bundle and back of tibia. Severity varies between individuals. Result of herniated outpouching (synoviocoele) of tarsal sheath that probably arises from a defect in the sheath wall. Distension of tarsal sheath itself is not usually present. Usually unilateral.

Cause
- Cause unknown.

Risk factors
- Uncommon.
- Any age/stage of training.

History
- Onset is usually over few days/weeks.

Signs
- Fluid-filled swelling above and forward of point of hock and Achilles tendon bundle; usually most prominent on outside of leg (**Figures 2.123a, b**).
- Distinguished from tarsal sheath effusion ('thoroughpin') by not being palpable through the tarsal canal into upper cannon region.
- Not usually associated with lameness or palpable pain, although may occasionally physically impair action if markedly distended.

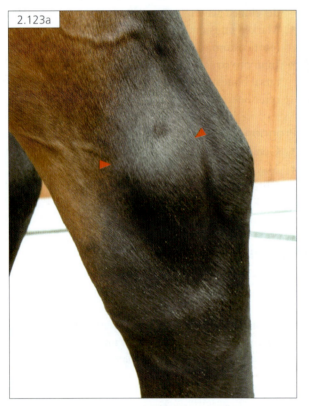
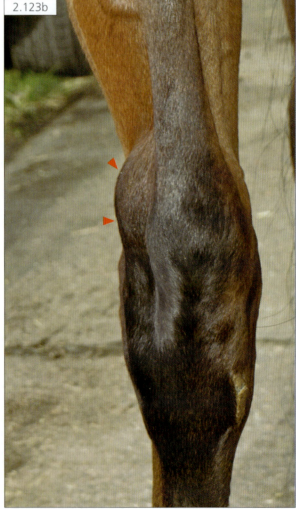

Figs. 2.123a, b False thoroughpin: (a) lateral, (b) caudal views. Note the distension of the acquired bursa (arrowheads) on the lateral aspect of the hock.

Diagnosis
- Clinical findings definitive.
- Diagnostic imaging not warranted.

Management
- Unless large, no treatment or rest necessary.
- If large and affecting action, intra-thecal medication (corticosteroid).
- Recurrence common in short/medium term and repeat medication often necessary.

Prognosis
- Excellent. Rarely interferes with training.

Lateral extensor tenosynovitis/ganglion

Effusion +/– synovial herniation ('ganglion') of the lateral extensor tendon sheath on the outside of the upper hock/lower tibia. Severity varies. Typically unilateral.

Cause
- Cause unknown.

Risk factors
- Uncommon condition.
- Any age/stage of training.

History
- Onset is usually acute.
- Initially develops as oedematous thickening over lateral aspect of hock +/– mild lameness; once acute inflammation subsides (days), discrete fluid-filled swelling remains.

Signs
- Fluid-filled swelling/pouch of variable size on lateral aspect of upper hock/lower tibia; may extend up along tendon sheath over lower tibia.
- +/– initial palpable focal thickening of extensor tendon mid hock.
- Usually without lameness/palpable pain after acute phase.

Diagnosis
- Clinical findings definitive.
- Diagnostic imaging not usually warranted; ultrasonography may reveal tenosynovitis/synovial thickening/dissecting fluid in lateral tarsal soft tissues.

Management
- Acute (initial days): topical and/or systemic anti-inflammatory therapy.
- Alteration of exercise not usually required.
- Intra-thecal medication (corticosteroid) may resolve effusion; long-term efficacy of methylprednisolone acetate appears greater than triamcinolone.

Prognosis
- Excellent. Interruption to training is unusual.
- May retain a non-painful swelling long term: cosmetic blemish only.

Curb

'Curb' is thickening/bowing of the soft tissues at the back of the hock and describes a clinical syndrome rather than a specific injury, as several structures can potentially be affected. Caused by enlargement/inflammation of one or more of the following: periligamentous/peritendinous tissue, long plantar ligament, SDFT and, less commonly, the DDFT. Should be distinguished from simple prominence of the head of the outside splint bone seen in some individuals. Most commonly unilateral but may be bilateral.

Cause
- Maladaptive response (or acute strain) of ligaments/tendons at back of hock to training/loading.

Risk factors
- Common condition.
- Any stage of training but most common in 2 YOs during early cantering phase.
- Horses with sickle/weak-hocked conformation at greater risk.

History
- Acute (most common) or chronic in onset.

Signs
- Soft-tissue thickening/bowing at back of lower hock/upper cannon (**Figure 2.124**).
- +/− pain response to palpation.
- Not always associated with lameness.
- Broad correlation between severity of clinical findings and presence of lameness: mild thickening less likely to be associated with lameness than extensive, oedematous and painful curb.

Diagnosis
- Clinical findings definitive.
- Diagnostic imaging rarely necessary; if required, ultrasonography is modality of choice.
- Ultrasonography: used to determine which soft-tissue structures are involved/extent of injury.

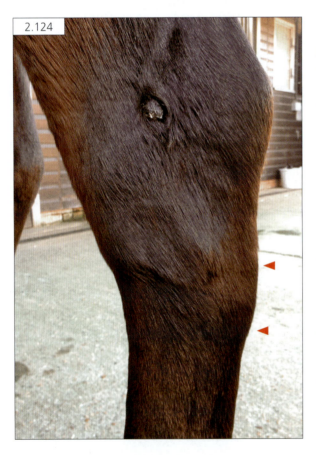

Fig. 2.124 Curb. Note the bowed/prominent profile of the caudal hock (arrowheads).

Management
- Management dictated by severity of clinical signs and is generally symptomatic.
- Mild thickening plus no lameness: no reduction in exercise required.
- Lameness: stable rest or walk until sound and free from palpable pain.
- Moderate–marked thickening plus moderate lameness: several weeks out of ridden exercise usually necessary.
- Topical +/− systemic anti-inflammatory therapy +/− local infiltration with corticosteroid in acute phase may assist recovery if combined with rest.
- Use of anti-inflammatory measures to facilitate continuation of training when rest is more appropriate may result in worsening of injury.
- Limited anecdotal support for counter-irritation (blistering/thermocautery) for recurrent/troublesome cases non-responsive to rest.

Prognosis
- Excellent prognosis for return to full use regardless of severity.
- Mild cases: no/minimal interruption to training.
- Moderate cases: duration of rehabilitation dependent on initial severity but unlikely to exceed several weeks.
- Once 'set', recurrence is rare.
- Rare cases of SDFT injury with fibre tearing may require lengthy convalescence.

Slipped tendon (subluxation of the superficial digital flexor tendon)

Lateral (rarely medial) displacement of the SDFT from its normal position on the point of the hock. Displacement may be partial or full, and in acute phase may slip off and on calcaneus with flexion of the leg. Most commonly unilateral but bilateral injury can occur (rare).

Cause
- Disruption of the calcaneal insertions of the SDFT +/− tearing of the tendon's fibrocartilagenous cap results in loss of stability of tendon on point of hock.
- Not known whether injury is preceded by degenerative change in affected calcaneal insertion/s.

Risk factors
- Rare condition.
- Any age/stage of training; more common in older horses.
- Risk factors unknown.

History
- Typically arises as acute injury at exercise.
- Occasionally preceded by some inflammation at site (distension of calcaneal bursa is a warning sign).

Signs
- Moderate–severe hindlimb lameness with unusual gait.
- Acute phase: may show considerable distress; sedation may be needed to facilitate examination.
- SDFT usually observed over lateral aspect of hock, but in acute phase may be obscured by secondary inflammation at site.
- SDFT may return to normal position during weight bearing or with manual assistance; palpation of point of hock and tendinous structures best performed with limb in flexion.
- Calcaneal bursal effusion.

Diagnosis
- Clinical findings definitive.

Management
- Goal of treatment is to permit SDFT to settle permanently into new position on side of hock.
- Conservative management: stable rest (8–16 weeks) followed by walking.
- Systemic anti-inflammatory medication in acute phase.
- Intermittent (unstable) displacement: tenoscopy of calcaneal bursa to permit resection of any torn fibrocartilage cap may offer improved prognosis for return to athletic function.
- Surgical repair to reposition SDFT on point of hock is not favoured.

Prognosis
- Guarded prognosis for return to full use with conservative management.
- Lameness resolves with rest but horses typically retain a gait abnormality due to new position of SDFT; in some cases this may prove performance-limiting for racing.
- Prognosis for non-racing athletic pursuits excellent.

Stringhalt
Acute-onset neuromuscular gait defect characterized by involuntary exaggerated flexion of one or both hocks. May resolve spontaneously or remain as chronic condition.

Cause
- 'Sporadic' form of condition usually affects one leg and can follow injury to front of hock or upper cannon.
- Neurotoxic form ('Australian' stringhalt): related to exposure to certain toxic pasture plants of the flatweed/dandelion group (esp. *Hypochoeris radicata*). Neurotoxicity causes a generalized nerve dysfunction (distal axonopathy) with resulting neurogenic muscle atrophy. Seen both in individuals and as outbreaks.
- Inciting cause in individual cases frequently unknown.

Risk factors
- Rare condition.
- Any age/stage of training.
- Recent/current grazing exposure to causative plants.

History
- Acute onset; no association with exercise.
- Signs may be worse in cold weather.

Signs
- Intermittent, exaggerated flexion of hock/s; sometimes to the point of striking belly.
- Generally observed when backing up or at walk/trot and not associated with lameness.
- Clinical examination of limb usually unremarkable.
- Chronic cases may display muscle atrophy of affected limb.

Diagnosis
- Clinical findings definitive.
- Radiography/ultrasonography of front of upper cannon/hock region may be warranted to determine underlying cause if sporadic form suspected.

Management
- Removal from pasture if toxicity suspected.
- Systemic corticosteroid medication warranted in acute phase.
- +/– phenytoin.
- Surgery (removal of lateral digital extensor tendon/muscle unit) in cases non-responsive to conservative/medical management.

Prognosis
- Continuation of training often possible.
- Many cases resolve spontaneously but not possible to predict course of condition and some remain affected long term.

THE UPPER HINDLIMB

Applied anatomy (Figure 2.125)
Tibia
The tibia articulates proximally with the femur at the stifle joint and distally with the trochlea of the talus at the hock. The fibula is a vestigial structure and articulates at its head with the lateral condyle of the tibia. The upper tibia is cloaked in muscle bellies on three sides, with only the medial aspect relatively exposed. The popliteus muscle inserts on the caudal surface of the proximal tibia and acts to flex the stifle and rotate the leg inward. The muscle bellies of the deep digital flexor arise in part from the roughened bone of the mid-caudal tibia, as well as the lateral condyle of the tibia. The deep head of this muscle lies on the caudal surface of the bone.

Stifle
The stifle is the largest joint in the horse and is the articulation between the tibia and the femur. The condyles of

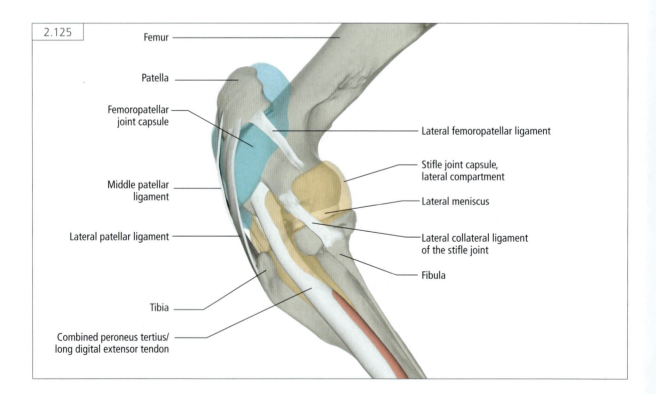

Fig. 2.125 Major structures of the stifle.

the femur do not conform in shape to the tibial plateau; two crescent-shaped menisci made of fibrocartilage provide congruency between the two bones and function to cushion the articular cartilage from the compression forces of weight bearing. The abaxial borders of the menisci are attached to the stifle joint capsule; the cranial ligament of each meniscus is anchored to the top of the tibia at the medial and lateral intercondylar eminences, respectively. There are two cruciate ligaments within the stifle: the cranial (CrCL) and caudal (CdCL). Although lying outside the joint space, they provide stability, with the CrCL being under tension when the leg is in extension and the CdCL in tension when the leg is in extreme flexion.

The patella is a large, rhomboid-shaped bone in the insertional tendon of the quadriceps femoris muscle. It articulates with the large medial and smaller lateral trochlear ridges of the femur. From its base, three patellar ligaments converge distally to attachments on the tibial crest. A large fat pad separates the patellar ligaments from the femoropatellar joint capsule.

The reciprocal ('stay') apparatus of the horse is the means by which it can remain standing with little muscular effort. This is achieved by a series of inter-related musculotendinous units, which ensure that the hock and stifle flex and extend in unison at all times, and by a functional peculiarity in which contraction of the quadriceps femoris muscle group hooks the patella over the medial trochlear ridge of the femur by way of the parapatellar fibrocartilage of the medial patellar ligament.

The stifle has three synovial spaces: the femoropatellar joint (FPJ) and the medial (MFTJ) and lateral (LFTJ) femorotibial joints. The femoropatellar joint at the front of the stifle is the articulation of the patella and the two trochlear ridges. The femorotibial joint spaces are distinct from each other and are found between each meniscus and its corresponding femoral condyle; the LFTJ is tightly constrained, while the MFTJ has a sometimes quite large pouch on the inner aspect of the limb.

Synovial communications
- FPJ and MFTJ: communicate directly in the majority (approximately 60–80%) of stifles.
- LFTJ and each of the other joints: communication is rare.
- Diffusion of local anaesthetic between the compartments occurs in a high proportion of stifles but it cannot be relied on for drug delivery.

Examination
Examination of the tibia is best undertaken with the limb raised. The medial surface of the bone is readily palpated, as it is largely free of muscle. Particular attention should be paid to the caudomedial aspect of the bone just above the hock; loss of the normal sharp definition of this site, focal thickening or palpable pain are strongly indicative of stress fracture. Response to percussion or torsion of the tibia may also provide clinical information, but should be interpreted with caution and compared with the opposite limb.

Palpation of the stifle is undertaken with the limb weight bearing. Apparent effusion of any joint compartment should be judged against the opposite limb and attention paid to stance, as limb position can influence perception of intra-articular pressure. Of the three compartments only FPJ effusion may be visible and is usually observed best with the leg in profile. MFTJ effusion is readily palpable on the inside of the groin just above the tibial plateau, while LFTJ effusion is rare and palpable only as a small pouch of fluid on the outside of the stifle.

Tibial stress fracture
Important and common racehorse injury. Three main predilection sites for injury exist: proximal (proximal caudolateral cortex), mid (mid-diaphysis, lateral cortex) and distal third (caudodistal cortex), with the latter being most common. Lameness when it develops is typically unilateral; however, pathology is commonly (up to one-third of cases) bilateral. Wide spectrum of severity but diagnosis is usually at incomplete fracture stage; catastrophic injuries very rare.

Cause
- Forces acting on the tibia are predominantly craniocaudal bending (with compression strain at back of tibia) with some superimposed torsion; torsional forces greatest in distal tibia.

- Cumulative microdamage from repetitive strains; mild or bilateral lameness may go unnoticed for considerable period before clinical lameness develops.
- Muscle fatigue may play role in overloading of tibia.

Risk factors
- The most common hindlimb stress fracture in many training centres.
- Unraced 2 and 3 YOs in cantering/early fast work stage of training at greatest risk.
- Typically in horses going through their first 'fast work' training cycle.
- Fillies may be at increased risk.
- Uphill training may increase risk: greater peak forces in hindlimb and increased stride frequency.
- Tibial morphology and relationship to BWT/type are risk factors in human athletes but have not been investigated in horses.

History
- Usually an acute-onset lameness.
- Commonly first detected on day following fast exercise.
- Less commonly as insidious mild lameness, worsening over days/weeks; also recent poor action/sudden loss of performance at canter/faster paces.

Signs
- Typically a unilateral hindlimb lameness of variable (typically moderate–marked) severity; usually a 'weight-bearing' lameness with low arc of foot flight and catching of toe.
- Bilateral lameness less common but characterized by close/plaiting hindlimb action at trot +/− poor hindlimb impulsion at canter.
- Usually without palpable abnormality of limb.
- Lameness usually resolves rapidly with short rest period but recurs on return to ridden exercise.
- Occasionally a painful bony thickening of medial aspect of lower tibia may be present.
- +/− pain response to percussion of exposed medial aspect of tibial shaft or forced torsion of tibia with the leg raised; however, manipulative tests have poor sensitivity and responses should be compared with opposite limb.
- Displaced or catastrophic injury: severe lameness/collapse; palpation of medial aspect of tibia may reveal pitting oedema/subcutaneous haemorrhage/instability.

Diagnosis
- Clinical findings and history are strongly indicative.
- Imaging usually undertaken in the first instance (before diagnostic analgesia).
- Radiography (LM, CdCr, PlMDLO projections of distal/midshaft/proximal tibia) has only moderate sensitivity but useful as initial imaging modality.
- Radiological signs often subtle: multiple projections and comparative images of opposite limb required.
- Distal tibia: ranges from subtle loss of corticomedullary definition through to caudal cortical thickening/periosteal reaction on LM projection (**Figures 2.126a–c**). Area of increased radiodensity +/− linear lucency may be present on CdCr/CdM-CrL0 projections (**Figure 2.127**).

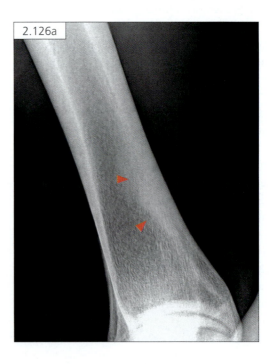

2.126a

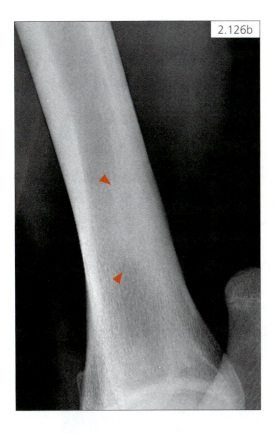
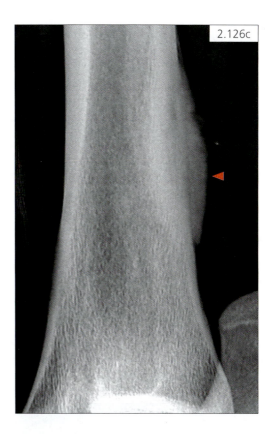

Figs. 2.126a–c Radiographs (LM) of distal tibial stress fractures. Note the endocortical (a, b) and marked periosteal (c) changes (arrowheads).

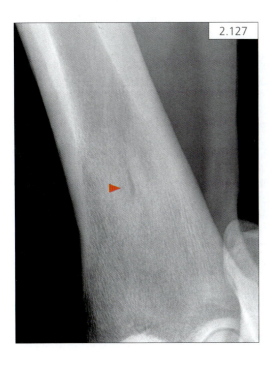

Fig. 2.127 Radiograph (CdM-CrLO) of a distal tibial stress fracture. Note the short lucent fracture line (arrowhead) in the distal tibia.

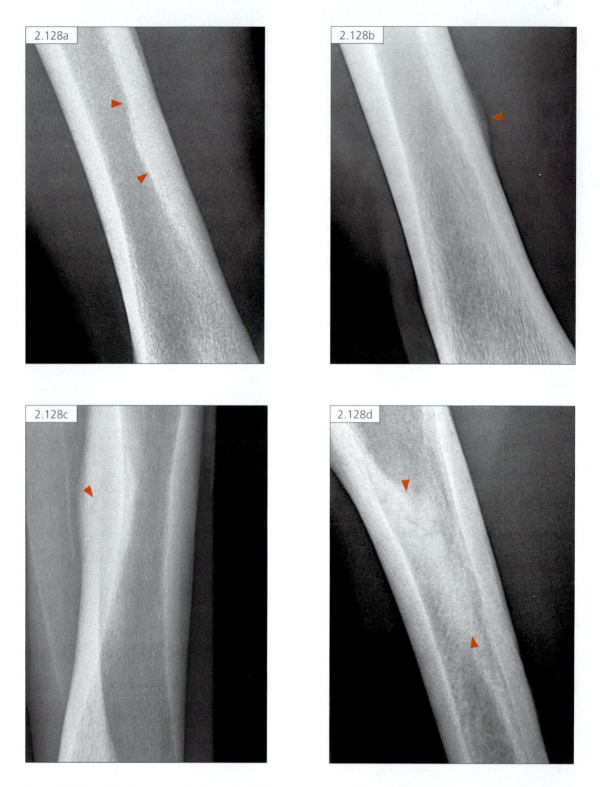

Figs. 2.128a–d Radiographs of mid-shaft tibial stress fractures. Note the endosteal (a) and periosteal (b) callus; radiolucent fracture line and periosteal change (c); and diffuse endosteal callus (d) (arrowheads).

- Mid tibia: poorly defined increased radiodensity through mid diaphysis +/− cortical thickening (**Figures 2.128a–d**).

- Proximal tibia: reactive bone/callus on proximolateral aspect of tibia (below articulation with fibula) on CdCr (+/− LM) projection (**Figures 2.129a, b**).

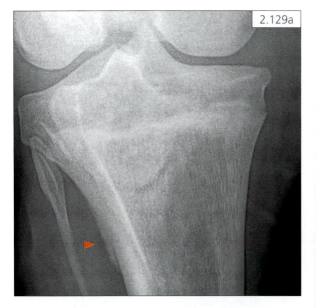
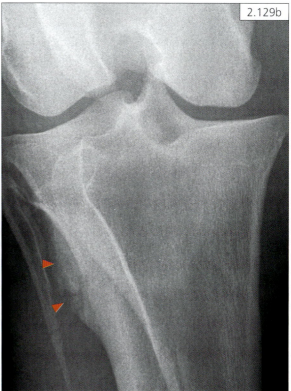

Figs. 2.129a, b Radiographs (CdCr) of a proximal tibial stress fracture. Note the early (a) and marked (b) periosteal changes (arrowheads) in the proximolateral tibia.

- Severe mid-shaft injuries (rare) with suspected cortical fracture frequently unremarkable on initial radiography or may have only indistinct increase in medullary opacity, with development of marked radiological findings over subsequent weeks (**Figure 2.130**).
- Bone scan: if radiography inconclusive; good sensitivity and distinctive patterns of IRU (**Figures 2.131a, b, 2.132a–c, 2.133**). Mid-shaft and distal lesions may be indistinct/subtle due to attenuation and if necessary, caudal/medial views should be obtained; patterns of normal radiomarker uptake in the proximal and distal tibial growth plates may also confound diagnosis.
- Ultrasonography: may permit detection of periosteal callus but rarely employed.

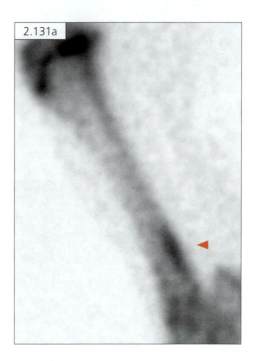

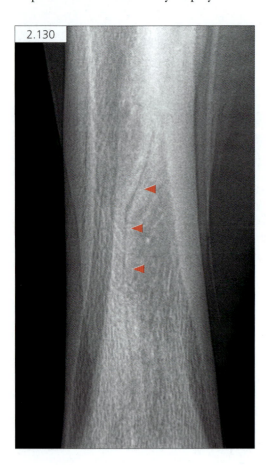

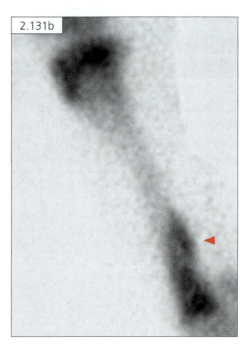

Fig. 2.130 Follow-up radiograph (CdCr) of an incomplete mid-shaft tibial stress fracture that was unremarkable at initial examination. Note the visible fracture line (arrowheads).

Figs. 2.131a, b Scintigrams (lateral) of tibial stress fractures. Note the focal IRU (arrowhead) (a) and the focal IRU with change in the caudal contour (arrowhead) (b) in the distal tibia.

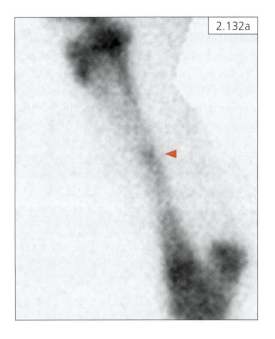 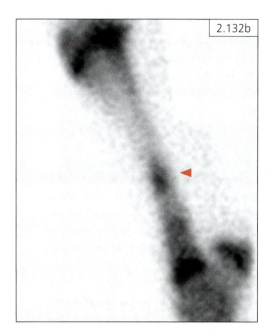

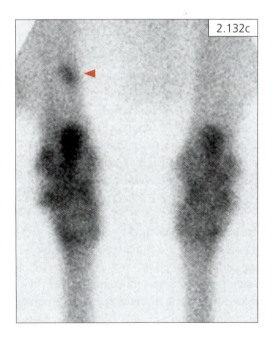 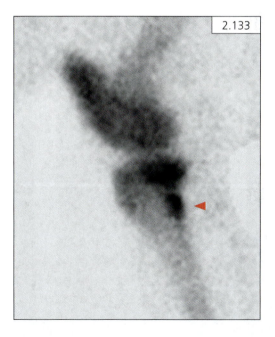

Figs. 2.132a–c Scintigrams of mid-shaft tibial stress fractures: mild (a) and moderate (b, c) focal IRU (arrowheads).

Fig. 2.133 Scintigram (lateral) of a proximal tibial stress fracture (arrowhead).

Management
- Rehabilitation programme determined by initial clinical and radiological severity (see Chapter 1, p. 23). Stable rest not always necessary.
- Typically require 6–10 weeks out of cantering exercise.
- Radiographic monitoring not necessary for majority of cases.
- Severe injury at high risk for displacement (rare): tying up or slinging (4–6 weeks) may be warranted; such management also carries risk of complications including pleuropneumonia. Radiographic monitoring to guide management.
- Complete fracture (**Figure 2.134**): euthanasia.

Prognosis
- Majority of tibial injuries (stress reactions to incomplete fracture) have excellent prognosis for return to full athletic soundness.
- Reinjury (same or opposite limb) is rare.

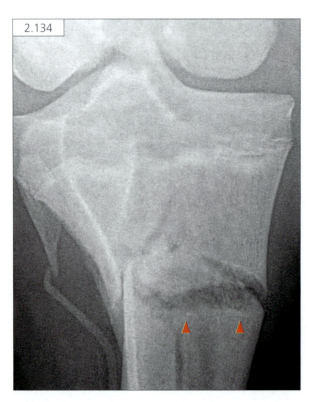

Fig. 2.134 Radiograph of a complete (catastrophic) proximal tibial stress fracture (arrowheads).

Stifle: subchondral bone cyst ('osseous cyst-like lesion'/OCL)
Osteochondrosis lesion of variable size predominantly found in mid-weight-bearing surface of the medial femoral condyle (MFC). Typically develops early in life and in the majority of cases remains clinically inactive throughout training. Very rarely found at other sites in the stifle (proximal medial tibia or lateral femoral condyle). Bilateral lesions occur in approximately 20% of cases.

Shallow subchondral lesion ('dimple') of medial femoral condyle thought to be a related condition arising from delayed/incomplete ossification; of uncertain significance in most horses. If associated with lameness, usually have articular cartilage defect.

Cause
- See Osteochondrosis (Other musculoskeletal conditions, p. 192).
- Arises from defect of endochondral ossification (less commonly following direct trauma to cartilage).

Risk factors
- Uncommon; prevalence of stifle cysts in sales yearlings approximately 2–6%.
- Greater prevalence of (non-cystic) subchondral lucencies of medial femoral condyle (approximately 10–16% of sales yearlings).
- Found in any age of horse, but most commonly first detected at yearling/2 YO stage when exercise increases or routine radiography undertaken.

History
- Most frequently an incidental finding at yearling pre-sales or pre-purchase radiographic examination.
- If associated with lameness (uncommon), usually first arises during early training (trotting/cantering phase).

Signs
- Not invariably associated with lameness.
- If lame: acute, unilateral lameness of moderate severity.
- +/– effusion of MFTJ; limb frequently without clinical abnormality.

Diagnosis
- Radiography: CdCr projection (+/− CdLCrMO projections). Variable appearance of lesion between individuals and over time: shape (semicircular to circular), definition (poorly to well-defined), articular communication (broad to narrow-necked) and presence/absence of sclerotic periphery (**Figures 2.135a–d**). Typically no concurrent radiological evidence of OA in the young horse.

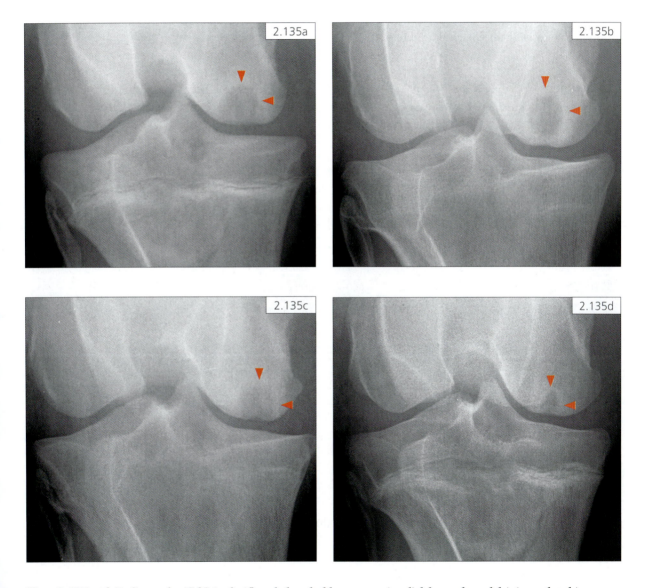

Figs. 2.135a–d Radiographs (CdCr) of stifle subchondral bone cysts (medial femoral condyle) (arrowheads).

- Non-cystic subchondral lesions characterized by flattening of MFC apex or wide/shallow subchondral radiolucency on CdCr radiographic projection (**Figures 2.136a, b**).
- Underexposed radiographs may partially/completely obscure lesion.
- Presence of even mild radiological abnormality often signifies cartilage damage.
- Diagnostic blocking (if lame): partial or complete response to blocking of the MFTJ.
- Ultrasonography: may be useful to investigate significance of shallow radiological defect (assessment of integrity of articular cartilage).
- Bone scan: usually unremarkable in clinically silent cases.

Management

- Management dependent on clinical activity/severity and stage of training. Goals of treatment are surgical removal of fibrous lining of cyst cavity or medical control of inflammatory mediators arising from the cystic lining.
- If subclinical: no treatment required.
- If lame, options are:
  - Intra-articular medication of MFTJ to facilitate continued training in short to medium term (only worthwhile if mild lameness).
  - Ultrasound-guided intralesional injection of corticosteroid, followed by rest (3–4 months out of ridden work).
  - Arthroscopic debridement of OCL, followed by rest (6–8 months out of ridden work). Surgical techniques are evolving and may include implantation of chondrocytes and growth factors to assist repair of cartilage defect overlying cyst cavity.
  - Surgical intervention is generally not recommended for shallow (non-cystic) subchondral lucencies ('dimples') as may result in worsening of lesion; surgical reattachment of cartilage has resulted in return to soundness in some individuals with extensive lesions.

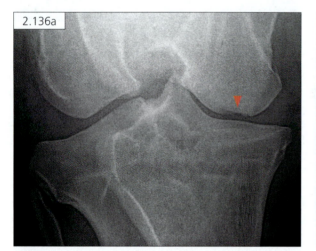
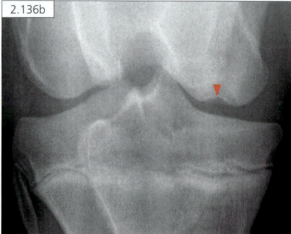

Figs. 2.136a, b Radiographs of a shallow (a) and a deep (b) subchondral lesion ('dimple') in the medial femoral condyle (arrowheads).

Prognosis
- Many cases never develop lameness and train without incident.
- If lameness develops, significant interruption to 2 YO season can be expected regardless of management.
- Accurate assessment of risk of lameness developing is not possible before horse has entered training (i.e. at yearling stage), although action/stride length may be useful indicators of clinical activity.
- When detected as incidental finding in horse that has raced ≥1 season, rarely considered a risk for future lameness.
- Clinical cases: good prognosis for return to full use (approximately 65–80%) with both arthroscopy and ultrasound-guided intralesional injections.
- Prognosis appears not to be related to depth/configuration of lesion, but may be worse for lesions with large/wide involvement of joint surface.
- Poorer success rate (for return to soundness) for older horses (≥3 YO), bilateral lesions or if radiological signs of OA at time of diagnosis; these cases may warrant surgical debridement plus chondrocyte implantation.
- Most non-cystic subchondral lesions do not deteriorate clinically/radiologically.

Stifle: osteochondritis dissecans
Within the stifle, the most common site for OCD lesions is the lateral trochlear ridge of the femur. Rarely, the medial trochlear ridge or patella may be involved. Bilateral lesions occur in approximately 30% of cases.

Cause
- See Osteochondrosis (Other musculoskeletal conditions, p. 192).
- Dynamic, multifactorial condition: lack of exercise/fast growth rate/nutritional/genetic factors in windows of susceptibility can cause abnormal cartilage development at certain articular predilection sites.

Risk factors
- Uncommon condition; prevalence in sales yearlings approximately 3–6%.

History
- May be detected as subclinical lesion at routine yearling radiography.
- Clinical entity of femoropatellar joint effusion +/− lameness at yearling/early 2 YO stage when exercise commences.

Signs
- Variable clinical signs.
- Often associated with considerable FPJ effusion.
- +/− lameness (mild–moderate severity).

Diagnosis
- Radiography: CdPrL-CrDiM oblique projection best for lateral trochlear ridge of femur (most common site of pathology).

- Radiological signs of OCD: flattening/irregular contour or changes in subchondral density of trochlear ridge (**Figure 2.137a**); radiopaque fragments may be present in adjacent affected sites (**Figure 2.137b**).
- Ultrasound: more sensitive than radiography but not used routinely. Useful when OCD lesions are suspected but not evident on radiography.

Management
- Management dependent on clinical/radiological severity and stage of training at detection.
- If detected as incidental finding when already in training and no lameness, no treatment necessary.
- If lame, surgery (arthroscopic removal or reattachment of defective cartilage) is only effective treatment.

Prognosis
- Prognosis for racing soundness determined by size of lesions.
- Unaffected by location of lesion or whether unilateral/bilateral.
- Horses with smaller lesions (total length <6 cm) undergoing surgery prior to their 2 YO season have similar trainability to normal horses.
- Horses with more extensive lesions (total length >6 cm) are less likely to race.

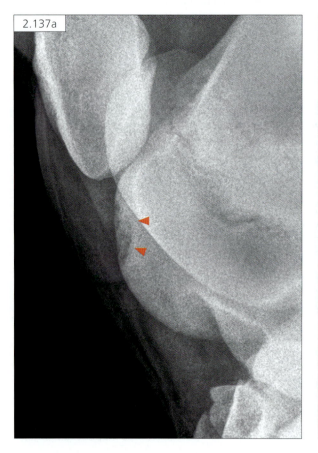 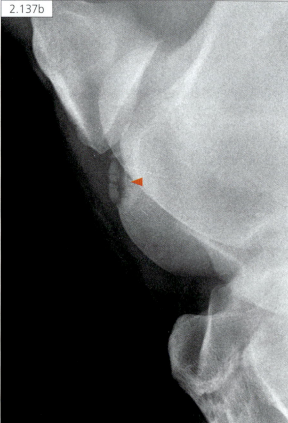

Figs. 2.137a, b Radiographs (CdPrL-CrDiMO) of stifle OCD: osteochondral lesions in the lateral trochlear ridge. (a) Irregular subchondral radiodensity. (b) Associated fragmentation (arrowheads).

Regional Musculoskeletal Conditions

Stifle: locking patella

Condition in which the patella fails to release correctly from its 'sleeping' position on the lower femur, thereby preventing the stifle from flexing. May be transient or require intervention to release.

Cause
- The 'stay apparatus' of the horse enables it to stand at rest with little muscular effort through hooking of the patella (parapatellar cartilage and medial patellar ligament) over the prominent medial trochlear ridge of the femur.
- Quadriceps femoris muscle helps to raise patella on and off the ridge.
- Failure to release the patella may result in stifle being 'locked' in extension.
- Certain movements (turning sharply) may precipitate.

Risk factors
- Common condition.
- All ages/stages of training.
- Main risk factors are loss of muscle tone and straight hindlimb conformation.

History
- May be encountered as sporadic or recurrent event.
- Commonly during phase of reduced exercise/stable rest.

Signs
- Affected hindlimb held straight and rigid, often with toe drawn slightly underneath the body (**Figure 2.138**). Reluctance to walk forward and, when forced to do so, leg will drag/knuckle over; when turned will pivot on locked leg.

Diagnosis
- Clinical findings definitive.
- Easily differentiated from injury: inability to flex limb.

Management
- Most cases readily unlocked through firm pressure from a hand placed above and lateral to the stifle (in the quadriceps muscle mass) directed down/forward in the direction of the opposite front leg. May be assisted by drawing lower leg forward with rope.

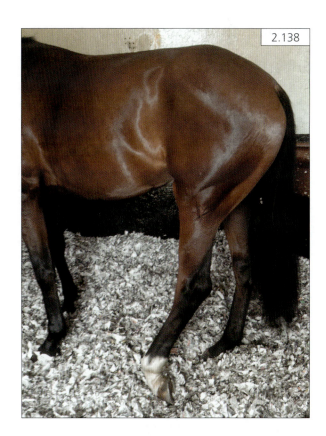

Fig. 2.138 Typical presentation of locked patella.

- Management of recurrent cases dependent on individual circumstances.
- Many resolve with strengthening/conditioning of the quadriceps (return to exercise/hillwork/ trotting on heavy/deep surface).
- Can be managed in short term with twice-daily administration of acepromazine +/− shoeing hind feet with raised lateral heels/wedges.
- Intraligamentous (medial patellar ligament) infiltration with iodine-based internal blister anecdotally beneficial but usually unnecessary.
- If arising from muscle wastage secondary to restricted exercise, may benefit from systemic anabolic steroid medication if permitted.
- Surgery rarely needed and considered a treatment of last resort for severe non-responsive cases.
- Surgical options: splitting or sectioning (desmotomy) of medial patellar ligament; complications of desmotomy include patellar instability/fragmentation.

Prognosis
- Good. Rarely interferes with training.

Stifle: trauma

Soft-tissue injuries of the stifle are typically acute and follow a fall or direct trauma. Damage is usually superficial with short-lived bruising/infection. Very rarely, supporting structures (menisci, cruciate, patellar or collateral ligaments) of stifle may be involved.

Cause
- The patellar and collateral ligaments are poorly protected by overlying soft tissue and vulnerable to direct trauma, particularly kicks.
- The menisci move over the tibia with flexion/ extension of stifle and may become torn during hyperextension of joint.
- Cruciate ligament tears arise from rotation or hyperextension of the stifle; injury to the CrCL is more common than to the CdCL.

Signs
- Following kick: soft-tissue swelling +/− skin abrasion or laceration to front or side of stifle.
- Acute, unilateral hindlimb lameness; moderate to marked severity in initial stages with reduced cranial phase to gait.
- Effusion of FPJ +/− MFTJ is common with injuries to supporting structures.
- Positive response to flexion test in most cases.

Diagnosis
- Acute stifle lameness is not specific for injury type.
- Diagnostic investigation generally only required if lameness persists beyond acute phase.
- Diagnostic blocking: response to blocking of stifle compartments varies with injury type.
- Ultrasound: good sensitivity for identifying meniscal/patellar/collateral ligament injury. Difficult to image cruciate ligaments satisfactorily.
- Radiography: indicators of injury are infrequent and not always specific. Meniscal injury: approximately one-third of horses have reactive new bone on the medial intercondylar eminence of the tibia. Cruciate injury: concurrent fragmentation of medial intercondylar eminence of tibia.
- Arthroscopy: along with ultrasound is only practical way to definitively diagnose a meniscal injury. Cruciate ligaments are largely extra-synovial and minor injuries difficult to detect.

Management
- Acute phase (no synovial infection): antibiotic/ anti-inflammatory therapy and walking exercise until lameness subsides.
- Meniscal/cruciate/patellar/collateral ligament injury: conservative management, guided by clinical progress. Stable rest (4–8 weeks)/walking (4–8 weeks).
- If poor response to initial rest, arthroscopy for further diagnosis/treatment.

Prognosis
- Simple wounds with no involvement of deeper structures: rarely interfere with training beyond few days.
- Damage to supporting structures: prognosis for return to racing dependent on severity of injury.
- Mild/moderate injury to menisci/cruciate ligaments: fair prognosis for racing soundness with extended period of rest.
- Marked tears/severe lameness/presence of radiological change associated with poor prognosis regardless of management.
- Patellar/collateral ligament injuries: good prognosis.

Stifle: tibial tuberosity fracture
Injury to front of stifle in which tibial tuberosity (top of tibia; point of attachment of the patellar ligaments) separates from the parent bone. Fracture fragment typically displaced cranially/proximally due to pull of quadriceps muscle. Usually non-articular.

Cause
- Arises from direct trauma (kick/jumping) or avulsion of quadriceps/biceps femoris muscle attachment following fall/slip.

Risk factors
- Rare condition.
- Any age/stage of training.

History
- Acute-onset lameness.

Signs
- Marked unilateral lameness.
- Local inflammation/pain on palpation of front of stifle.

Diagnosis
- Radiography: LM projection most useful (**Figure 2.139**); differentiate from proximal tibial physis (open in 2 and 3 YOs).
- Ultrasonography: permits assessment of concurrent damage to soft-tissue structures (patellar ligaments/menisci).

Management
- Non-articular fractures: conservative management: stable rest (8–12 weeks)/walking (4–8 weeks). Surgical reduction offers little advantage in most cases.
- NSAID medication during acute phase.

Prognosis
- Non-articular fractures: good prognosis for return to racing with conservative management (approximately 80%) regardless of fragment size/displacement; average time to return to racetrack 6–7 months.
- Concurrent soft-tissue damage to supporting structures of stifle can have a negative impact on prognosis.

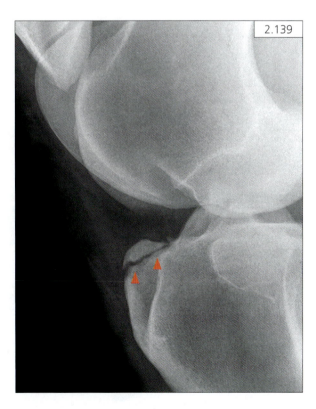

Fig. 2.139 Radiograph (LM) of a tibial tuberosity fracture. Note the displaced fracture fragment (arrowheads).

THE PELVIS

Applied anatomy

The pelvis comprises several fused bones (ilium, pubis and ischium) and articulates with the axial skeleton and both hindlimbs (**Figure 2.140**). The ilium is the largest bone on each side of the pelvis: the broad wing of the ilium is largely covered by the gluteal muscles and only lies close to the skin laterally at the tuber coxa ('point of hip') and axially at the tuber sacrale ('jumper's bump'). The wing is continued caudally by the ilial shaft, which runs back to form part of the hip socket (acetabulum), where it terminates. The ischium forms the back of the pelvic floor and is palpable on both sides of the tail base as the tuber ischium, to which the 'hamstring' caudal thigh muscles attach (biceps femoris, semitendinosus and semimembranosus). The pubis is the smallest of the pelvic bones and forms part of the acetabulum and pelvic floor, fusing with its counterpart at the midline. Important muscles include the large gluteal muscles that connect the ilium to the femur and act to abduct the limb and flex/extend the hip joint, and the biceps femoris muscle, which is complex in form and acts to extend the limb in propulsion. The pelvis is not a rigid structure and mild deformation occurs in response to limb loading and sacroiliac joint movement.

The sacroiliac joints (SIJs) are the articulations between the ilial wings of the pelvis and the wings of the sacrum on each side. They have an important role in transmitting the forces generated by the hindlimbs up through the rest of the axial skeleton. Each SIJ is a broad, flat attachment that houses very little joint fluid; movements are small and are predominantly axial rolling and shear actions (rather than compression) in response to limb loading. The joints are supported by several pairs of strong ligaments on both their dorsal

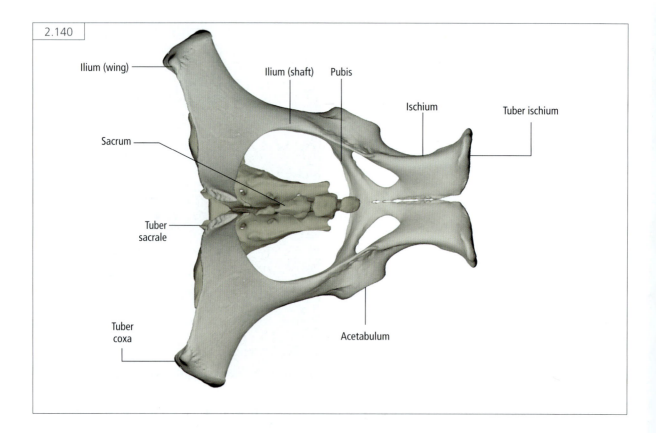

Fig. 2.140 Major structures of the pelvis (dorsal view).

and ventral surfaces and are in close proximity to important neurovascular structures (sciatic and cranial gluteal nerves, cranial gluteal blood vessels).

The hip joint is a ball-and-socket articulation between the head of the femur and the acetabulum of the pelvis (formed from the convergence of the ilium, ischium and pubis). Although its configuration permits some rotation, the main movements are extension/flexion. The cavity of the acetabulum is extended by a fibrocartilaginous rim that, along with the strong accessory femoral and short round ligaments, keeps the head of femur in place. The joint is large but not accessible to palpation because of the overlying musculature.

Examination

The pelvis should be assessed for both skeletal and muscular symmetry, with the horse positioned squarely on a level surface. The large muscle bellies of the quarters cloak the pelvis in such a way that only the bony promontories (tubera sacrale, tubera coxae and tubera ischii) close to the skin are directly palpable. Pelvic skeletal asymmetry is usually readily distinguished from muscular atrophy. Asymmetry in the region of the tubera sacrale is often an incidental finding and may arise from either relative enlargement of the dorsal sacroiliac ligament or gluteal muscle atrophy rather than skeletal deformation *per se*; however, asymmetry of the tubera coxae almost invariably signals current or previous injury. The tubera ischii either side of the tail base, and their associated 'hamstring' caudal thigh muscles, should also be examined for visible or palpable abnormality.

Direct or translated movement of the pelvis through depression of the tubera sacrale/coxae may elicit a pain response. Lumbar epaxial and/or gluteal muscle spasm may be an indication of underlying skeletal pain or may be present in isolation. Manipulation of the hindlimb (flexion/adduction/abduction) rarely causes pain in cases of pelvic fracture, but if undertaken with care in cases of suspected pelvic instability it may provide useful audible or palpable evidence of crepitus. Horses with SIJ pain may resent the contralateral hindlimb being flexed/abducted. Rectal examination of the internal borders of the pelvis may also be appropriate to assist diagnosis of pelvic fractures, and firm digital palpation of internal soft-tissue structures (lumbosacral disc, iliopsoas muscles) can be informative.

Ilial stress fracture

This is a stress injury affecting one or both sides of pelvis. The spectrum of pathology (and severity at time of detection) ranges from subtle/subclinical to catastrophic. The most common predilection site for injury is the axial part of the ilial wing, overlying the SIJ. The fracture line generally propagates forwards from the caudal margin of the wing as a single or forking crack. Ilial stress fractures less commonly involve the shaft of ilium; these are generally considered to be more serious, as close proximity to the iliac artery can result in catastrophic internal bleeding if displacement occurs.

Cause
- Stress/fatigue fracture.
- Main stresses are tensile forces on caudal ilial border and bending at sacroiliac joint.

Risk factors
- Uncommon condition.
- Develops during cantering/fast exercise phase of training.
- All ages but more common in horses ≥3 YO.
- Other risk factors unknown.

History
- Acute-onset hindlimb lameness that often develops during or immediately after exercise (either on track or upon return to yard).
- Some cases (particularly if pathology is mild or bilateral) present with poor performance/poor hindlimb action/reluctance to train over several days or weeks, rather than overt lameness; may be mistaken for muscle soreness/exertional rhabdomyolysis (p. 190).
- Occasionally catastrophic (non-weight-bearing or recumbent) injury encountered on track.

Signs
- Vary considerably; determined by pathological stage at which injury tips over from subclinical to clinical.
- Lameness ranges from none/subtle to severe.
- Bilateral injury: plaiting, short-striding hindlimb gait (at walk or trot) is typical.
- If mild lameness, there may be few or no localizing signs.

- If marked lameness, reluctance to move or weight bear on affected leg. Frequently accompanied by muscular spasm ('guarding') over gluteals +/− pain on depression of tuber sacrale on affected side.
- Displaced ilial wing fracture: asymmetry of pelvis (tubera sacrale +/− tubera coxae) may develop within 1–2 weeks of injury; lower on affected side. May be accompanied by gluteal muscle atrophy of variable severity.
- Displaced ilial shaft fracture: crepitus +/− pelvic instability may be noted with external or internal examination. Catastrophic internal bleeding may occur at any time during initial weeks following injury: collapse/shock/death.

Diagnosis
- Clinical findings strongly indicative (but not specific for location of injury).
- Blood analysis (muscle enzymes: AST/CK) may be useful to differentiate from exertional rhabdomyolysis ('setfast', p. 190), although elevation of muscle enzymes does not preclude concurrent presence of stress fracture and clinical judgement should take precedence over laboratory findings.
- Ultrasound (transcutaneous): used as initial screening aid. Discontinuity/callus in upper face of ilial wing (**Figures 2.141, 2.142**) easily detected (non-displaced ilial shaft injuries more difficult); however, absence of abnormality does not preclude presence of injury. Both sides of pelvis should be imaged.
- Ilial shaft injuries: internal haematoma may be palpable on rectal examination.
- Bone scan: definitive diagnostic modality; however, patterns and degree of IRU highly variable (**Figures 2.143a–f, 2.144a, b**).

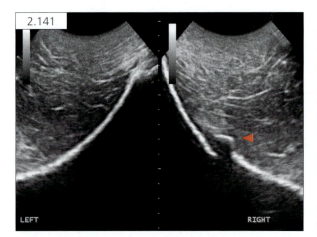

Fig. 2.141 Ultrasonogram (transcutaneous) of an ilial wing stress fracture. Note the normal and injured sides of the pelvis, with disrupted contour of the ilium and callus (arrowhead).

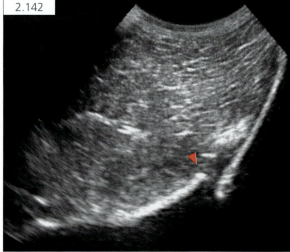

Fig. 2.142 Ultrasonogram (transcutaneous) of an ilial wing stress fracture. Note the displaced fracture (arrowhead).

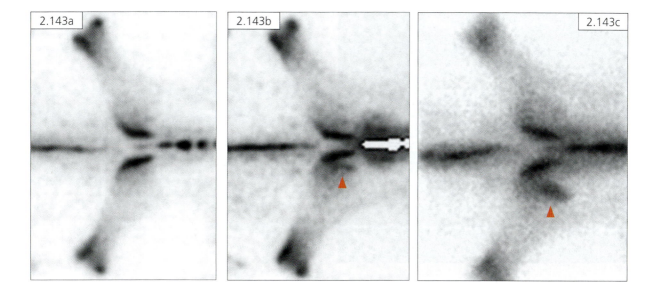
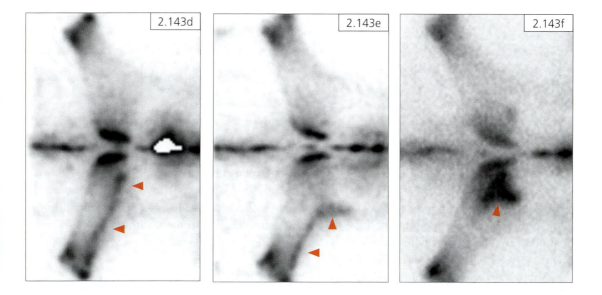

Figs. 2.143a–f Scintigrams showing the normal dorsal scintigraphic appearance of the pelvis (a) and examples of patterns of IRU (arrowheads) seen with ilial wing stress fracture (b–f) on dorsal views.

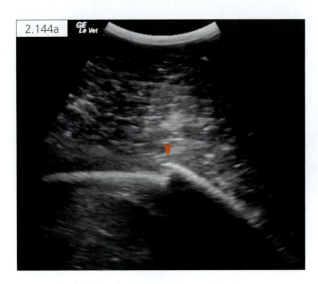
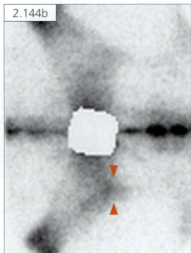

Figs. 2.144a, b Complete ilial shaft stress fracture. Transcutaneous ultrasonographic image (a) showing disruption of bone contour (arrowhead), yet subtle IRU (arrowheads) on dorsal scintigram (b).

Management
- Rehabilitation programme determined by initial clinical and imaging severity, and risk of further displacement (see Chapter 1).
- Ultrasonography may be used in some cases to monitor healing (**Figure 2.145a, b**).
- Severely lame horses (at training/racetrack): avoid lengthy travel; hospitalization also often best avoided as may result in 'stranding' for initial high-risk phase (weeks). Risk assessment in field and transportation to local stable is preferable.
- Subtle/subclinical injuries detected through screening bone scan may require little time out of cantering; continued bone scan activity beyond clinical resolution is common.
- Marked lameness +/or ultrasonographic evidence of possible displacement: tie up for 4–10 weeks (determined by severity and location of injury) with ultrasonographic monitoring to guide management. Measures to limit risk of supporting limb laminitis and pleuropneumonia (Chapter 3, p. 233). Return to ridden exercise in 3–6 months.
- Moderate/marked lameness and non-displaced fractures: stable rest (4–6 weeks)/walking (4–6 weeks) usually sufficient; ultrasonographic monitoring to guide management.
- Subtle/mild lameness and non-displaced fracture: 3–4 weeks walking/3–4 weeks trotting often sufficient (+/– ultrasonographic monitoring).
- Catastrophic displacement with arterial disruption is sudden, cannot be halted and invariably results in death

Prognosis
- Non-displaced wing or shaft fractures: prognosis for racing is good.
- Displaced wing fractures: retain some pelvic asymmetry but action unaffected; prognosis for racing is good.
- Displaced shaft fractures: risk of catastrophic haemorrhage in initial days/weeks after injury in small number of cases. Guarded to fair prognosis for racing depending on degree of resulting pelvic asymmetry.

- Reinjury (same or contralateral side) may occur on return to full work/racing, but rare.
- Prognosis for breeding: pelvic asymmetry following displaced fracture does not usually preclude breeding career for fillies.

Tuber coxa fracture

Commonly known as 'knocked down hip'; involves the bony prominence of the ilium, which is largely unprotected by overlying muscle. Fracture may either be complete (transverse or oblique) with caudolateral displacement of the tuber coxa, or partial with caudoventral or cranioventral distraction of fragments. Unilateral.

Cause
- May occur either as result of direct trauma (such as catching point of hip on doorway) or as muscular avulsion or stress fracture at exercise.

Risk factors
- Uncommon condition.
- Any age/stage of training.
- Risk factors unknown.

History
- Acute-onset lameness; initially noted either in stable or following exercise.

Signs
- Unilateral hindlimb lameness of moderate–marked severity.
- May be more severe at walk than at trot.
- May display 'tracking off' gait.
- Palpable and visible asymmetry of tubera coxae when examined from rear: affected side is lower or may appear absent with loss of normal bony landmarks +/− palpable bony fragment in paralumbar fossa.
- Haematoma +/− crepitus may be noted below point of tuber coxa.
- Pain on palpation/'guarding'/muscle spasm at site in acute phase.

Diagnosis
- Clinical findings usually definitive.
- Ultrasonography (transcutaneous): not always definitive due to normal irregular bony margin of tubera coxae.

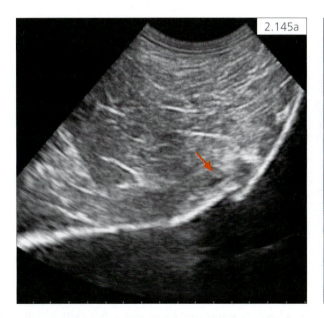 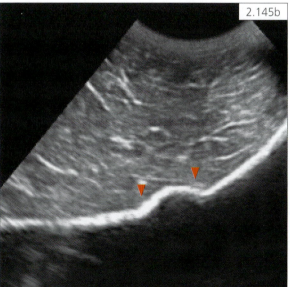

Figs. 2.145a, b Ultrasonograms (transcutaneous) of an ilial wing stress fracture. Note acute disruption (arrow) (a) and healing injury with smoothing of callus (arrowheads) (b).

- Radiography (standing dorsomedial–ventrolateral 50° oblique projection): possible but rarely necessary or practical.
- Bone scan: rarely necessary but if performed, asymmetry of tubera coxae readily seen on dorsal and lateral images. Bone activity increased for many months following injury.

Management
- Conservative management.
- Partial fractures: stable rest (4-6 weeks)/walking (4-6 weeks).
- Complete fractures: stable rest (6–8 weeks)/walking (4-8 weeks).

Prognosis
- Good prognosis for return to full athletic soundness.
- Permanent pelvic asymmetry is inevitable; some abnormality of gait (particularly at walk) may result but unlikely to affect faster paces.
- Rarely, skin penetration by the fractured parent bone may result: requires surgical resection.

Tuber ischium fracture
Injury to the bone promontory at the back of the pelvis from which the caudal thigh muscles originate. Usually unilateral.

Cause
- Usually direct trauma or avulsion injury following a backward fall/slip.
- Occasionally as a spontaneous avulsion injury sustained at exercise.

Risk factors
- Rare condition.
- Any age/stage of training.

History
- Causative incident not always observed and lameness may be reported to have arisen at exercise.
- Often presented for examination as chronic low-grade lameness rather than during acute phase.

Signs
- Mild–moderate unilateral hindlimb lameness; reduced cranial phase of stride +/− reluctance to weight bear on heels.
- Flattened appearance to affected tuber ischium.
- Acute phase: pain on palpation +/− visible dimpling of muscle/focal sweating over affected site. Associated hamstring muscles may be palpably tight.
- Chronic injuries: visible asymmetry of tubera ischii +/− atrophy of caudal thigh muscles (semimembranosus/semitendinosus). Rarely, a hamstring 'strain' will result in swelling/pain in these muscles in the subacute phase and can be detected ultrasonographically.

Diagnosis
- Clinical findings usually definitive.
- Ultrasonography: obvious 'step' in tuber ischium usually visible (**Figure 2.146**), although bone margin has irregular appearance in normal horses.
- Bone scan: may be required for diagnosis in chronic/low-grade cases.

Management
- Conservative management: stable rest (4–6 weeks)/walking (4-6 weeks).
- Insufficient initial rest may result in chronic/recurrent lameness.

Prognosis
- Excellent prognosis for return to racing soundness.
- Affected side remains flattened but action unaffected.

Acetabular/pubic fracture
Fracture of one or more of the pelvic bones that form the hip socket (acetabulum) is typically an injury that occurs in the stable and is unrelated to exercise, although it can also be associated with ilial shaft fracture. Severity varies and instability of hip joint may result. Unilateral.

Cause
- Usually a traumatic injury arising from slip or fall.
- Occasionally due to caudal propagation of ilial shaft stress fracture (p. 169).

Risk factors
- Rare condition.
- Any age/stage of training.
- Predominantly occurs in fillies.
- Fractures through the growth plate occur in juveniles.

History
- Usually found with acute severe lameness in stable.
- May be evidence of a fall or having been cast.

Signs
- Severe hindlimb lameness.
- Reluctance to move.
- Guarding response +/– pelvic crepitus to manipulation/movement of affected limb.
- +/– pelvic asymmetry, visible prominence of hip region due to swelling/haemorrhage in acute phase.

Diagnosis
- Rectal examination: internal haematoma may be palpable on affected side.
- Ultrasonography (transcutaneous and transrectal): obvious 'step' in contour of acetabular bone; may be overriding of fragments +/– focal haematoma (**Figure 2.147**).
- Full assessment of extent of injury difficult due to frequently complex fracture configuration.

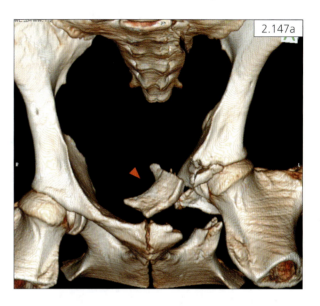

Fig. 2.147a Postmortem CT image (volume rendered). Cranial view of comminuted fracture involving left acetabulum. Note the displaced pubic fragment (arrowhead).

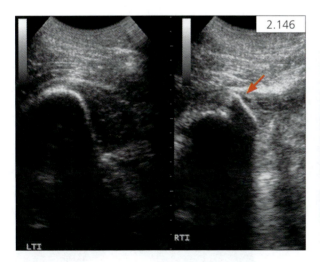

Fig. 2.146 Ultrasonogram (transcutaneous) of a tuber ischium fracture. Note the normal tuber ischium (left) and the fractured (arrow) tuber ischium with fragment displacement (right).

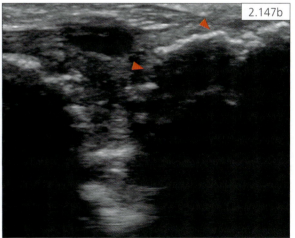

Fig. 2.147b Transrectal ultrasound image of an acetabular fracture showing callus and loss of continuity (arrowheads) of the axial bone margin.

- Bone scan examinations have greater sensitivity for detecting acetabular fracture than ultrasound, but rarely practical (transport inadvisable). Standing radiography is usually definitive in cases of displaced fractures in lightly muscled horses but also rarely practical (not feasible with ambulatory radiographic equipment).

Management
- Management dependent on clinical/ultrasonographic severity.
- Tie up for initial 6–12 weeks; ultrasonographic monitoring to assess stability and guide management.
- Analgesics/deep bedding to minimize risk of supporting limb laminitis (p. 46), although many will weight-bear satisfactorily when stationary. Pleuropneumonia is a risk (Chapter 3, p. 233).
- Persistence of severe lameness/pelvic instability beyond initial phase may warrant euthanasia.

Prognosis
- Moderate risk of catastrophic displacement or supporting limb laminitis in initial weeks.
- If survival beyond period of pelvic instability, fair prognosis for paddock soundness.
- Prognosis for athletic soundness: guarded/poor and dependent on degree of resulting pelvic asymmetry. Return to training is possible in some individuals.
- Prognosis for breeding soundness: guarded and dependent on degree of derangement of internal pelvic architecture.

Sacral/caudal vertebral fracture
Fractures involving the sacrum are rare and usually the result of direct trauma. They may be associated with (or mistaken for) other fractures of the pelvic girdle, including the hip. Fracture is usually at the S2/S3 site with variable displacement; this site is the last of the sacral vertebral junctions to fuse and may be predisposed to injury. Specific fracture configuration is often difficult to determine, but is characterized by callus with concurrent/secondary reactive bone change occurring at the sacral facet joints. Acute or chronic (through callus impingement) damage to nerve roots in the proximity of the fracture site may lead to associated neurological signs (neurogenic muscle atrophy, urinary +/or faecal incontinence).

Fractures of the caudal vertebrae (particularly the tail base) also result from direct trauma and generally cause short-lived pain/inflammation and loss of tail tone.

Cause
- Generally considered to be traumatic injury arising from fall (stress/fatigue fractures of sacrum may occur).

Risk factors
- Rare condition.
- Any age/stage of training.

History
- Sacral fracture: loss of hindlimb action +/− rapid-onset focal/generalized muscle loss over pelvis/sacrum.
- Recent history of fall/slip.

Signs
- Sacral fracture: marked 'hollow' focal/generalized muscle atrophy over caudal pelvis/sacrum (unilateral or bilateral) (**Figure 2.148**).
- Urinary/faecal retention and/or incontinence may occur if neural damage is a feature.

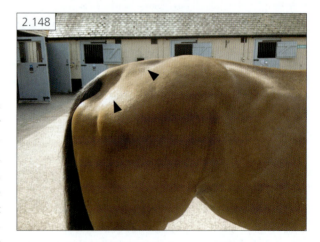

Fig. 2.148 Sacral fracture. Note the focal neurogenic muscle atrophy over the caudal gluteal region (arrowheads).

- Marked pain on palpation +/− muscular guarding of sacral/tail base region.
- +/− diminished tail tone/anal reflex.
- +/− hindlimb lameness; reduction/loss of caudal phase of stride with injuries involving hip.
- Tail base fractures characterized by localized pain (often severe) and loss of tail tone; +/− urine/faecal scalding as unable to raise tail.

Diagnosis
- Clinical findings strongly indicative but sacral fractures also may resemble bilateral pelvic (ilial wing) stress fracture.
- Ultrasonography (transrectal and percutaneous): detection of displacement/bone callus at fracture site.
- Bone scan: may be useful to characterize injury and involvement of other pelvic structures.

Management
- Anti-inflammatory medication in acute phase.
- Conservative management: 4–6 weeks stable rest with return to light exercise guided by ultrasonographic monitoring.
- May require intensive supportive care if incontinent. If urine retention: catheterization or regular manual decompression of bladder +/− evacuation of faeces per rectum until neurological improvement.
- Persistence of neuromuscular signs beyond acute phase may justify ultrasound-guided perineural anti-inflammatory medication (corticosteroid).

Prognosis
- Displaced sacral fractures: varies with severity but generally poor prognosis for full neuromuscular normality (commonly retain some muscular atrophy).
- Guarded–fair prognosis for return to full use.

Sacroiliac and lumbosacral pain

Despite their importance to locomotion, conditions of the sacroiliac/lumbosacral region are poorly understood and difficult to investigate. Diagnostic imaging is limited by access and specificity. Postmortem surveys suggest that a high proportion of 'normal' racehorses probably have degenerative changes of both SIJs; however, it is generally considered that true sacroiliac 'pain' is more common in other disciplines (showjumping, dressage) than in flat racing.

The lumbosacral junction is the articulation of the lumbar spine with the pelvis (ilial wings) and sacrum (**Figure 2.149**). Degenerative arthropathy may affect the lumbosacral and intertransverse joints; severity varies and pathology may not be symmetrical.

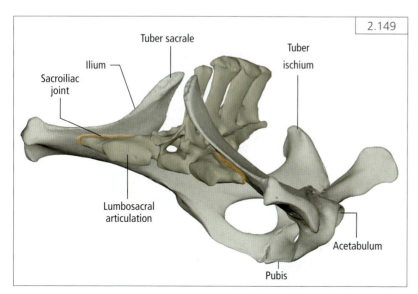

Fig. 2.149 Lumbosacral anatomy.

Cause
- Chronic/degenerative condition.

Risk factors
- Uncommon; true prevalence unknown; probably underdiagnosed as a cause of poor performance/lameness.
- All ages/stages of training.
- Risk factors unknown.

History
- Presenting signs are typically mild and chronic.
- Include poor hindlimb impulsion, back stiffness and poor muscling over thoracolumbar spine.
- May display resistance behaviour (bucking/kicking/unwillingness to jump off at start of canter).

Signs
- +/− mild bilateral hindlimb lameness with toe drag (unilateral lameness not usually a feature).
- The tubera sacrale ('jumper's bumps') are usually level; variable response to manual pressure on these structures.
- Reluctance to flex and extend the lumbosacral region.
- May resent opposite leg being picked up.

Diagnosis
- Not possible to definitively diagnose sacroiliac or lumbosacral pain from clinical examination alone.
- Clinical signs non-specific and similar to many conditions (plantar osteochondral disease/tibial stress fracture/kissing spines).
- Should be considered a diagnosis of exclusion: comprehensive nerve blocking +/− imaging (bone scan and ultrasonography) to rule out other potential problems.
- Ultrasonography: callus on ventral margin of SIJ or lumbosacral joints (transrectal scan) or disruption/enlargement of dorsal and/or ventral sacroiliac ligaments (transcutaneous scan).
- Bone scan: generally non-specific; bone scan appearance of normal horses varies considerably with age, muscling and symmetry of hindquarters.
- Trial medication (corticosteroid) of SIJ and intertransverse joint (combination of three approaches: cranial/cranial midline/caudal) may assist diagnosis.
- Only possible to block via the cranial midline approach due to recognized risks of temporary ataxia through inadvertent blockade of major nerves in the region (sciatic and cranial gluteal) and (rarely) clostridial myositis (frequently fatal).

Management
- In absence of viable intra-articular techniques, treatment usually consists of periarticular deposition of anti-inflammatory drug (corticosteroid) +/− sclerosing drugs (prolotherapy).
- Efficacy of periarticular medication has not been substantiated.
- Prolonged drug detection times may be experienced with deposition of corticosteroid in ligamentous tissue.
- Horses should be kept in work to maintain muscular fitness.

Prognosis
- Prognosis for continued training hinges on severity of clinical signs and response to medication.
- Rarely curtails racing career.

THE NECK AND BACK

Applied anatomy

The spinal column serves both to protect the spinal cord and to be the axis upon which the limbs act to generate motion. The column consists of vertebrae, intrinsic musculature and longitudinal and intervertebral ligaments (**Figure 2.150**). Although the vertebrae vary in form throughout the neck and back, their basic structure consists of a cylindrical vertebral body surmounted by a vertebral arch through which the spinal cord passes, and vertebral processes that act as attachment points for muscles and ligaments. Each vertebra articulates with its neighbours through 'ball and socket' fibrocartilaginous joints (with intervertebral discs) at the vertebral body and at the dorsolateral cranial and caudal synovial (facet) joints on each side of the vertebral arch. The orientation of the synovial articular facets changes along the spine, reflecting different ranges of motion of particular spinal segments. Stability and movement of the spinal column come from longitudinal and intervertebral muscle units and from longitudinal ligaments that traverse the dorsal spinous summits (nuchal and supraspinous ligaments), the vertebral canal (dorsal longitudinal ligament) and the vertebral bodies (ventral longitudinal ligament). Movement between adjacent vertebrae is limited but overall range of movement is sometimes considerable. Segmental movements are complex and vary with location and gait.

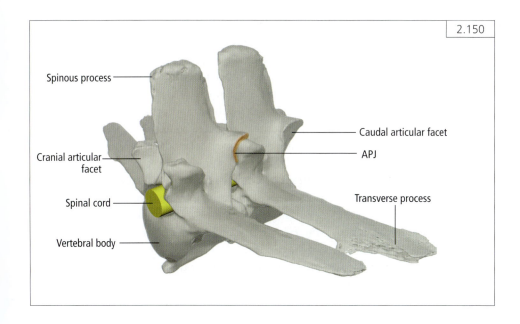

Fig. 2.150 Lumbar vertebral anatomy

Neck

There are seven vertebrae in the neck. The first two vertebrae are specialized in form: C1 (atlas) articulates with the skull and has broad wings that are palpable behind the poll; and C2 (axis) has a large dorsal spinous process that serves as an attachment point for the nuchal ligament. The nuchal ligament extends from the skull to the withers. Movement at the neck–skull articulation is primarily flexion/extension, while that at C1/C2 is rotation. Through the remainder of the neck lateral bending predominates. The muscles of the neck lie largely lateral and ventral to the spinal column and have a role in locomotion.

Back

The back is made up of 18 thoracic and six lumbar vertebrae, although individual variation in numbers of particular vertebrae occurs. The thoracic vertebrae have large dorsal spinous processes (most prominent in the withers: highest at T4–T6) and each articulates with a pair of ribs, while the lumbar vertebrae are notable for their relatively wide transverse processes. The dorsal spinous processes are oriented caudally through the thoracic spine to the 'anticlinal' vertebra (T16), beyond which they proceed to angle cranially. The spinal column continues into the fused sacrum, which by articulating with the pelvis at the SIJs links the trunk to the hindlimbs. The junction of the lumbar spine and sacrum is an important site for mobility of the back and comprises the lumbosacral joint (between L6 and S1) and the paired lumbar sacral facet and intertransverse joints.

The supraspinous ligament continues on from the nuchal ligament of the neck and attaches to the dorsal spinous summits to limit flexion of the back. The interspinous ligament joins the caudal aspect of a dorsal spine to the cranial margin of its neighbour. Epaxial muscles lying above and hypaxial muscles below the transverse processes facilitate lateral flexion and also provide dynamic stability to the back. The major epaxial muscle is the longissimus dorsi, with the multifidus muscles also playing a large role in stability. A thick thoracolumbar fascia serves as the origin of several muscles important to hindlimb impulsion and hip flexion.

The vertebral segments are each capable of dorsal flexion/extension, lateral bending and axial rotation to various degrees. Movement (dorsoventral) is greatest at the lumbosacral articulation, while lateral bending and axial rotation are greatest in the mid-back (around T11).

Examination

Examination of the neck includes observation of muscular symmetry and palpation to detect obvious deformation or guarding of the vertebral column. Lateral and dorsoventral flexibility are tested actively and passively for resentment or restriction of movement. Local skin reflexes and jugular vein patency are also assessed.

Examination of the back begins with an assessment of symmetry of the musculature, spine and pelvis. There is great variability between horses in their response to palpation/manipulation of the back and findings should be interpreted in the context of clinical presentation. Note should be made of asymmetry or atrophy of epaxial musculature as well as areas of visible tack contact. Palpation of epaxial muscles and dorsal spinous summits may permit localization of pain or muscular spasm/fasciculation. Stimulation of movement can also allow for assessment of flexion, extension and lateral bending in the thoracolumbar and lumbosacral regions. Generally, restricted motion may indicate skeletal pathology and hypermobility/aggression may indicate superficial muscle 'soreness' or simply skin sensitivity. Back pain typically results in reduced dynamic back flexibility and stride length due to guarding; assessment of gait in hand and ridden (to determine any influence of weight of rider) may be useful.

Cervical vertebral (neck) fracture

Fractures of the neck may involve the vertebral body or arch (most common in mid-neck region C3–C6) or the facet joints (most common in lower neck C5–C7) of the cervical vertebrae. The spinal cord is not always affected. Spinal cord involvement in the acute phase can be due to direct bone impingement or local haemorrhage/oedema. In some cases with no acute involvement of the spinal cord, subsequent encroachment of inflammatory pannus or bony callus during the healing phase may result in delayed onset of neurological signs.

Cause

- Usually the result of a traumatic incident such as rearing over, diving under the starting stalls, pulling back or fall at exercise.

Risk factors
- Any age/stage of training.

Signs
- Determined by configuration/location/severity of fracture and involvement of spinal cord.
- Range from mild neck stiffness to marked neurological deficits or recumbency.
- Neck may be held abnormally low +/− stiffness/guarding/swelling/patches of sweating.
- +/− ataxia: varies in severity and may be transient or persistent.
- Assessment of voluntary or passive ability to flex neck to each side (avoid if concern over unstable fracture) may reveal pain or restriction.

Diagnosis
- Radiography: laterolateral projection (**Figure 2.151**) most useful for displaced vertebral body fractures; oblique projections essential for full assessment of lateral processes/facet joints. Fracture line not always evident. Projections from left and right sides essential for comparison.
- CT useful for assessment/prognosis in some cases.

Management
- 'Treat the patient not the radiograph'.
- Fractures with severe or deteriorating neurological signs or recumbency: may warrant euthanasia (surgical stabilization has been reported but rarely practical or justifiable).
- Cases with no or few neurological signs: conservative management. Duration of stable rest dependent on clinical/radiological progress; typically 6–8 weeks.
- No return to ridden exercise while neurological signs persist.
- Anti-inflammatory medication in acute phase, although local swelling/muscle guarding limits movement and may be protective.
- +/− use of a cradle to splint the neck.
- Hay/feed/water provided at height to avoid lowering of neck; avoid tying up.

Prognosis
- Depends on initial clinical and radiological severity and any resulting neurological deficit caused by compression of spinal cord.
- Horses with no or minimal neurological signs: good prognosis for racing; return to ridden exercise usually possible within 3–6 months.

Dorsal spinous process impingement ('kissing spines')

Close apposition, impingement or overriding of dorsal spinous processes (DSPs) of thoracic or lumbar vertebrae is widely known as 'kissing spines'. May affect one or multiple sites: most commonly in saddle region (T13–18). Pathology may also involve interspinous ligaments and associated bone interface. Rarely clinically active or cause interruption to training but occasionally associated with back pain.

Cause
- May reflect a combination of factors including conformation, age and heritability.

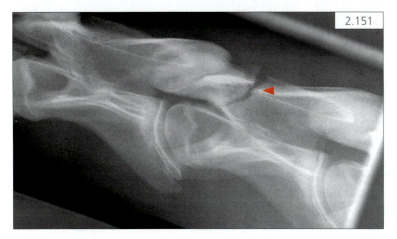

Fig. 2.151 Radiograph (laterolateral) of a cervical fracture. Note the fracture line (arrowhead) through the cranial articular process of C4.

Risk factors
- Most (60–90%) horses free from signs of back pain have kissing spines.
- Factors determining severity and significance of lesions are unknown.

History
- Frequently first detected during imaging of back (radiography/bone scan) as part of investigation into suspected orthopaedic injury; in these circumstances may be an incidental finding.
- When clinically active: may have history of being cold-backed, displaying poor action under tack, uncoupled canter, or lack of hindlimb impulsion.

Signs
- Clinical findings usually non-specific and cannot be readily distinguished from other forms of pelvic/thoracolumbar pain (or some hindlimb injuries).
- +/– palpable focal back pain or epaxial muscle spasm (non-specific).
- Not typically associated with lameness.

Diagnosis
- Clinical examination not definitive in isolation: requires radiographic/ultrasonographic imaging.
- Radiography: lateral projections of entire thoracolumbar region (placement of markers to assist future blocking/medication). Radiological severity ranges from narrowing of interspinal space +/– densification of adjacent bone margins (**Figure 2.152a**) to marked bony modelling/cystic change (**Figure 2.152b**).
- Determining significance is problematic: exclusion of other potential injuries +/– regional analgesia/medication of suspected sites.
- Ultrasonography: assessment of thoracolumbar articulations and supraspinous ligament.
- Bone scan: presence and intensity of radiomarker uptake at sites of DSP impingement is variable (**Figure 2.153**).
- Defining relevance of radiological/bone scan findings may require diagnostic local anaesthesia and/or trial medication.
- Genuine thoracolumbar back pain more likely with greater severity/extent of radiological signs of impingement, presence of concurrent arthritis of facet joints and/or increased bone scan activity.

Management
- Due to relatively short career and lack of necessity for racehorses to work in an outline, kissing spines rarely require significant input (unlike the situation in sport horses).
- Local infiltration of local anaesthetic/corticosteroid/pitcher plant extract on both sides of impingement sites can be used as presumptive treatment or diagnostic measure.
- Prolonged drug detection times may be experienced with deposition of corticosteroid in ligamentous tissue.

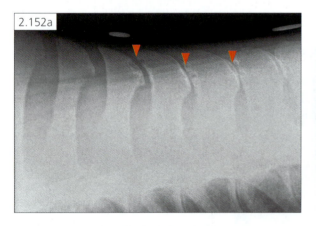
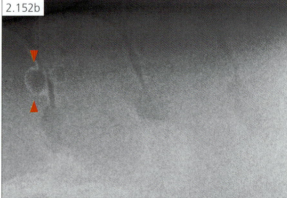

Figs. 2.152a, b Radiographs (laterolateral) of dorsal spinous process impingement. (a) Close apposition of thoracic DSPs. (b) Associated focal radiolucencies at interspinous ligament attachment (arrowheads).

- Physical therapies such as ESWT, manipulative/massage techniques and hot-packs may assist relief of muscle spasm.
- In rare cases of firm diagnosis plus poor response to above treatments plus continued interference with training: surgery can be considered. Surgical resection of the most affected spinous summits; return to ridden exercise generally after 3–6 months.

Prognosis
- Highly unusual for kissing spines to interfere with training.
- Response to medication frequently indicative of strength of initial diagnosis.
- Corticosteroid infiltration +/– physical therapies carry a fair prognosis for improvement in signs and continued training. Repeat medication usually necessary.
- Surgery: fair prognosis for return to full use.

Thoracolumbar vertebral stress injury

Stress injuries of the spinal column are common in the lower back of racehorses; however, most go undetected because of indistinct/mild clinical signs that generally do not interfere with training. The spectrum of injury includes arthropathy of the articulating process joints (APJs or 'facet joints') and stress fracture involving the vertebral bodies or articulations, with these generally considered clinically indistinguishable. It is common for several sites in the back to be involved. Stress fractures are often unilateral and involve the lumbar vertebrae (particularly at the lumbosacral junction) but are also found in mid- and caudal thoracic vertebrae. Modelling or fracture typically occurs at the cranial aspect of the vertebral lamina, between the cranial articular and dorsal spinous processes, with extension to the adjacent APJ also observed (**Figure 2.154**).

As with some other abnormalities of the back (see 'kissing spines'), it is likely that detection of arthritic facet joints is not always clinically significant and should be interpreted in the context of a full diagnostic workup.

Cause
- Stress/fatigue injury.
- Some degeneration of facet joints probably occurs with age/training but progression poorly understood.

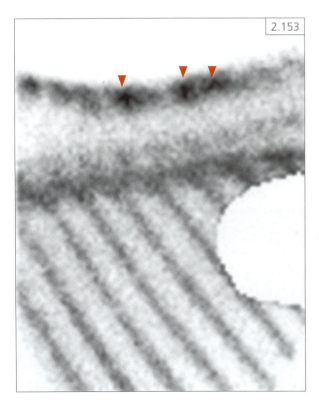

Fig. 2.153 Scintigram (dorsolateral) of dorsal spinous process impingement. Note the focal IRU (arrowheads).

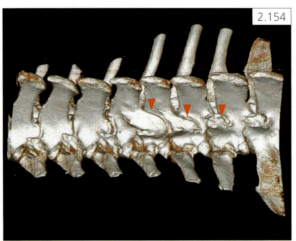

Fig. 2.154 Postmortem CT image (volume rendered) showing lumbar facet arthropathy. Note the long-standing articular modelling (arrowheads).

Risk factors
- Prevalence in racehorse population not known but appears to increase with age.
- Risk factors unknown but conformation, training and concurrent orthopaedic disease likely to play role in development.

History
- May present with history of suspected back pain, loss of action (shortened stride/tracking off line) or loss of performance.
- May be encountered when imaging the back in isolation or along with other abnormalities.
- May be subclinical.

Signs
- As with other potential sources of back pain, clinical findings not specific or definitive.
- When clinically active: may display back stiffness, restricted gait at walk/trot, tracking off line at trot, reduced thoracolumbar epaxial muscle bulk and focal muscle spasm.

Diagnosis
- Bone scan: focal IRU (mild to marked intensity depending on activity and soft-tissue attenuation) associated with one or more vertebral lamina/body/APJ (**Figure 2.155**).
- Ultrasonography (transcutaneous): modelling/enlargement of facet joints with loss of definition of the joint margins and variable amount of callus formation (**Figure 2.156**) depending on aetiology (stress injury or degenerative arthropathy). Mild 'rounding' of the joint contour may be only sign in the latter. Essential to compare left with right and with neighbouring joints.
- Radiography: frequently unrewarding due to superimposition of ribs and depth of tissues in lower back (high-quality radiographs required).

Management
- Dependent on severity of clinical/imaging findings.
- Suspected stress fracture (acute presentation): rest (stable rest/walking for 8–12 weeks) +/− anti-inflammatory medication.
- Facet joint arthropathy (mild signs/subclinical injury): continuation of training +/− ultrasound-guided intra-articular medication (corticosteroid) usually feasible, with awareness that any deterioration may warrant rest period.

Prognosis
- Stress fracture: good; usually settle with rest and recurrence rare.
- Facet joint arthropathy: guarded. Recurrence of clinical signs is common; may cause persistent poor performance.

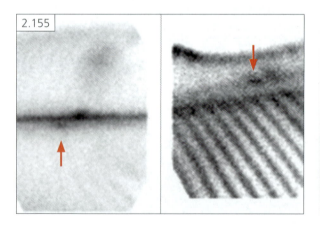

Fig. 2.155 Scintigrams (dorsal/dorsolateral) of lumbar facet arthropathy. Note the focal IRU associated with the articulating process joints (arrows).

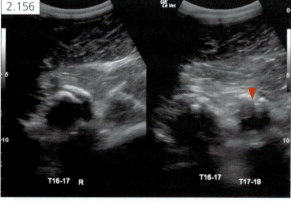

Fig. 2.156 Ultrasonograms (transcutaneous) of thoracic facet arthropathy. Note the (arrowhead) callus and enlargement of the articular facet.

Rib fracture

Rib fractures are an uncommon and sporadic cause of poor performance or lameness. Usually involves a single rib but can be multiple; fractures may be complete or incomplete. The 1st rib is most frequently affected, with injuries occurring at/near the costochondral junction or higher in the shaft. Fractures further back in the ribcage usually involve the mid-portion of the rib.

Cause
- Fractures involving the exposed mid- and caudal ribs of the trunk are usually attributed to direct trauma (e.g. following a fall), but can be stress injuries.
- 1st rib is well protected by muscles of upper forelimb/chest; the underlying mechanism of injury at this site is not known but likely to be repetitive (stress fracture) or acute overload (single incident at exercise) by muscular forces acting on the ribcage.

Risk factors
- Rare condition.
- Usually in horses in fast exercise/racing phase of training.
- Underlying risk factors poorly understood; gait characteristics or incidents at high speed (interference) may contribute.

History
- 1st rib fractures: typically present as insidious forelimb lameness that worsens over several days, but may be acute/severe in onset. May follow incident during fast exercise/racing.
- Mid- to caudal rib fractures: history of poor performance/poor action under tack/anxiety when girth tightened/reluctance to train. Delay between incident and onset of clinical signs may obscure exact origin of injury.

Signs
- 1st rib fractures: unilateral forelimb lameness of moderate severity, with abduction of limb and reduced cranial phase of gait at walk. Forced extension of limb may be resented. Frequently with guarding/spasm of muscles of shoulder girdle (especially triceps) on affected side. Neck lateroflexion may be resented/restricted.
- Mid- to caudal rib fractures: +/– localized pain on palpation but frequently without obvious sign of injury; bone callus occasionally palpable/visible.

Diagnosis
- Radiography: cranial ribs difficult to image but complete 1st rib fractures usually visible on mediolateral shoulder projection (**Figures 2.157a, b**).

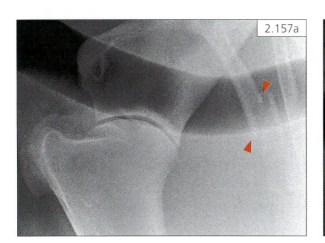
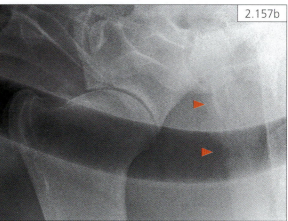

Figs. 2.157a, b Radiographs (ML) of a rib fracture. Acute stage (a) and 2-month follow-up (b) appearance of a complete fracture of the 1st rib (arrowheads), showing development of callus.

- Ultrasonography: useful to confirm fracture (discontinuity of bone margin) when palpable abnormality of mid- to caudal ribs is present.
- Bone scan: most useful imaging modality, although not all cases show increased activity in acute phase. IRU from cranial rib fractures may be masked by upper forelimb, and non-standard views required (**Figure 2.158**).

Management
- Conservative management: stable rest (4–8 weeks)/walking (4–6 weeks).
- Radiographic monitoring useful to guide management.

Prognosis
- Good prognosis for return to full use.
- Non-union and secondary nerve palsy may follow 1st rib fractures in people but have not been reported in horses.

Fractured withers
The prominence of the vertebral DSPs of the withers makes them susceptible to blunt injury. Fracture typically involves the dorsal third of several (≥3) adjacent DSPs but can be solitary; most commonly from T5–T7 (highest point of the withers). Complete fracture with marked displacement +/− vertical impaction of fracture fragments is typical. Rarely, open fractures may occur.

Cause
- Injury arises from direct trauma: fall/rearing over.

Risk factors
- Any age/stage of training.

History
- Invariably associated with recent history of falling/rearing over.
- Injury may not be immediately apparent.
- Stiffness of gait and/or resentment of saddle may prompt examination.

Signs
- Stiff/shuffling forelimb gait at walk.
- Withers usually flattened in profile with shoulder blades the highest point.
- Dorsal spinous summits may be palpably out of line or absent.
- 'Guarding' of withers, hypersensitivity of local skin and pain on palpation are characteristic (may resemble infection/abscess).

Diagnosis
- Clinical findings usually definitive.
- Radiography: (lateral projection) sometimes useful to determine severity (**Figure 2.159**). Fracture fragments should not be confused with separate centres of ossification associated with summits of T2–T7/8.

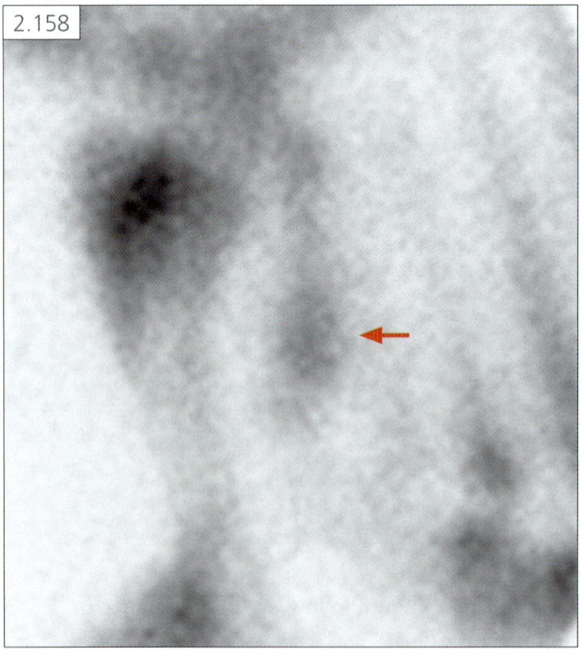

Fig. 2.158 Scintigram (lateral [ipsilateral limb protracted]) of a rib fracture. Note the IRU associated with the 1st rib (arrow).

Management
- Anti-inflammatory medication during acute phase.
- Conservative management: varies between individuals but 2–4 weeks stable rest/6–8 weeks walking is typical.
- Management guided by resolution of palpable pain/lameness.
- Open fractures treated with debridement and antibiotic therapy.

Prognosis
- Excellent prognosis for return to full racing function.
- Permanent flattening of withers can be expected; non-union/fibrous union of fractures is usual outcome.
- Resulting deformity/asymmetry of withers may necessitate use of fitted saddle (to minimize saddle rubs) in small proportion of cases.
- Once site has settled, has no impact on soundness or trainability.

Injection abscess/reaction
IM injections occasionally result in septic abscessation of affected side of neck. Non-septic inflammation can also occur (most commonly following vaccination) and is typically transient.

Risk factors
- Use of non-sterile medications or needle/syringe most common cause of infection.
- No apparent link with injection site disinfection.
- Some horses appear susceptible to vaccine-specific non-septic adverse reactions.

History
- Neck stiffness that develops in days following IM injection.

Signs
- Stiffness/thickening/hypersensitivity/guarding of neck.
- Reluctance to lower head to eat.
- +/− subcutaneous oedema at injection site.
- Infection: affected site in neck progressively larger/more painful over several days and may 'point' into abscess.

Diagnosis
- Ultrasonography: in the case of infection, IM fluid cavity develops over course of several days; measured depth useful to assist treatment.

Management
- Non-septic inflammatory (adverse drug) reaction: anti-inflammatory medication usually results in remission of signs in 1–2 days.
- Infection/abscessation: anti-inflammatory medication to manage clinical signs until abscess ready to lance; followed by open drainage or catheter lavage (sterile saline) plus systemic antibiotic medication.
- If infection suspected but little ultrasonographic evidence of fluid accumulation, systemic broad-spectrum antibiotic medication may be warranted in early stages to prevent abscess formation.

Prognosis
- Excellent prognosis but may interfere with training for short period.

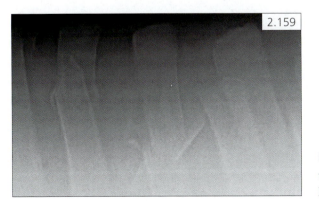

Fig. 2.159 Radiograph (LM) of fractured withers. Note the complete fracture of several thoracic DSPs with lateral displacement/comminution.

Poll injuries

Injuries to the poll are sustained by rearing over or throwing head up and catching doorway/ceiling. Most injuries are simple lacerations immediately behind the poll (nuchal crest). Full-thickness wounds may be deep and fragmentation of the nuchal crest may occur.

Tension/torsion/rotation injury due to pulling back from chain/tether may cause avulsion of the semispinalis capitis tendon +/− nuchal ligament injury. Less commonly, momentum of fall and hyperextension of neck may cause muscle avulsion injury to the base of the cranium (rectus capitis/longus capitis muscles). This is a more severe injury, with resulting guttural pouch/retropharyngeal haemorrhage, neurological signs and high mortality.

Cause
- Direct or dynamic trauma to poll region.

Risk factors
- Any age/stage of training.

Signs
- Simple poll wound: may resent examination. Small transverse laceration (**Figure 2.160**); anatomical dead space ensures wound usually deep. Reluctance to raise neck/head immediately after injury. Neurological signs not a feature. May develop head shyness due to local pain.
- Skull base fracture: profuse bilateral epistaxis +/− neurological deficits/collapse +/− respiratory distress.

Diagnosis
- Uncomplicated poll injuries require no diagnostic imaging.
- Soft-tissue injuries are readily detected by experienced ultrasonographer.
- Suspected skull base injuries: radiography (LM projection for detection of avulsion fragment) +/− endoscopy of guttural pouches. CT is imaging modality of choice but practical limitations for acutely ataxic horse.

Management
- Simple poll injuries: wound management (clip/lavage) +/− antibiotic/anti-inflammatory medication.
- Failure of poll wound to heal may indicate nuchal crest fragmentation/sequestrum: surgical removal or prolonged antibiotic medication.
- If neurological signs or suspected skull base fracture, hospitalization. Care with handling to minimize risk to personnel.

Prognosis
- Simple poll injuries: rarely interfere with training beyond acute phase (may preclude bridle use for several days).
- Skull base fractures: risk of mortality or serious neurological complications is high.

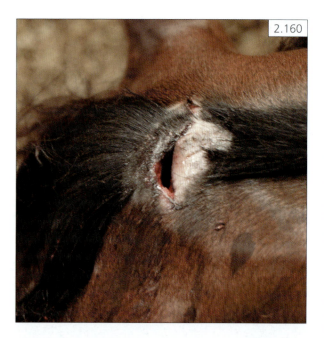

Fig. 2.160 Typical horizontal skin wound associated with direct trauma to the poll.

Saddle sores

Bruising, rubs or infection secondary to pressure from tack may occur at any site from the withers to the mid-back; usually found on midline, although sores may develop on either side of the withers.

Cause
- Peak pressures on back are greatest at back-of-saddle region when trotting and at withers during cantering and galloping.
- Treeless saddles tend to put pressure on mid-saddle region, while full-tree saddles impact further back.

Risk factors
- Poor fitting or unhygienic tack.
- New rider.
- Prominence/shape of topline may predispose to tack pressure.

Signs
- Focal dermatitis (**Figure 2.161a**)/subcutaneous bursa (seroma) +/− surrounding oedema in saddle region (**Figure 2.161b**).
- +/− pain on palpation.
- +/− open wound/broken skin/exudative dermatitis/subcutaneous abscess (**Figure 2.161c**).

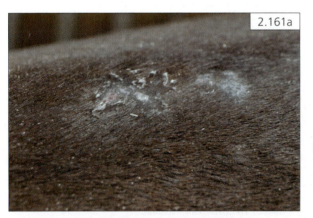
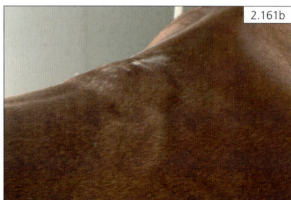
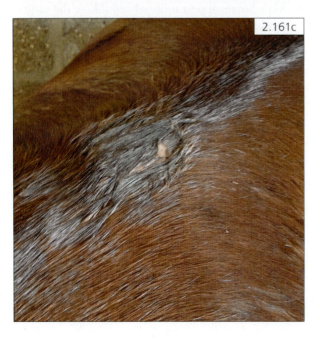

Figs. 2.161a–c Typical saddle sores. (a) Non-infected focal dermatitis; (b) seroma; (c) exudative dermatitis.

Diagnosis
- Clinical findings definitive.
- Non-infected bruising/seroma: relatively painless on palpation.
- Infection associated with presence of broken skin +/– intense pain +/– lymphatic 'runners'.

Management
- Management determined by severity/presence of infection.
- Infection/broken skin: topical +/– systemic antibiotic medication (typically 3–5 days).
- Bruised/inflamed without infection: topical emollient or anti-inflammatory ointment.
- Avoid further pressure at site from tack in short term; rest from ridden exercise may permit most rapid resolution.
- If rest not feasible, cut out hole in saddle pad over site.
- Focal seroma: consider intralesional corticosteroid.
- Muscular bruising: daily application of hot packs useful.

Prognosis
- Interference with training usually minimal (days).
- Recurrence uncommon, although some horses appear predisposed or may develop semi-permanent seroma.

OTHER MUSCULOSKELETAL CONDITIONS

Exertional rhabdomyolysis ('setfast'/'tying-up')
Episodic muscle disorder characterized by stiffness, muscle cramping and discomfort during or following exercise. Predominantly affects the hindlimbs but occasionally may involve muscles of the forelimb or flank.

Cause
- Underlying abnormality of muscle contraction/relaxation: disruption of normal calcium transport in muscle cell.
- Unrelated to raised lactic acid levels.
- Heritable component: autosomal dominant inheritance pattern, with variable expression.
- Affected genes appear to be those involved in energy regulation and calcium regulation of skeletal muscle.
- Possible that selective breeding for race performance has led to trait becoming commonplace.

Risk factors
- Common; affects approximately 5% of horses in training.
- Susceptibility to condition is inherited, but severity varies between individuals due to influence of other factors such as sex, temperament, exercise and diet.
- Fillies, 2 YOs and horses with nervous/excitable temperament at greater risk.
- Most episodes follow simple management errors that expose susceptible horses to a risk factor (e.g. oversupply of energy ration relative to expenditure/rapid step up in exercise/stress).
- Recurrently affected horses likely to be those with greater genetic expression of muscle abnormality and for whom the threshold for clinical disease is lower.
- No direct link with oestrus in fillies but possibly a factor in some individuals.
- Male horses appear more susceptible to the rarer forelimb expression of the condition.

History
- Episode occurs during/after training.
- Horse usually trains without incident but gait stiffens while walking in.
- Can follow training at any pace (walk/trot/canter/gallop).
- Typically occurs when exercise is being stepped up following a period of relative inactivity (i.e. start of week, or following rest period for lameness/illness/weather).
- Episodes during racing are rare: horse may shorten in final stages of race or develop stiffness post race.

Signs
- Typical presentation is restricted/stiff hindlimb gait (bilateral) at walk, but trot freely and without lameness.
- Tightness/cramping of gluteal +/− caudal thigh musculature a variable feature and not always obvious.
- Moderately/severely affected horses may sweat.
- May mimic colic (scraping floor/flank-watching); however, recumbency is rare and horses typically stand over pile of scraped-up bedding (rather than moving around stable).
- Rarely, may affect forelimb/s: restricted protraction of limb (sometimes profound) at walk, although lameness typically absent at trot. Mild–moderate lameness occasionally at both walk and trot, but not typical.

Diagnosis
- Clinical presentation usually definitive.
- Blood analysis: elevations of muscle-derived enzymes CK and AST confirm diagnosis, severity and timing of episode.
- CK: 'acute' enzyme and peaks at 4–6 hours after episode, dropping to normal levels by 3–4 days.
- AST: peaks later at 1–2 days, and takes longer to return to baseline level depending on severity of episode.
- CK higher than AST usually means episode occurred on day of sampling.
- Subclinical episodes occur and most likely to be associated with acute CK levels of 1,000–2,000 IU/l.
- Muscle biopsy of little practical use for either diagnosis or management.

Management: acute case
- Most episodes simply require management of acute pain: single dose of NSAID (+/− acepromazine if distressed).
- Severe episodes (rare) with recumbency: intensive support with IV isotonic fluids and diuretics to limit renal damage from myoglobinuria.
- Rest period following episode should be avoided in all but severe cases.
- No necessity to allow muscle enzyme levels to normalize before return to exercise: rest from ridden exercise simply prolongs risk period for further episodes.
- Resumption of normal training on day/s following episode aided by prophylactic use of skeletal muscle relaxant dantrolene sodium.
- Oral dantrolene sodium given 45 minutes to 4 hours pre-exercise (blood levels peak at approximately 4 hours): initial treatment 1.5–2 mg/kg; tapering (halving) of dose over subsequent days as normal exercise resumed.
- Episode of mild–moderate severity does not preclude racing in short term; horses may perform satisfactorily with muscle enzymes (CK and/or AST) above normal reference ranges.
- 'Fitness to race' best determined by clinical severity of episode rather than absolute blood levels.

Management: chronic case
- Avoidance of 'no exercise' days (affected horse should do some exercise every day of the week: level of exercise required determined on individual basis).
- Use of horsewalker exercise +/− daily turnout in addition to regular ridden work.
- May benefit from extended 'warm-up' (walk/trot) prior to regular exercise.
- Prophylactic use of dantrolene sodium for susceptible horses on 'high risk' days such as following period of relative inactivity.
- Maintenance on low-dose dantrolene sodium throughout training may be necessary for severely affected horses; successful maintenance level varies between individuals and determined by trial and error.
- +/− prophylactic use of low-dose acepromazine in excitable horses.
- Dietary management: partial replacement of carbohydrate with a high oil/fat diet may be beneficial, although wholesale replacement of starch in diet usually incompatible with maintenance of satisfactory body condition in full work.

- High-fat (15–20%) diet well tolerated and may act by reducing excitability.
- Assessment of diet to ensure adequate potassium intake: 1.5–2% BWT/day good-quality forage advisable.
- Little/no benefit of supplementation with sodium bicarbonate or vitamin E/selenium.

Prognosis
- Majority of cases easily managed with greater attention to feeding and exercise.
- Additional prophylactic use of dantrolene sodium +/− acepromazine permits training of more troublesome cases.
- Effect on racing performance thought to be minimal in most cases.
- Many fillies affected as 2 YO show reduced susceptibility later in career.
- Very small minority of affected horses fail to respond satisfactorily when managed as above and retirement considered if racing performance repeatedly affected.

Osteochondrosis (overview)

Osteochondrosis is a collective term for developmental defects of cartilage/subchondral bone: includes subchondral bone cysts ('OCLs') and OCD. The majority of subchondral bone cysts and OCD lesions found in the young racehorse are present from an early age. Defective differentiation of articular cartilage can lead to cartilage or cartilage/bone flaps (OCD), which may become detached, or cystic lesions in subchondral bone. Lesions can also develop following trauma to cartilage or subchondral bone. Osteochondrosis is a dynamic condition and particularly in the case of OCD, lesions may develop then heal early in life with little external sign of joint disease. Subchondral bone cysts typically remain visible radiologically long term, although size and appearance can also vary over time: progressive enlargement when it occurs is the result of inflammation within the cyst cavity. Lameness, if present, may result from synovitis or, in the case of subchondral bone cysts, increased intracystic or intra-osseous pressures.

Both OCD and subchondral bone cysts have certain predilection sites within joints, with cysts in particular often being found in association with high load-bearing joint surfaces. Predilection sites are:
- OCD: most common sites are in fetlock (sagittal ridge), hock (distal intermediate ridge and medial malleolus) and stifle (lateral trochlear ridge).
- Subchondral bone cyst: most common sites are stifle (medial femoral condyle) and carpus (ulnar carpal bone) but also encountered sporadically at many other sites including fetlock, pastern, foot, elbow, shoulder and other carpal bones.

Causes
- Multifactorial: nutritional and exercise factors can act in windows of susceptibility (foal/yearling) to cause development of focal areas of abnormal cartilage at predilection sites.
- Heritability: genetic component to OCD lesions but contribution unknown at present.

Risk factors
- Growth rate and body size: high-energy (not high-protein) diets, fast growth rates and nutritional imbalances of some trace elements are risk factors.
- Mechanical loading of joints: restricted exercise at early age increases risk of osteochondrosis (normal paddock exercise as foal important for appropriate cartilage development).

History
- Frequently first detected at routine yearling radiography.
- May be incidental finding or clinically active (joint effusion +/− lameness).

Signs
- Clinical findings vary widely with lesion type and location.
- Many lesions are subclinical.
- Generally considered that subchondral bone cysts beneath high load-bearing joint surfaces are more likely to display lameness.

Diagnosis
- Radiography: most OCD and subchondral bone cyst lesions are visible radiologically. Small lesions may not be obvious and secondary arthritic change or alternative imaging may be required for diagnosis.
- Ultrasonography: useful for detection of radiologically silent lesions in hock and stifle.
- MRI: useful if radiological findings are equivocal. Imaging modality of choice for detection and assessment of lesions in DIPJ and PIPJ.
- Bone scan: generally poor sensitivity. Of little use for most OCD lesions, and activity of subchondral bone cysts is highly variable.

Management
- Management dependent on lesion type, location, appearance and clinical relevance.
- Many lesions cause no/few problems in training.
- Goal is usually maintenance of acceptable degree of soundness (rather than improved radiological appearance of lesion).
- OCD: surgical debridement (if required) best undertaken at yearling stage for minimal interruption to training.
- Subchondral bone cysts: treatments aim to limit growth of lesion and promote healing of associated cartilage defect in order to improve integrity of joint surface. Intralesional medication (corticosteroid) or surgical debridement +/− bone or cell grafting are the usual treatment paths. Bisphosphonate therapy in developmental phase may have some merit, although efficacy not established.

Prognosis
- OCD: fetlock and hock lesions rarely interfere with training. Stifle/elbow/shoulder lesions: vary with location and appearance.
- Subchondral bone cysts: risk of developing lameness is generally low (regardless of location) but unquantifiable, and when clinically active may be career threatening. Aside from stifle lesions, little objective information available on prognosis for racing or likelihood of remaining sound in training.

Peritarsal/inguinal infection (lymphangitis)
Acute and painful lymphatic infection of hindlimb. Typically affects front of hock and/or inner thigh/groin region. Generally of unknown origin but presumed to seed from site in lower limb. Associated with acute severe lameness that can be mistaken for injury or synovial infection.

Cause
- Infection arises in lower leg, often from small/long-standing skin lesion.
- Spread of infection through lymphatic system, with localized inflammation commonly at front of hock or inner thigh/groin.
- Severity of pain/lameness in cases of peritarsal infection likely to be due to inflammation in anatomical region tightly constrained by retinaculae.

Risk factors
- Uncommon condition.
- Any age/stage of training.

History
- Acute onset and progression (hours).
- Usually found lame in stable; no association with exercise.

Signs
- Severe unilateral hindlimb lameness.
- Lameness improves with forced walking (not the case if orthopaedic injury or synovial sepsis are responsible).
- +/− mild fever in acute phase.
- Profound pain response to palpation of front of hock or groin: may cause marked flexion/abduction of leg.

- +/− raised lymphatic vessel or ridge/plaque of oedematous filling on inner thigh (**Figure 2.162**).
- +/− secondary effusion of tarsocrural joint: may resemble synovial infection.
- Typically no generalized filling of leg in acute phase but develops within 1–2 days.

Diagnosis
- Clinical findings usually definitive.
- Blood analysis: inflammatory response may permit differentiation from orthopaedic injury (but rarely needed).
- Differentiate from orthopaedic fracture and synovial sepsis (tibiotarsal joint): synoviocentesis usually best delayed for 1–2 days to determine efficacy of treatment/avoid inoculation of infection into joint.

Management
- Broad-spectrum antibiotic and anti-inflammatory medication.
- Forced exercise assists recovery and limits filling of leg.
- Level of exercise limited by lameness severity: twice daily walking/trotting in acute phase, return to cantering usually possible within 2–5 days.

Prognosis
- Excellent.
- Early diagnosis and prompt, aggressive management usually results in minimal interruption to training.
- Rarely (with delayed or inappropriate management): semi-permanent thickening of limb (disrupted lymphatic drainage) or extension of infection to associated splint bones/synovial structures (requires hospitalization).

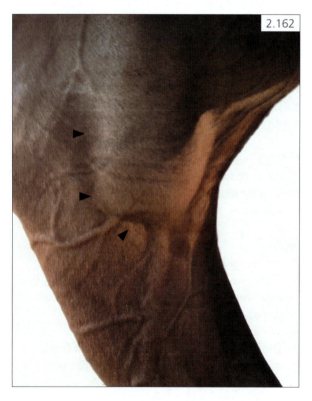

Fig. 2.162 Peritarsal/inguinal infection. Note the raised oedematous thickening on the medial aspect of the thigh (arrowheads).

Enostosis-like lesions ('bone islands')
Unusual condition in which focal proliferation of bone occurs within the medullary cavity of one or more long bones, with characteristic location in the vicinity of nutrient vessel foramen. Lesions occur most commonly in the cannon and tibia, and less frequently in other long bones including the radius, femur and humerus. Forelimbs and hindlimbs affected. Most cases have concurrent lesions in 1–3 bones. Lameness is a variable feature and in many cases the lesions are clinically silent.

Cause
- Cause unknown.
- Location of intramedullary lesions in close proximity to nutrient foramen suggests possible link with raised intramedullary pressure or vascular occlusion.

Risk factors
- Rare condition.
- Risk factors unknown.

History
- In many cases lesions are unrelated to lameness and detected as incidental finding during radiographic/scintigraphic screening.

- Lameness when present is often intermittent/transient and of unusual character; may occur at/after exercise and diminish within minutes/hours.

Signs
- Affected limb palpably normal.
- May be clinically silent.
- +/− unilateral and frequently inconsistent lameness of moderate severity.

Diagnosis
- Diagnostic blocking: if located in cannon, blocking pattern may be similar to that for suspensory ligament desmopathy (p. 98).
- Radiography: characteristic focal smooth-margined endosteal radiopacity in mid-diaphysis, generally opposite/adjacent nutrient foramen (**Figure 2.163**). Multiple lesions common. Radiological definition more difficult for lesions in proximal limb (humerus/femur).
- Bone scan: focal IRU at lesion site (**Figure 2.164**); may sometimes resemble stress fracture.

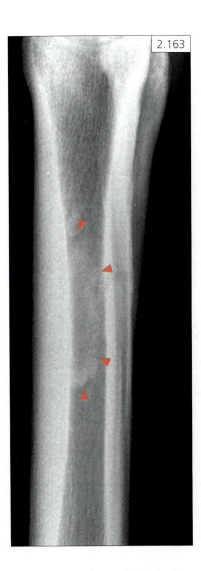

Fig. 2.163 Radiograph (LM) of an enostosis-like lesion. Note the medullary/endocortical radiopacity (arrowheads) opposite the nutrient foramen in the mid-shaft of the metacarpus.

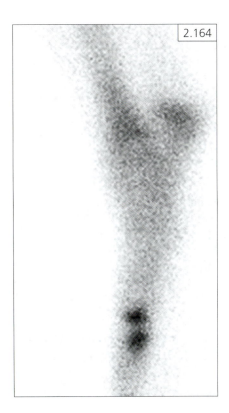

Fig. 2.164 Scintigram (lateral) of an enostosis-like lesion. Note the intense IRU.

Management
- Clinically silent lesions: no treatment necessary.
- Clinically active lesions: lameness generally resolves with rest (removal from ridden exercise for 6–8 weeks). Anecdotal support for bisphosphonate (tiludronate) therapy in clinical cases; return to training dependent on abolition of lameness but typically 1–3 weeks.

Prognosis
- Excellent prognosis for return to full use.
- Radiological/bone scan appearance returns to normal with time/rest.
- Recurrence is rare.

Haematoma
Haematomas usually develop at the back of the thigh and are presumed to arise from tearing of a muscle belly or its fascial lining. Subsequent fluid accumulation forms a subcutaneous pouch; severity varies between individuals.

Cause
- Cause rarely determined.
- Most frequently arises from exercise or following a slip or fall.
- Less commonly: direct trauma (kick) to pectoral muscles of chest.

Risk factors
- Uncommon condition.
- Any age/stage of training.

History
- Acute onset, although may enlarge over initial few days.

Signs
- Unilateral fluid-filled, fluctuant swelling typically at back or side of thigh (**Figure 2.165**).
- Size variable but frequently large.
- Generally no lameness.
- Usually painless to palpate (mild inflammation of haematoma edges in acute phase).

Diagnosis
- Clinical findings definitive.

Management
- Reduced exercise level (removal from cantering) for initial few days recommended to minimize final extent of swelling.
- Moderate–large haematomas: may be lanced. Small (2–5 cm) vertical incision at lowest extent of swelling; wound management over subsequent 1–2 weeks to facilitate drainage +/– local or systemic antibiotic medication. No rest required.

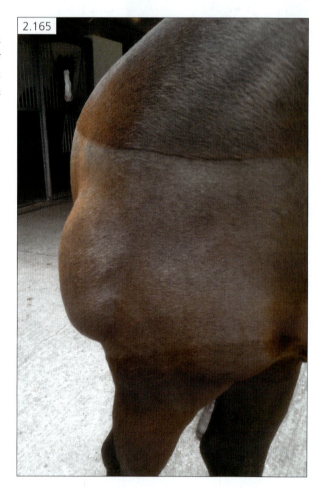

Fig. 2.165 Typical haematoma; note the fluctuant swelling over the caudal thigh.

Prognosis
- Excellent.
- Any interruption to training is usually brief.
- Heals with minimal cosmetic blemish.

Idiopathic recurrent haemarthrosis
Rare condition characterized by recurrent joint filling and lameness secondary to articular haemorrhage. Antebrachiocarpal and tibiotarsal joints are most commonly affected.

Cause
- Unknown.

Risk factors
- Rare condition.
- All ages/stages of training but more frequent in horses in fast exercise.
- Risk factors unknown.

History
- Acute initial onset.
- Intermittent recurrence despite rest/medication.

Signs
- Moderate–marked unilateral joint effusion.
- +/– restricted or painful flexion of affected joint.
- Lameness usually a feature but severity varies.

Diagnosis
- Typically a diagnosis of elimination of other (more common) pathology.
- Frank haemorrhage within joint revealed by synoviocentesis.
- Radiography/scintigraphy/MRI should be undertaken to rule out presence of fracture or osteochondral injury.

Management
- Marked improvement in joint filling/lameness usually results following initial synoviocentesis and systemic anti-inflammatory medication.
- Short rest +/– intra-articular medication (corticosteroid) usually undertaken initially.
- Recurrent cases: surgery (diagnostic arthroscopy) in attempt to determine underlying lesion and permit synovectomy, followed by prolonged rehabilitation (2–6 months out of ridden exercise).

Prognosis
- Guarded prognosis for return to full use.
- Unpredictable course of condition; recurrence is common (approximately 50% of cases).
- Retirement may be necessary in severely affected individuals that are non-responsive to treatment.

Part 2
OTHER BODY SYSTEMS

CHAPTER **3** Respiratory conditions

CHAPTER **4** Cardiovascular conditions

CHAPTER **5** The head

CHAPTER **6** Gastrointestinal conditions

CHAPTER **7** Urogenital conditions

CHAPTER **8** Neurological conditions

CHAPTER **9** Skin conditions

CHAPTER **10** Miscellaneous conditions

CHAPTER **11** Infectious diseases

CHAPTER 3
RESPIRATORY CONDITIONS

UPPER AIRWAY OBSTRUCTIONS

Applied anatomy
Nasal passages
The nostrils are large, mobile and dilated by muscular action during exercise. The left and right nasal passages are separated by the nasal septum and partitioned further on each side by scrolls of thin bone lined by vascular mucosa (dorsal and ventral nasal conchae). The air passages around these conchae communicate and converge in the pharynx. The lowermost passage (ventral nasal meatus) is the largest and the one commonly used during routine endoscopy and nasogastric intubation.

Larynx
The larynx (**Figure 3.1**) is made up of several cartilages (epiglottis, cricoid, thyroid and paired arytenoids) linked by joints and moved by intrinsic and extrinsic muscles. It functions to both protect the airway from aspiration

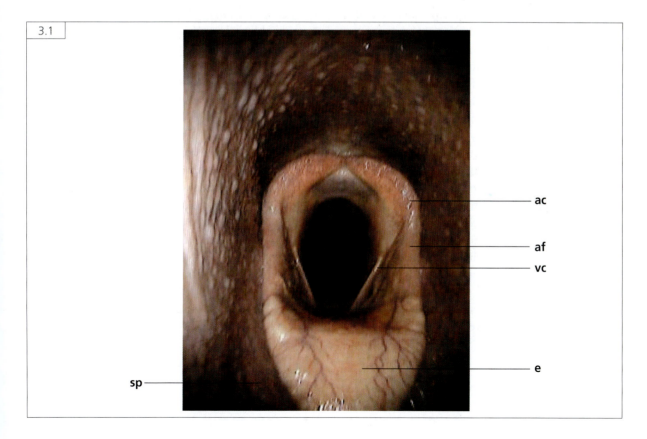

Fig. 3.1 Endoscopic view of the nasopharynx/larynx: epiglottis (e); left arytenoid cartilage (ac); left vocal cord (vc); left aryepiglottic fold (af); soft palate (sp).

of food during swallowing and facilitate unobstructed passage of air into the trachea and lungs during breathing. The key muscle relevant to laryngeal function during exercise is the cricoarytenoideus dorsalis (CAD) muscle, which opens (abducts) the arytenoid cartilages and is the major dilating muscle of the laryngeal opening. The epiglottis is a prominent triangular-shaped cartilage. Size and relative stiffness/flaccidity can vary between individuals. Its only muscular attachment is the hypoepiglotticus, which serves to tense the epiglottis down onto the soft palate. On each side of the epiglottis, a fold of mucosa confluent with the corniculate process of the arytenoid cartilage forms the aryepiglottic fold. Within the opening of the larynx, connecting the arytenoids to the thyroid cartilage, are the vocal folds, which border blind-ended lateral ventricles.

Pharynx

Between the rigid nasal passages and the semi-rigid trachea, the airway traverses the muscular tube of the pharynx. The pharynx is the intersection between the respiratory and digestive tracts and must perform diverse functions. To accommodate swallowing it must constrict in order for the food bolus to move back towards the oesophagus, yet to permit free flow of air during exercise it must remain dilated in the face of the strongly negative pressures of inspiration.

During exercise the soft palate (which separates the oral from the nasal portions of the pharynx) must remain anchored below the epiglottis and the larynx be firmly seated in the airtight 'buttonhole' of the pharyngeal ostium, otherwise respiratory obstruction will ensue. Correct soft palate and pharyngeal function is dependent on many factors including the relative position of the larynx and hyoid apparatus and coordinated action of the intrinsic and extrinsic muscles. Hyoid apparatus movements are determined by contributions of the tongue muscles as well as the strap muscles of the neck (sternohyoideus and sternothyroideus), while tensing of the soft palate itself is the function of the intrinsic palatal muscles (levator veli palatini, tensor veli palatini, palatinus and palatopharyngeus).

Guttural pouches

The paired guttural pouches are located between the pharynx and the base of the skull and are accessed through a slit-like opening on each side of the pharynx. The pouches contact each other on the midline but do not communicate. Each pouch is partially divided into a large medial and smaller lateral compartment by the stylohyoid bone. Important neurovascular structures traverse the inside of each pouch including the internal and external carotid arteries and several cranial nerves; the function of the guttural pouch is uncertain but one role is likely to be thermoregulation of the cranial vasculature.

Overview

Oxygen utilization by the racehorse during exercise is considerable and respiratory function is one of the key limiting factors to performance. Energy is expended in overcoming airway resistance, and even small obstructions have a disproportionately large impact on resistance and the work of breathing. The majority of airway resistance in the normal horse derives from the upper airway (nostrils, nasal passages and throat).

The horse is anatomically and functionally adapted to breathing solely through the nostrils whether at rest or during exercise. Major swings in intraluminal pressure of the airways occur between expiration and inspiration to facilitate movement of large volumes of air between nostril and lung. At strenuous exercise (and peak airflow) the negative pressures of inspiration have the potential to cause airway collapse. While this has little effect on the rigid/semi-rigid parts of the respiratory tract (nasal passages and trachea), the nostrils, pharynx and larynx must rely on muscular activity to remain dilated and have the greatest potential to weaken and impede airflow.

It is failure to maintain full function in the face of peak physiological demand (rather than structural abnormality) that characterizes the most important upper airway obstructions of racehorses. The manifestations of neuromuscular disorders, such as recurrent laryngeal neuropathy (RLN) and palatal displacement, vary considerably between rest and high-intensity exercise and this has ramifications for both diagnosis and treatment. Dynamic airway collapse is also frequently complex in nature, with more than one anatomical structure involved at different stages of exercise.

The relative significance of any upper airway obstruction to athletic performance differs between horses and interpretation of findings may be influenced by age, racing form and stage of career, as well as the severity of the condition. It is preferable that treatment decisions take into account individual circumstances rather than being prescriptive, and they should be based on appropriate diagnostic information.

Assessment of upper airway function

Upper airway assessment is performed during the investigation of respiratory noise or poor performance and during pre-purchase examinations. Traditionally, assessment has been based on the presence and character of respiratory noise at exercise ('wind testing') and resting endoscopy. While these modalities continue to have roles, direct visualization of upper airway function during exercise (overground/treadmill endoscopy), supplemented by ultrasonography, is now the method of choice due to the dynamic nature of many conditions.

Respiratory noise

Respiratory noise at exercise may be the first sign of impaired airway function and although not diagnostic in isolation, it may be used to guide further investigations. Inspiratory noise in particular implies dynamic airway obstruction. Noises may vary in character depending on pathology, exercise intensity and whether exercised on a lunge or in straight lines. Relevant history that assists interpretation includes:

- Whether noise is reported by trainer or jockey/rider.
- Length of time that noise has been noted.
- Intensity of exercise (training canter/training gallop/race) and point during exercise (throughout/under pressure/pulling up) at which horse usually makes noise.
- Previous use (and effect) of headgear such as a crossed noseband or tongue-tie.

Wind testing should be arranged to occur under conditions in which the horse is most likely to make any reported noise. Abnormal noises are categorized as inspiratory, expiratory or pan-respiratory; at a canter/gallop, exhalation begins when the leading leg hits the ground. Inspiratory 'whistle' or 'roar' is suggestive of RLN and expiratory 'gargle' of palatal displacement, but respiratory noise is not perfectly condition-specific. 'High blowing' expiratory noise is common and usually due to vibration of the alar fold (nostril).

Resting endoscopy

Resting endoscopy allows assessment of upper airway anatomy and resting laryngeal function. Sedative drugs may negatively influence laryngeal movements and should be avoided; if a nose twitch is used for restraint while passing the endoscope, it should be released for assessment of the throat.

The pharynx and larynx are examined for anatomical flaws and evidence of previous surgery. Laryngeal function is assessed through observation of natural movements of the laryngeal cartilages and by provoking opening (abduction) of the arytenoid cartilages by swallowing and/or blocking of nostrils (**Figures 3.2a–c**). Laryngeal function is graded according to symmetry at rest, synchrony of movement and ability to achieve/maintain full symmetric abduction (*Table 3.1*) (**Figures 3.3, 3.4**). Asynchronous movement of the arytenoid cartilages may include tremor, hesitation or flutter.

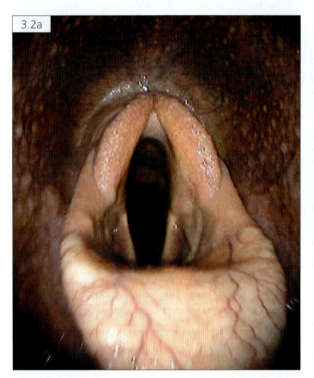

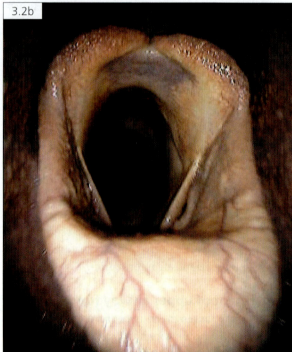

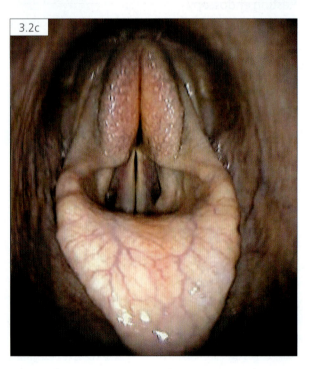

Figs. 3.2a–c Normal laryngeal function: (a) at rest, (b) full abduction of arytenoid cartilages, (c) full adduction/closure (during swallowing).

Respiratory Conditions

Table 3.1 Endoscopic grading of resting laryngeal function

	HAVEMEYER	LANE
Resting symmetry and full arytenoid abduction can be achieved and maintained; all movements (adductory and abductory) synchronized	1	1
Full arytenoid abduction can be achieved and maintained with some asymmetry/asynchrony at times:	2	2
(1) Transient asynchrony	(2.1)	
(2) Asymmetry much of time at rest but occasions (swallowing/nasal occlusion) when full symmetrical abduction is achieved and maintained	(2.2)	3
Full abduction can be achieved but not maintained; asymmetry/asynchrony of cartilage movements much of time	3.1	
Full abduction cannot be achieved; obvious resting asymmetry	3.2	4
Full abduction cannot be achieved; marked resting asymmetry with little arytenoid movement	3.3	
Complete immobility/paralysis of arytenoid cartilage	4	5

Adapted from Dixon PM, Robinson NE, Wade JF (2003) (eds) Proceedings of a Workshop on Equine Recurrent Laryngeal Neuropathy, Havemeyer Foundation Monograph Series No. 11. R&W Publications, Newmarket.

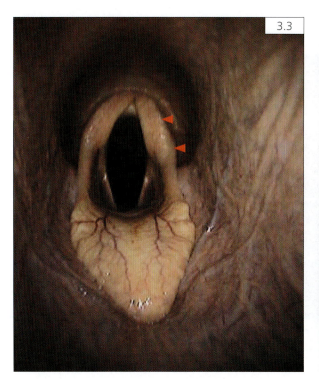

Fig. 3.3 Recurrent laryngeal neuropathy (resting): moderate resting asymmetry with left arytenoid cartilage (arrowheads) closer to midline.

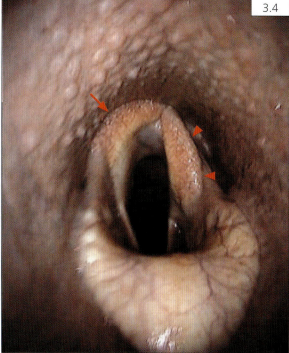

Fig. 3.4 Recurrent laryngeal neuropathy (resting): complete left-sided paralysis with left arytenoid cartilage slumped to midline (arrowheads) while right arytenoid cartilage (arrow) fully abducted on nasal occlusion.

Intermittent dorsal displacement of the soft palate (DDSP) during resting endoscopy is commonplace and is not an indicator of palatal function at exercise.

Overground and treadmill endoscopy

Overground or treadmill endoscopy permits a more complete assessment of airway function than resting endoscopy and is necessary for diagnosis of dynamic conditions (*Table 3.2*). Exercise tests should replicate as close as is practicable the circumstances in which it is suspected that the obstruction occurs: testing over shorter distances or slower speeds may not elicit the dysfunction. At submaximal exercise, head carriage (poll flexion) can worsen dynamic respiratory obstructions

Table 3.2 Endoscopic grading of laryngeal function at exercise

A	Full abduction of arytenoid cartilages during inspiration (**Figure 3.5a**)
B	Partial abduction of affected arytenoid cartilages (between full abduction and the resting position) (**Figure 3.5b**)
C	Abduction less than resting position including collapse into the contralateral half of the rima glottidis during inspiration (**Figure 3.5c**)

Adapted from Rakestraw PC, Hackett RP, Ducharme NG *et al.* (1991) Arytenoid cartilage movement in resting and exercising horses. Vet Surg **20(2)**:122–127.

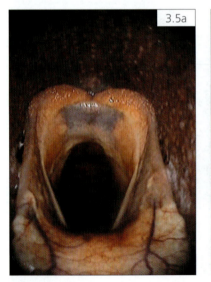 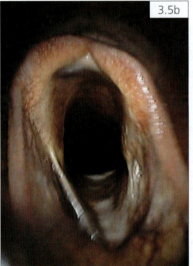 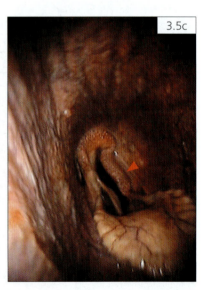

Figs. 3.5a–c Laryngeal function at exercise: (a) grade A, (b) grade B, (c) grade C: collapse of left arytenoid (arrowhead) at exercise, with concurrent right vocal and aryepiglottic fold collapse resulting in a markedly occluded airway.

by raising airway pressures and provoking laryngeal or pharyngeal collapse. Concurrent information on speed and heart rate may assist in interpretation of findings.

Ultrasonography

Transcutaneous ultrasonography permits imaging of some intrinsic muscles important to laryngeal function. Neurogenic atrophy results in increased echogenicity of the cricoarytenoideus lateralis/CAD/vocalis muscles (**Figure 3.6**) and, combined with assessment of left–right symmetry, provides objective information on the presence of pathological change. Sensitivity and specificity for RLN is high and is a useful supplementary technique to resting endoscopy.

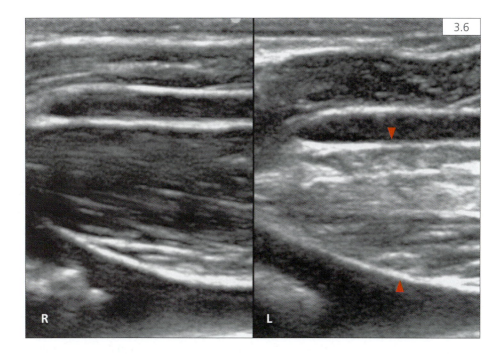

Fig. 3.6 Ultrasonographic images of right (R) and left (L) sides of the larynx with relative hyperechogenicity of the left-sided cricoarytenoideus lateralis intrinsic muscles (arrowheads).

Recurrent laryngeal neuropathy ('roaring'/laryngeal hemiplegia)

RLN is an important cause of dynamic respiratory obstruction. The arytenoid cartilages of the larynx are highly mobile and during exercise are normally maintained fully open by the action of intrinsic muscles. Neuromuscular dysfunction can lead to failure to achieve/maintain full abduction, particularly in the presence of negative pressures acting during inspiration at exercise. Collapse of the cartilage and/or associated vocal cord into the airway during breathing is responsible for the characteristic inspiratory noise (whistle/roar) and has the potential to affect performance. Most commonly left-sided; right-sided weakness is rare. Range of severity encountered ranges from mild to complete paralysis and the condition is frequently progressive, although the rate of deterioration is highly variable.

Cause
- Disease of the recurrent laryngeal nerves, which innervate important paired intrinsic muscles of the larynx.
- Progressive 'dieback' of affected nerves causes first loss of adductor, then abductor function: wastage of CAD muscle is of greatest importance.
- Cause/s uncertain; however, length (longest motor nerve in body) and complicated path of left nerve may be implicated.
- Nerve lies close to jugular vein; some cases may arise secondary to perivascular injection of irritant drugs.

Risk factors
- Approximately 2–3% of yearlings and 3–4% of horses in training have true left-sided laryngeal paralysis detectable with resting endoscopy; prevalence of dynamic collapse in these populations is not known.
- May be encountered at any age/stage of training.
- More common in colts than fillies.
- Large/tall horses at greater risk.
- Genetic factors: relatively low heritability, although some bloodlines appear to be particularly affected. Mode of inheritance is complex and multiple genes probably responsible.

History
- May be an incidental finding at routine or pre-purchase endoscopy.
- Characteristic inspiratory noise (whistle/roar) may be heard during cantering/galloping.
- +/– poor performance.

Diagnosis
- Resting +/or overground/treadmill endoscopy to visualize range of laryngeal movements.
- Resting endoscopy: practical screening aid but provides only an approximation of likely function at exercise (*Table 3.1*).
- Overground/treadmill endoscopy: assessment of dynamic function (*Table 3.2*).
- Sedative drugs (acepromazine/detomidine/xylazine) can cause or exacerbate resting laryngeal weakness. Tends to affect left side only: not known whether this feature is predictive for future RLN in some individuals. Assessment of laryngeal function should be postponed 24 hours if sedation has been administered.
- Palpation of larynx: may reveal prominence of muscular process of left arytenoid cartilage (due to loss of overlying muscle) with advanced disease.
- Laryngeal ultrasound: high sensitivity and specificity for RLN and useful adjunct to endoscopy in 'borderline' cases.

Relationship between resting and exercising function
- Only moderate correlation between resting and exercising function.
- Most horses that fail to achieve full abduction at rest (nasal occlusion/swallowing: Havemeyer G3.2/Lane G4) display dynamic collapse at exercise.
- Most horses with good (symmetric) resting grades show good function at exercise.
- Exceptions to both rules occur: small proportion (3–7%) of resting G1 and G2 throats display dynamic collapse at exercise, and some Havemeyer G3.2/Lane G4 throats achieve full abduction at exercise.
- Horses with some asymmetry but adequate resting function (Havemeyer G2.2/Lane G3) can be considered 'normal' but are more likely to

display dynamic collapse at exercise than 'better' (Havemeter G2/Lane G2) graded throats.

Effect on performance
- Dynamic laryngeal function is only one factor influencing athletic potential.
- Just under 20% of yearlings have moderate resting asymmetry and some asynchrony of movement but are capable of full abduction (Havemeyer G2.2/3.1; Lane G3).
- Horses with weak resting grades (Havemeyer >G3.1/Lane G4) are less likely to be successful athletes.
- Deterioration in resting laryngeal function can occur over time: speed and degree of progression cannot be predicted and may affect all grades.

Management
Treatment decisions should be based on appropriate assessment of laryngeal function (preferably overground endoscopy/ultrasonography). Surgical procedures are directed at reducing inspiratory noise and/or preventing dynamic laryngeal collapse. Age, stage of career, severity of laryngeal dysfunction and race form determine choice of procedure. Surgical options include:
- Ventriculectomy ('Hobday'): ablation of lining of ventricle/s; reduces severity of vocal fold collapse and respiratory noise. For milder cases. Typically 3–4 weeks rest.
- Ventriculocordectomy: ablation of ventricle and vocal cord (usually unilateral) (**Figure 3.7**); considered more effective than ventriculectomy but in common with it does little to restore overall airway function and is reserved for milder cases. Typically 3–4 weeks rest.
- Prosthetic laryngoplasty ('tie-back'): placement of sutures to 'pin back' left arytenoid cartilage and emulate action of CAD muscle (**Figure 3.8**); goal is to stabilize arytenoid cartilage and prevent dynamic collapse (rather than 'opening up'). For moderately severe cases. Commonly combined with ventriculocordectomy. Restores upper airway

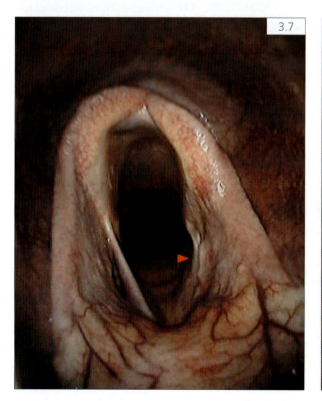

Fig. 3.7 Prior ventriculocordectomy: absence of left vocal cord (arrowhead).

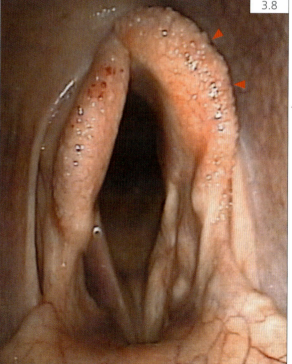

Fig. 3.8 Prior prosthetic laryngoplasty ('tie-back'): full abduction of left arytenoid cartilage (arrowheads) with right arytenoid cartilage at rest.

function, but not invariably successful due to implant failure and dynamic collapse of other structures. Treated horses are more prone to coughing (food inhalation), inflammatory airway disease and significant exercise-induced pulmonary haemorrhage (EIPH) (p. 229), including epistaxis, through remainder of career. Typically 6 weeks stable rest post surgery.
- Partial arytenoidectomy: removes some of the respiratory obstruction but return to function not equal to tie-back. Similar risk of food inhalation to tie-back. Typically 6 weeks rest.
- Laryngeal reinnervation: rarely performed due to duration of time required for healing (up to 12 months).
- Semi-permanent tracheostomy: surgical insertion of tube into windpipe bypasses throat altogether. Daily wound management required but generally good outcome. Use dependent on regulatory approval.

Prognosis
- Disease is chronic and generally progressive; however, deterioration is not always linear or predictable.
- Up to 15% of horses show deterioration in laryngeal function over time; it is also possible to encounter horses that 'improve' in resting grade.
- Efficacy of surgery in restoring/improving athletic potential in any individual is difficult to quantify.

Palatal displacement/instability
During exercise the soft palate and palatopharyngeal arch form an airtight seal around the larynx. Displacement of the caudal free border of the soft palate from its regular position below the epiglottis (**Figure 3.9**) occurs during swallowing of food, but if it takes place during exercise this seal is disrupted, creating an obstruction to airflow. A loud expiratory noise ('gargling'/'choking') typically results and may be accompanied by immediate interruption of athletic effort as the horse breaks stride. Displacement is transient but variable in duration between episodes, sometimes returning to normal position within the same stride and at other times lasting until cessation of exercise.

DDSP is an intermittent and unpredictable condition with considerable variation in severity both between individuals and over time. Episodes most commonly occur during peak exertion; it may also be precipitated by neck flexion on pulling up at the end of exercise. Palatal instability (PI) ('billowing' of caudal or rostral parts of the soft palate) is considered part of the syndrome and often precedes DDSP at exercise (**Figures 3.10a, b**).

Cause
- Multifactorial neuromuscular dysfunction.
- Failure of coordinated control of intrinsic and extrinsic musculature to maintain palatal tension and counteract negative pressures of inspiration.
- Structures potentially involved: extrinsic muscles controlling positioning of tongue/hyoid apparatus; intrinsic 'tensing' muscles of soft palate; pharyngeal branch of vagus nerve, hypoglossal nerve.

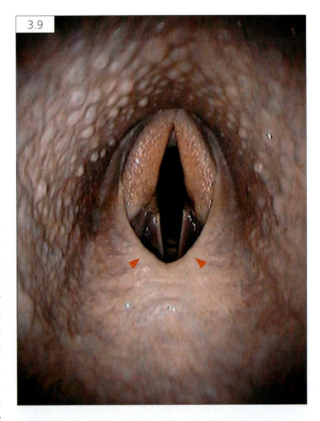

Fig. 3.9 Dorsal displacement of soft palate; free margin of palate (arrowheads) temporarily dislocated above the epiglottis.

- Potential role of respiratory inflammation/infection (particularly in young horses) due to close proximity of neural structures to lymphoid tissue in retropharyngeal region.

Risk factors
- Prevalence unknown but is the most common dynamic respiratory obstruction encountered in racehorses.
- Any age/stage of training but may be more common in 2 YOs.
- Risk factors poorly understood.
- Unlikely to be heritable.
- Role of epiglottis size/function uncertain.

History
- 'Performance limiting' DDSP: typical history of sudden cessation of athletic effort during race/gallop in association with loud/expiratory ('gargling') noise.
- Up to 30% of affected horses do not make a noise: in these cases poor performance may be primary presenting complaint.

Diagnosis
- Overground/treadmill endoscopy is sole means of definitive diagnosis.
- Exercise test conditions should replicate as closely as possible those in which horse usually displays problem (typically at fast gallop).
- Resting endoscopy not useful in diagnosis of DDSP/PI; palatal displacement occurs during most resting examinations and is not predictive for future development of palatal problems.
- If overground/treadmill endoscopy unavailable, abolition of respiratory noise by application of tongue-tie or Cornell collar may be indicative (but not diagnostic).

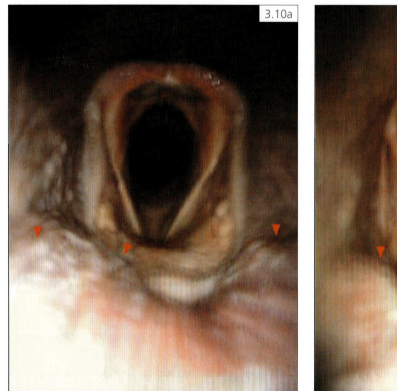
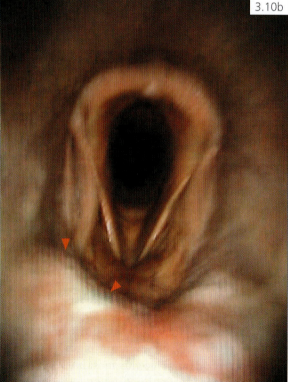

Figs. 3.10a, b Palatal instability: billowing (arrowheads) of rostral soft palate at exercise.

Management
- 2 YOs: many cases of suspected DDSP resolve with maturity/improved fitness; investigation/treatment best reserved for horses displaying exercise intolerance.
- Recommended that conservative measures are tried initially: tongue-tie (anchors tongue to mandible, moving larynx and hyoid apparatus forward); crossed noseband (prevents opening of mouth); Cornell collar (positions larynx in similar fashion to laryngeal tie-forward surgery, see below); spoon bit (may stabilize tongue).
- Surgical intervention if conservative measures unsuccessful.
- Multiple surgical procedures available: lack of scientific consensus on the most appropriate surgical technique and likely that no current procedure is particularly efficacious.
- Surgical options include one (or combination of several) of the following:
  - Laryngeal tie-forward: suture placed to emulate function of thyrohyoid muscle; positions larynx further forward and higher in throat. 3–4 weeks rest from ridden exercise post surgery.
  - Thermocautery: firing of nasal or oral surfaces of soft palate often in combination with other surgical procedures: induces scarring/stiffening of palate.
  - Tension palatoplasty: surgical procedures intended to 'tighten' the mid and caudal soft palate.
  - Myectomy/tenectomy: removal or cutting of insertional tendon/s of strap muscles of neck; thought to limit caudal retraction of larynx.
  - Staphylectomy: resection of the free border of palate.

Prognosis
- 50% of affected horses respond favourably to conservative measures such as use of tongue-tie.
- Reported improvements in performance with current surgical techniques occur in approximately 50–70% of horses; however, true efficacy undetermined (until recently most horses treated without definitive diagnosis/overground endoscopy).
- Currently considered that most appropriate surgical procedure for horses that respond favourably to a Cornell collar is the laryngeal 'tie-forward'.
- Small proportion of affected horses cannot be managed successfully and are retired.

Axial deviation of the aryepiglottic fold/s (ADAF)
Dynamic collapse of the aryepiglottic folds can occur during exercise and may be associated with an inspiratory noise. Intermittent and sometimes transient condition. Usually bilateral, but may be unilateral. Severity of respiratory obstruction varies. Can occur in isolation, or in combination with other upper respiratory tract conditions such as PI, DDSP and RLN. There does not appear to be a causal relationship with these conditions; however, the greater the severity of ADAF the more likely it is that other upper airway problems will be present.

Cause
- Cause unknown.
- No muscular tissue in fold so may represent stretching of tissue or altered position/function of arytenoid/epiglottis.

Risk factors
- Any age/stage of training.
- Overall prevalence unknown but primary diagnosis of moderate–severe ADAF in <10% of racehorses investigated for dynamic respiratory obstructions.

History
- Inspiratory noise during cantering/galloping exercise.
- Noise frequently similar in character to that associated with RLN.

Diagnosis
- Overground/treadmill endoscopy is sole means of diagnosis.
- Severity graded as mild/moderate/marked depending on degree of axial deviation (**Figures 3.11a–c**) relative to position of vocal cord.

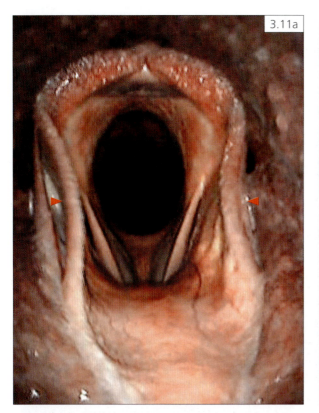
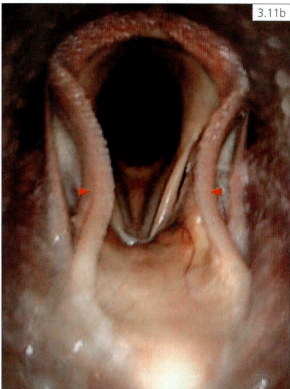
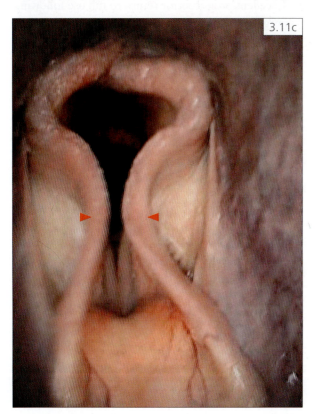

Figs. 3.11a–c Axial deviation of the aryepiglottic folds (arrowheads): (a) mild, (b) moderate, (c) marked (latter with concurrent vocal fold collapse).

Management
- Mild deviations rarely interfere with training.
- Treatment warranted if moderate–severe ADAF considered to be affecting performance or responsible for respiratory noise.
- Surgery: thermoablation (laser) of aryepiglottic fold/s. Require 2–4 weeks out of ridden exercise.
- Concurrent treatment of other respiratory problem/s.

Prognosis
- Rarely interferes with training.
- Spontaneous resolution in some horses without treatment.
- Surgery resolves ADAF in most cases but may not have any effect on other components of complex dynamic collapse (if present). Recurrence of ADAF following surgery may occur.

Epiglottic entrapment
Condition in which epiglottis becomes temporarily or semi-permanently enveloped in a fold of subepiglottic tissue. Usually observed at resting endoscopy but also occurs less commonly as a purely dynamic condition at exercise only (**Figures 3.12a, b**). Not usually associated with poor performance and frequently subclinical.

Cause
- Underlying cause unknown.

Risk factors
- Any age/stage of training.
- Incidence reported as 0.06–1.3% of yearlings and horses in training.
- Some affected horses have small epiglottic dimensions; however, not a universal feature.

History
- Most make a harsh but non-specific inspiratory and expiratory respiratory noise at exercise.
- Many cases detected as incidental finding at routine endoscopy (no respiratory noise).

Diagnosis
- Resting endoscopy: epiglottis appears sheathed in close-fitting 'glove' of tissue; this tissue may be ulcerated/thickened (**Figure 3.12c**).
- Determining whether entrapment is intermittent or fixed is important for management.

Management
- Generally not associated with poor performance; however, as it is readily corrected treatment is usually advised.
- Treatment is elective and can be planned to fit with training programme/racing engagements.
- Surgical release of entrapping tissue is treatment of choice and usually performed as a standing/sedated procedure. Requires little time out of training (1–3 weeks).
- If entrapment is intermittent, surgical resection of subepiglottic tissue may be required.
- Conservative management (rest and anti-inflammatory throat spray) also effective but less favoured.

Prognosis
- Uninterrupted training (no treatment) possible in horses without respiratory noise/poor performance.
- Excellent prognosis for return to full use following surgery.
- Approximately 5–10% of cases recur.
- Rare complications of surgery include development of DDSP and scarring of epiglottis.

Epiglottic retroversion
Dynamic condition in which epiglottis 'flips' up and occludes airway during inspiration at exercise (**Figure 3.13**). Frequency increases with speed and may be exacerbated by neck flexion.

Cause
- Unknown but likely to be a neuromuscular disorder.
- May arise from damage to hyoglossal nerve or to hyoepiglotticus or geniohyoideus muscles.

Risk factors
- Rare.
- Any age/stage of training.
- Recent upper airway surgery or inflammation may predispose.

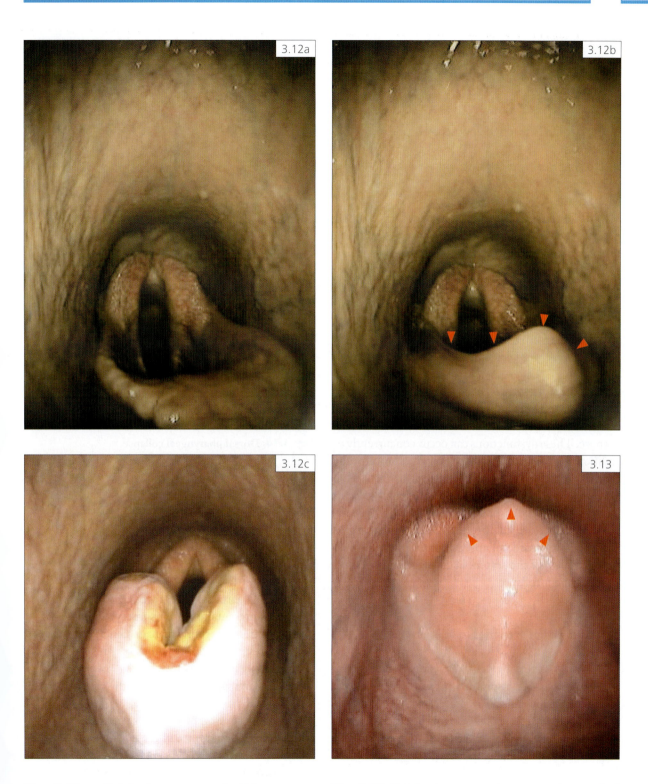

Figs. 3.12a–c Epiglottic entrapment: (a, b) images from a horse with intermittent epiglottic entrapment (arrowheads) at exercise; (c) chronically thickened/ulcerated subepiglottic tissue cloaking the epiglottis.

Fig. 3.13 Epiglottic retroversion at exercise: vertical tipping of epiglottis (arrowheads) and occlusion of airway.

History
- Loud respiratory noise (inspiratory) and exercise intolerance.

Diagnosis
- Overground/treadmill endoscopy is sole means of diagnosis.
- No abnormality on resting endoscopy.

Management
- No current effective treatment.
- Rest +/− anti-inflammatory medication if post-surgical inflammation thought to be responsible.
- Surgical procedure has been reported but efficacy unknown.

Prognosis
- Limited information available; prognosis for athletic recovery considered to be poor.

Complex dynamic upper airway collapse

Many horses display dynamic collapse of more than one anatomical structure of the upper airway during exercise. These dysfunctions can occur concurrently or at different stages of exercise, or may emerge following surgical correction of other respiratory obstructions.

Conditions that may occur in various combinations include RLN, ADAF, epiglottic retroversion, palatal displacement or instability (DDSP/PI), pharyngeal collapse, vocal cord collapse, subluxated corniculate process (apex) of the arytenoid cartilage and cricotracheal ligament collapse.

Cause
- Unknown but presumed to be neuromuscular dysfunction.
- Normal functioning of upper airway in the face of large negative inspiratory pressures requires complex neuromuscular control.
- Dorsal pharyngeal collapse may be caused by pressure differential between guttural pouches (above pharynx) and nasopharynx (**Figure 3.14**).

Risk factors
- Any age/stage of training.
- Risk factors unknown.

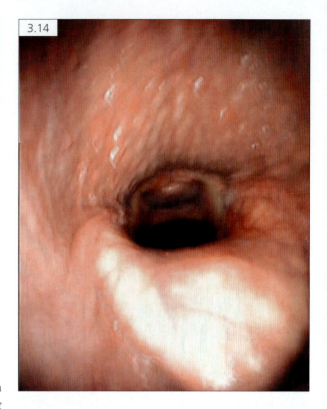

Fig. 3.14 Dorsal pharyngeal collapse.

Diagnosis
- Overground/treadmill endoscopy is sole means of diagnosis.

Management
- Individual circumstances (age/stage of career/clinical presentation/prior surgery) and type of obstruction determine management.
- Some respiratory obstructions may respond favourably to conservative management (rest +/− anti-inflammatory medication); this does not apply to RLN.
- Choice of surgical procedure/s determined by relative significance of each diagnosed dysfunction, with goal being long-term improvement in upper airway stability.

Prognosis
- Information on prognosis not available.

Pharyngeal lymphoid hyperplasia (juvenile pharyngitis)

The mucosa lining the dorsal/lateral walls and floor of the nasopharynx is rich in lymphoid tissue and is the equivalent of the human tonsil. It plays an important role in immune defence, priming the rest of the body against bacterial and viral challenge. Enlargement of this lymphoid tissue is a normal finding in yearlings and 2 YOs. Severity varies between individuals. When pharyngeal lymphoid hyperplasia is marked or persistent, it may have an effect on upper airway function but generally has no impact on performance.

Cause
- Part of the natural priming of immune system and represents adaptation to microbes found in the training environment.

Risk factors
- Almost ubiquitous in young (yearling/2 YO) horses in training.

History
- Usually an incidental finding at routine endoscopy.
- May display harsh respiratory noise at exercise.

Diagnosis
- Resting endoscopy: enlarged lymphoid patches in walls/roof of nasopharynx (**Figures 3.15a, b**).

Management
- Treatment is not required in majority of horses (normal phase of immune system maturation).
- If associated with dynamic airway collapse/respiratory noise: treatment with topical/systemic anti-inflammatory (corticosteroid) +/− antibiotic medication may be justified, although efficacy undetermined.

Prognosis
- Excellent. Invariably resolves with maturity.

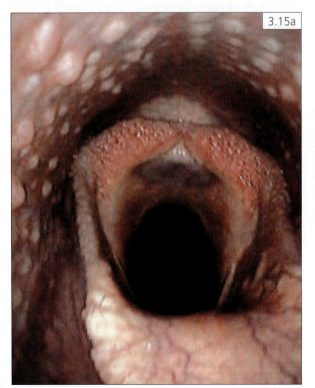
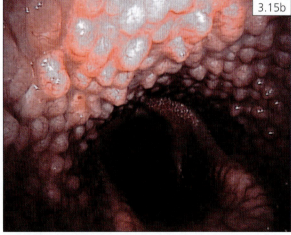

Figs. 3.15a, b Pharyngeal lymphoid hyperplasia: (a) mild, (b) marked.

Arytenoid ulceration/chondritis

Ulceration/erosions occasionally occur on the medial aspect of one or both arytenoid cartilages of the larynx. Most lesions involve only the mucosa and resolve spontaneously; however, a small proportion go on to develop more advanced disease at the site including granulomas or (rarely) infection of cartilage (chondritis). Chondritis most likely to be left-sided but can be bilateral or right-sided.

Cause
- Underlying cause unknown in most cases.
- May be multifactorial: infection, trauma (from nasogastric intubation or endoscopy) or 'kissing' lesions from dynamic airway collapse.
- When associated with RLN, is assumed to be secondary; however, mechanical arytenoid dysfunction from enlargement/distortion of cartilage also possible.

Risk factors
- Any age/stage of training.
- Prevalence of ulcers/small granulomas in yearlings: approximately 0.6%.
- Prevalence of chondritis in yearlings: approximately 0.2%.
- Training on dirt/all-weather tracks may be associated with increased risk.

History
- Usually detected at routine endoscopic examination.
- Generally no outward sign of disease.
- No respiratory noise at exercise unless a concurrent dynamic respiratory obstruction is present.

Diagnosis
- Resting endoscopy: mild disease seen as localized ulceration (+/− small granuloma) at rostral margin of vocal process of one or both arytenoid cartilages. Chondritis appears as thickening/inflammation of affected cartilage (**Figure 3.16**), often with superficial erosions; +/− reduced movement of cartilage.
- Ultrasonography: useful to determine extent of cartilage involvement and assist treatment planning.

Management
- Ulcers and small granulomas: most require no treatment and usually resolve spontaneously, although surgical removal of granulomas may be warranted.
- If secondary to dynamic collapse of arytenoid cartilage: consider treating underlying RLN.
- Arytenoid chondritis: rest (removal from ridden exercise) and medical treatment; systemic antibiotic and anti-inflammatory medication +/− anti-inflammatory topical throat spray. Endoscopic monitoring guides return to ridden exercise.

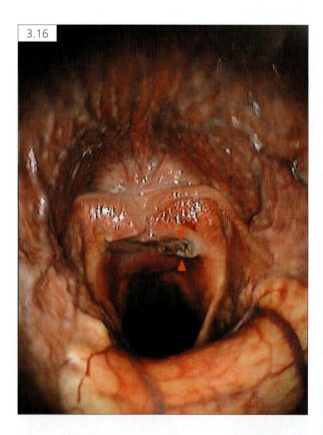

Fig. 3.16 Arytenoid chondritis: ulcerated lesion (arrowheads) on thickened left arytenoid cartilage.

- Rarely, large lesions or those that respond poorly to medical treatment may require surgical resection of affected tissue (partial/total arytenoidectomy). Require several weeks out of ridden exercise (until mucosa heals).

Prognosis
- Ulcers/granulomas: not associated with performance loss and heal without complication in most cases.
- Occasionally, progression to arytenoid chondritis will occur, requiring more aggressive treatment.
- Arytenoid chondritis: can disrupt training for weeks/months depending on severity and response to treatment; surgery is an uncommon but possible outcome. Prognosis for return to full use is good.

Laryngeal dysplasia (4th and 6th branchial arch defects; 4-BAD/6-BAD)

Syndrome of congenital defects of the cartilages and muscles of the larynx:
- 4-BAD may involve the cricothyroid articulation, the thyroid cartilage or the cricothyroideus and cricopharyngeus muscles; individuals may be affected to varying degrees and defects may be present on one or both sides of the larynx. Also known as 'rostral displacement of the palatopharyngeal arch' because absence of the cricopharyngeal sphincter muscle may cause the apex of the corniculate processes of the arytenoids to be obscured by the palatal pillars (**Figure 3.17**), although this feature is not universal.
- 6-BAD: muscular process of the right arytenoid cartilage is affected. Most affected individuals display varying degrees of laryngeal weakness: most commonly (65%) right-sided.

Cause
- Incomplete development of embryological derivatives of the 4th (most commonly) or 6th branchial arches.

Risk factors
- Rare condition; prevalence approximately 0.2% in unselected yearlings.
- Risk factors unknown.
- Not considered to be heritable.

History
- Majority make respiratory noise at exercise.
- Many cases detected for first time at routine yearling endoscopy.
- Affected horses commonly 'swallow air' due to incomplete upper oesophageal sphincter and 'hiccups'/'belching' and intermittent colic may be features.

Diagnosis
- Palpation of larynx usually reveals a gap between the thyroid and cricoid cartilages (should normally overlap).

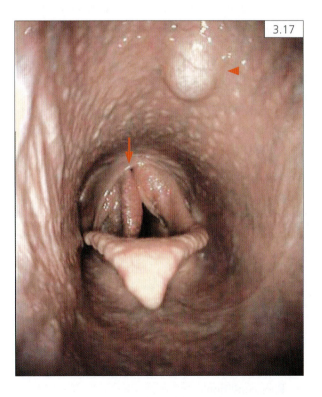

Fig. 3.17 Rostral displacement of the palatopharyngeal arch (arrow) seen with 4-BAD laryngeal dysplasia; dorsal pharyngeal cyst also present (arrowhead).

- Resting endoscopy: inability to visualize corniculate process apices of arytenoid cartilages (due to a band of soft tissue) +/− right (+/− left)-sided laryngeal weakness indicates laryngeal dysplasia.
- Other imaging modalities rarely needed; however:
  - Radiography: presence of column of air from pharynx into oesophagus is confirmatory (insufficiency of upper oesophageal sphincter).
  - Ultrasonography: lack of cricothyroid articulation on affected side; dorsal extension of thyroid cartilage; +/− muscular abnormalities.
  - CT and MRI: may be used to better define specific defects present in an individual.

Management
- Considered surgically irreparable at present; laser thermoplasty may be used to correct rostral displacement of the palatopharyngeal arch but cannot address underlying anatomical fault. Partial arytenoidectomy may be considered.
- Laryngeal prosthetic surgery generally unsuccessful due to abnormal cricoarytenoid articulation.

Prognosis
- Many affected horses do not enter training due to culling at yearling stage.
- Of those that do: reasonable prognosis for racing, although few are considered effective athletes.

Epiglottitis
Inflammation/infection of the epiglottic cartilage.

Cause
- Unknown.
- In some cases may be seen secondary to epiglottic entrapment (or its surgical management): possible effect of avascular necrosis/direct trauma.

Risk factors
- Rare condition.
- Any age/stage of training.
- Sometimes associated with other upper airway conditions (DDSP, epiglottic entrapment).

History
- Respiratory noise.
- Coughing.
- Exercise intolerance.

Diagnosis
- Resting endoscopy: inflammation/thickening/scarring of tip of epiglottis.

Management
- Acute phase: removal from ridden exercise plus anti-inflammatory (systemic +/− topical) and antibiotic therapy.
- Chronic phase (scarring/deformity): surgical resection may be warranted depending on severity.

Prognosis
- Most cases resolve with medical therapy.
- Some permanent deformation of epiglottis usually results.
- Occasional development of DDSP or epiglottic entrapment.

Pharyngeal cysts
Solitary cystic masses in the pharynx may be found at several sites but most commonly occur in subepiglottic position or in dorsal pharyngeal wall. Present from early in life (foal or yearling). Not invariably progressive.

Cause
- Developmental, arising from remnants of embryonic ductal tissue.

Risk factors
- Rare condition.
- Usually present from early age.

History
- Dorsal pharyngeal cysts typically an incidental finding at routine endoscopy.

- Subepiglottic cysts most commonly detected as an incidental finding at routine yearling endoscopy. Clinical signs more common in horses in ridden work: may cause dynamic respiratory dysfunction and can present with respiratory noise (+/− DDSP), coughing, poor performance and, less commonly, dysphagia.

Diagnosis
- Resting endoscopy: smooth, thin-walled cystic mass of variable size (**Figure 3.17**).
- Subepiglottic cysts: smooth mass below epiglottis that usually results in asymmetric elevation of the epiglottis above the soft palate. Mass may be concealed by soft palate and only visible intermittently; stimulation of the swallowing reflex or use of an epiglottic elevator usually results in visualization (**Figure 3.18**). Endoscopy from oropharynx and/or CT may be required in some cases.

Management
- Treatment of incidental or small dorsal pharyngeal cysts not necessary unless respiratory function affected.
- Surgical/laser/formalin ablation if cyst removal desired.
- Several surgical techniques for removal of subepiglottic cysts: laryngotomy or oral approaches most commonly employed.

Prognosis
- Good prognosis for return to racing.
- Recurrence following surgical removal is rare.
- Interruption to training minimal (4–6 weeks for subepiglottic cyst).

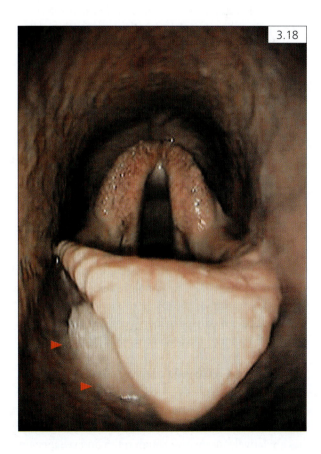

Fig. 3.18 Subepiglottic pharyngeal mass (arrowheads).

LOWER AIRWAY DISEASE

Applied anatomy
Lower airways
The primary function of the respiratory tract is gas exchange; however, this only occurs in the terminal alveoli, with the remainder of the airways serving to deliver, humidify, warm and filter inspired air. The tracheobronchial tree is largely composed of cartilaginous tubes, with only the terminal airways being free of cartilage and surrounded by smooth muscle. The trachea and the bronchi that branch from it are lined with mucosa that both secretes mucus and mobilizes it in the direction of the larynx through the 'beating' action of epithelial cilia.

Mucus
Mucus is composed primarily of water, mucins and inflammatory cells and is largely produced by glands in the lining of the small airways. It plays an important role in maintaining airway health by trapping inhaled matter and bacteria and clearing it from the respiratory tract up the ciliary 'escalator'; it also contains immunologically active factors important to respiratory defence.

The amount of mucus present in the lower airways depends on both the rate of production and the rate of clearance (speed of removal by trachea is normally around 20 mm/minute). Inflammation and infection can increase mucus secretion as well as inhibit mucus clearance (through damage to the cells lining the airway). The presence of inflammatory cells and debris increases the purulence of mucus and can change its viscoelasticity, also leading to reduced clearance.

Coughing
Coughing clears mucus and foreign material from the large (but not small) airways and is an important defence mechanism. The cough reflex can be stimulated by irritation of the lining of the larynx or lower trachea, and is mediated by nerve endings that are sensitive to both mechanical and chemical stimuli.

Assessment of lower airway disease
Coughing
Coughing during or after exercise is commonly used as a marker of disease by trainers; however, the horse has a relatively insensitive cough reflex and reliance on coughing for the detection of lower airway disease is inherently inaccurate. Many horses with increased tracheal mucus or blood do not cough at all. Regardless of this, coughing can contribute useful information that may assist respiratory investigations:
- Horses that cough several (≥4) times at or after exercise generally do have increased mucus; this can be used as a threshold to select horses for endoscopy.
- Overall prevalence and severity of coughing in a yard can be a reasonable indicator of group health status.
- Uncharacteristic coughing (few coughs) immediately after fast exercise may indicate EIPH.
- Very high (>15–20) and uncharacteristic cough frequency after exercise can sometimes be associated with inhalation of track material ('kickback').

Physical examination
Nasal discharge is an unreliable indicator of lower airway disease. Bilateral purulent nasal discharge may accompany lower airway infection but can also arise from upper airway inflammation such as rhinitis. Haemorrhage from the nostril/s (epistaxis) may originate in the nasal passages as well as the lungs and, when associated with EIPH, correlates poorly with severity of tracheal blood accumulation. Observation of breathing rate, respiratory effort and auscultation of the lung fields for increased or diminished respiratory sounds is indicated in cases of suspected pneumonia or respiratory distress in the systemically ill horse (but not generally for routine investigation of coughing).

Endoscopy
Resting endoscopy is the most useful diagnostic technique for the detection of lower airway disease in the racehorse. It is preferably performed immediately/within 30 minutes following exercise to permit the most representative observation/sampling of lower airway secretions. Most horses can be examined with simple restraint and sedation is rarely necessary. Note is made of inflammation/discharge within the nasal passages and pharynx during passage of the endoscope. Grading systems for the quantification of increased tracheal mucus (*Table 3.3*) and blood (*Table 3.4*) are reproducible (low inter-observer variability) and are useful to assess/

Respiratory Conditions

Table 3.3 **Endoscopic grading of tracheal mucus**

GRADE	
0	No visible mucus (**Figure 3.19a**)
1	Single small drops (**Figure 3.19b**)
2	Mild: multiple partly confluent drops (**Figure 3.19c**)
3	Moderate: thin continuous stream or several large accumulations (**Figure 3.19d**)
4	Marked: broad continuous stream (**Figure 3.19e**)

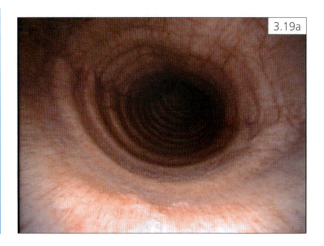

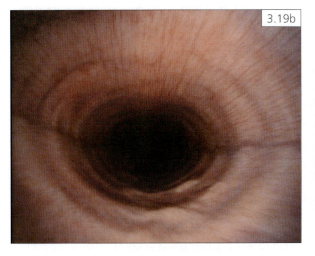

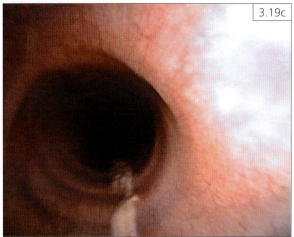

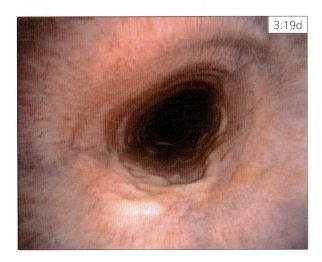

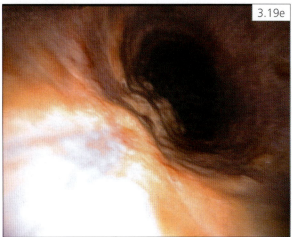

Fig. 3.19a–e (a) Tracheal mucus grade 0. (b) Tracheal mucus grade 1. (c) Tracheal mucus grade 2. (d) Tracheal mucus grade 3. (e) Tracheal mucus grade 4.

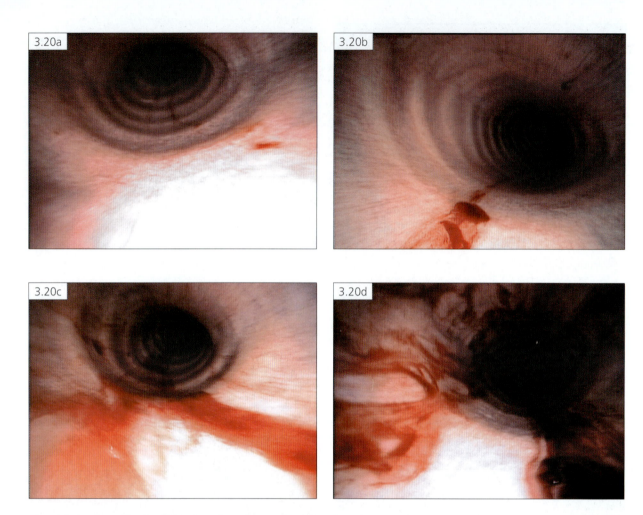

Fig. 3.20a–d (a) Tracheal blood grade 1. (b) Tracheal blood grade 2. (c) Tracheal blood grade 3. (d) Tracheal blood grade 4.

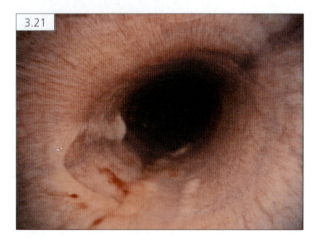

Fig. 3.21 Tracheal mucus and blood.

Table 3.4 **Endoscopic grading of tracheal blood**

GRADE	
0	No blood
1	One or more flecks of blood, or ≤2 short, narrow (<10% trachea) streams of blood (**Figure 3.20a**)
2	One long (narrow) stream of blood (less than half the length of trachea) or >2 short streams occupying less than one-third of the tracheal circumference (**Figure 3.20b**)
3	One long stream or multiple streams of blood occupying more than one-third of the tracheal circumference. No blood pooling at the thoracic inlet (**Figure 3.20c**)
4	Multiple, coalescing streams of blood covering >90% of the tracheal circumference. Blood pooling at the thoracic inlet (**Figure 3.20d**)

Note: Concurrent tracheal mucus and blood is shown in **Figure 3.21**.

record severity of disease. Additional observations that may assist diagnosis include quality (viscoelasticity/colour) of the mucus and inflammation (vascularity/oedema) of the tracheal lining.

Endoscopic sampling

The only practical and rapid method of sampling lower airway secretions is transendoscopic tracheal lavage ('tracheal wash'). Mucus and inflammatory cells accumulate in the natural 'sump' of the trachea at the thoracic inlet; instillation of 10–30 ml isotonic saline into the lower trachea through a catheter passed from the working channel of the endoscope allows harvesting of this material. Sampling is not always representative and may depend on mucus viscosity and coughing during the procedure. Tracheal lavage samples can be subjectively assessed for turbidity (*Table 3.5*) or submitted for laboratory analysis (cytology and bacteriology):

- Cytology may permit some differentiation of infection from non-septic causes of airway disease based on neutrophil morphology.
- Samples can also be used for bacteriological culture to assist treatment planning.
- Bacterial culture should be interpreted with caution: many affected horses have no significant bacterial growth, the distal trachea of the normal horse is not sterile and passage of an endoscope may cause contamination of retrieved sample with pharyngeal bacteria.
- Pure growth of a single pathogenic organism, or quantitative culture (>10^3 cfu/ml), more likely to indicate true infection

Table 3.5 **Grading of tracheal lavage visual turbidity**

GRADE	
0	Clear; occasional small spot of flocculent material
1	Clear with mild levels of flocculent material (**Figure 3.22a**)
2	Slightly cloudy/opaque (**Figure 3.22b**)
3	Turbid; moderate–marked flocculent material (**Figure 3.22c**)
4	Thick mucopurulent material, often difficult to aspirate (**Figure 3.22d**)

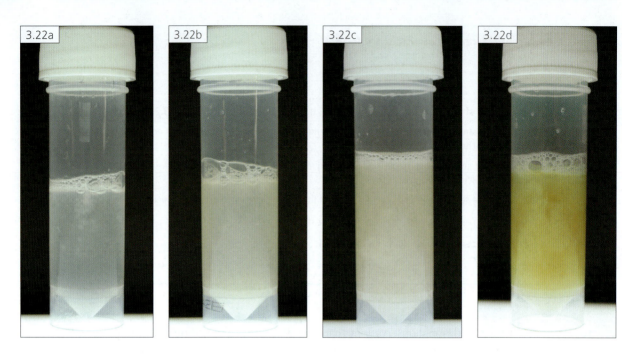

Fig. 3.22a–d (a) Tracheal lavage grade 1. (b) Tracheal lavage grade 2. (c) Tracheal lavage grade 3. (d) Tracheal lavage grade 4.

Other examinations
- Blood sampling is of no use in the detection of inflammatory airway disease or EIPH, but may have a role in the investigation of suspected respiratory infection in the systemically ill animal.
- Ultrasonography of the chest permits detection of fluid/gas in the pleural cavity and consolidation of lung, and is therefore an important aid in the investigation of suspected pleuropneumonia/pulmonary abscess.
- Radiography of the chest is similarly reserved for cases of suspected pleuropneumonia/pulmonary abscess or chronic/severe 'bleeders' (p. 229).

Endoscope disinfection
- Biosecurity to safeguard individual and herd health is important when conducting respiratory endoscopy.
- Sterilization/high-level disinfection between individual examinations not always feasible during routine racetrack rounds.
- Protocol used is guided by assessment of horse-to-horse infection risk.
- Disinfection between horses in a single group or training yard is generally acceptable for routine endoscopy, while between training yards sterilization/high-level disinfection should be standard practice.
- Disinfection should be undertaken as soon as possible after endoscope use.
- Immersion is preferable to wipe/spray (all parts in contact) but not always possible in ambulatory practice.
- Pre-cleaning with enzymatic detergent to remove organic matter (mucus/blood): effective soak times relatively short (approximately 1 minute).

- Follow by disinfection with liquid chemical disinfectant +/− rinsing with sterile water: minimum effective concentration and soak/contact times differ between products and are specified by manufacturer; may be temperature-dependent:
  - Glutaraldehyde (2%): broad efficacy but long contact times required and human health implications.
  - Orthophthalaldehyde: broad efficacy; 5 minutes soak time at 25°C.
  - Ethanol (70% v/v): fast-acting and good efficacy in absence of organic matter.
  - Quaternary ammonium compounds not recommended due to limited efficacy against many pathogens.
- Gas (ethylene oxide) sterilization or automated high-level disinfection of endoscope following high-risk examinations. Good practice to perform on regular basis in combination with leakage testing.

Lower airway infection/inflammation

Lower airway inflammation, characterized by increased tracheal mucus, coughing and poor performance, is widespread in racehorses worldwide. It is a syndrome rather than a single disease, and factors such as bacterial and viral infection, air quality and individual immune status may contribute. Young immunologically naïve racehorses entering the training environment and exposed to respiratory challenge (mixing populations, housing and exercise) are susceptible to opportunistic pathogens and may develop lower airway infection. The condition is usually self-limiting (average duration 2 weeks); however, some horses remain affected by persistent or recurrent disease and appear particularly sensitized to inhaled particulate matter and further infections. Most horses typically experience several episodes during a training career, with unidentified bacterial or viral infections usually responsible.

Cause
- Multifactorial: causative factors include infection (bacterial and viral) and poor air quality.
- Bacterial infection generally more important in onset (and spread) than viral infection.
- Main bacterial species involved (*Streptococcus zooepidemicus*, *Streptococcus pneumoniae*, *Pasteurella* spp.) occur widely in normal racehorse populations but particular strains may act as opportunistic pathogens.
- Other bacteria (e.g. *Bordetella* spp.) may be primary pathogens.
- Herpesvirus and influenza virus may cause lower airway disease: compromise respiratory defences and predispose to secondary bacterial infection.
- Exposure to airway irritants such as dust, fungal spores and endotoxin may exacerbate or prolong disease.

Risk factors
- Any age/stage of training but most prevalent in 2 YOs.
- Risk of developing lower airway disease decreases with age and time in training (as immunity to common bacterial and viral pathogens develops).
- Influence of vaccination history (influenza/herpesvirus) and air hygiene on risk is unquantified.

Effects on performance
- Presence of mucus in airways can interfere with oxygen exchange and increase energy expenditure during breathing.
- Many horses train and race satisfactorily despite mild–moderate levels of tracheal mucus.
- Moderate–severe grades of tracheal mucus often linked to poor racetrack performance.
- Link with EIPH (p. 229) uncertain: common perception that fast work/racing may precipitate pulmonary haemorrhage in a 'dirty' horse but likely to be true in only small proportion of cases.

History
- Coughing at exercise is main presenting sign but is an insensitive indicator of disease and not always present (approximately 40% of affected horses cough).
- +/− poor racetrack performance.
- Increased tracheal mucus frequently an incidental finding at routine endoscopy.

Signs
- Most affected horses appear outwardly healthy.
- +/− coughing at/after exercise.
- Nasal discharge ('dirty nose') +/− fever only in small proportion of cases.

Diagnosis
- Tracheal endoscopy (best performed immediately/within 30 minutes following exercise): excessive tracheal mucus defines the condition.
- Grading of mucus accumulation in trachea (*Table 3.3*) correlates well with severity but does not provide information on duration or likely cause.
- Clinical history often a good guide to origin/progression of disease: age of horse/cough frequency and duration/previous medications/yard health.
- Transendoscopic tracheal lavage can permit sampling of respiratory secretions for subjective evaluation (turbidity/mucus viscosity/colour) or laboratory analysis.
- Resting breathing rate and effort, auscultation of lung fields and blood analysis generally unremarkable.

Laboratory aids
- Cytology and bacteriology of tracheal lavage sample may be used to assist management in troublesome individual cases or yard health planning.
- Laboratory findings should be interpreted with caution; consider primarily as an adjunct to clinical history and endoscopy.

Management
Individual
- Endoscopic findings and clinical history determine whether to treat as primarily an infectious or an inflammatory condition.
- Management influenced by age/stage of racing season/proximity to race targets/economic constraints.
- Treatment may not be necessary or desired for young horses (yearling/early 2 YO) or those not currently in full exercise.
- Aggressive treatment usually reserved for horses in fast exercise when poor performance or interruption to training is undesirable.
- If active infection suspected: broad-spectrum systemic antibiotic medication (to effect; typically 7–10 days). Fluoroquinolones, third-generation cephalosporins and oxytetracycline have greater efficacy than potentiated sulphonamides for common respiratory pathogens.
- Exercise: guided by clinical severity; avoidance of fast exercise/racing during course of disease usually recommended. Validated protocols do not exist; however, cantering may generally continue.
- Periodic endoscopic review useful to monitor resolution/progression.
- Persistence of tracheal mucus after initial treatment: consider further anti-inflammatory +/− mucoactive therapy.
- 'Mucoactive' agents can modify clearance of mucus from lower airways: 'expectorants' (increase water volume of airway secretions so that more readily coughed up), 'mucolytics' (reduce mucus viscosity), and 'mucokinetics' (increase clearance rate by directly acting on ciliary cells). Commonly used mucoactive agents include clenbuterol, dembrexine and sodium/potassium iodides.
- Corticosteroids (systemic or inhaled), air hygiene (soaked/steamed forage, stable ventilation), mucolytic or expectorant drugs or treatments (e.g. nebulization with inhaled hypertonic saline) and nebulized antibiotics may have a role in individual therapy.
- Decision-making regarding whether to permit an affected horse to race is influenced by severity of endoscopic findings, history of coughing/performance/treatment and trainer-influenced factors such as expected level of performance/aversion to risk of under-performance. Excessive tracheal mucus does not necessarily preclude satisfactory racetrack performance.

Group
- Generalized increase in coughing or poor racing performances may warrant wider investigation and/or treatment within yard.
- Assess incidence of disease in the group through endoscopy of a sample of horses (including those thought to be healthy).
- Bacterial opportunistic pathogens naturally circulate in racing yards; biosecurity measures intended to eradicate infection are unrealistic but minimizing shedding, spread and exposure may be beneficial.
- Treatment of choice is dependent on stage of season/level of disease in yard/suspected cause.
- Mass treatment of at-risk group (e.g. 2 YOs) justifiable in some circumstances if applied responsibly and appropriately.
- Endoscopic monitoring of horses with race targets in order to lower risk of poor racetrack performances.

Prevention
- Inevitable that a large proportion of 2 YOs will be affected at some point in season.
- Goal is to reduce susceptibility to disease (vaccination programme/biosecurity/air hygiene) and speed recovery time (medication/exercise modification) so that total lost training days are minimized.
- Timing of influenza/herpesvirus vaccinations to account for high-risk periods.
- Preferable to introduce yearlings to yard only after end of main racing season (if there is to be close proximity to older horses).
- Timing of influenza/herpesvirus vaccinations to account for high-risk periods.
- Quarantine protocol for new entrants during racing season.
- +/− use of immunostimulants (*Parapox ovis* virus/*Propionibacterium acnes*-derived products) in selected horses prior to high-risk periods: some evidence of improved non-specific immune response/reduced disease severity.

Prognosis
- Most episodes are self-limiting and regardless of management resolve within several weeks.
- Small proportion of horses display persistent disease due either to recurrent infections or to non-septic lower airway reactivity. Usually resolves during following racing season.

Exercise-induced pulmonary haemorrhage ('bleeding')

EIPH is a condition in which bleeding occurs into the small airways of the lung, typically during strenuous exercise. Caused by rupture of small capillaries in the dorsocaudal lung lobes. Severity varies between individuals and regardless of severity usually goes unnoticed; blood rarely appears at the nostrils (**Figure 3.23**). In the majority of horses EIPH causes no significant

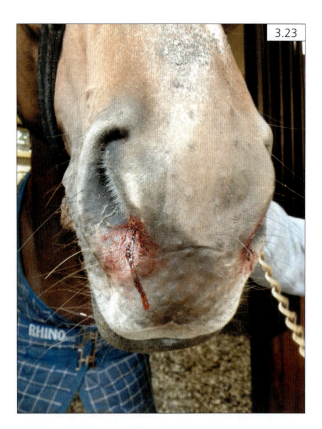

Fig. 3.23 Mild epistaxis.

problems, but in a small proportion can lead to loss of performance when severe. Physiological adaptations of the Thoroughbred (high cardiac output, pulmonary arterial pressures and very large gas exchange capacity) may predispose to the condition.

Cause
- Stress failure of pulmonary capillary wall occurs when pressure across wall exceeds wall strength. Forces arise from disparity between very high blood pressure during fast exercise and subatmospheric pressure in alveolus during inspiration.
- Chronic exercise-induced hypertension in dorsocaudal lung leads to remodelling (thickening of walls and reduced compliance) of the pulmonary veins, which in turn causes local increases in pulmonary capillary pressure.
- Subsequent haemorrhage causes small airway inflammation and has potential to lead to fibrosis in lung.
- Interface between normal and fibrosed lung tissue is mechanically more prone to further stress failure, such that repeated episodes of EIPH may result in further damage to lung.
- Involvement of progressively larger areas of lung tissue increases risk of more severe episodes.
- Impact of forelimbs striking the ground creates shear waves that are focused in dorsocaudal lung fields and may contribute to the condition.

Risk factors
- Risk factors summarized in *Table 3.6*.
- May be encountered in any horse in cantering/fast exercise.

Table 3.6 **Risk factors for epistaxis (from EIPH)**

Age	Risk of epistaxis greater in older horses (≥4 YO).
Heritability	Heritability not fully known; strong genetic component to more severe forms of the condition (epistaxis).
Upper airway function	No direct link with upper airway obstructions (including RLN and DDSP), although previous laryngeal 'tie-back' surgery may predispose to EIPH and epistaxis.
Lower airway disease	No direct link with respiratory infection, although lower airway inflammation may predispose to EIPH during fast exercise. Bleeding itself causes a non-septic lower airway inflammatory response.
Air quality	In the stable: no difference in risk between bedding on paper or straw.
	At the track: some anecdotal indication that poor air quality (dust/pollution) may increase the incidence of EIPH but firm evidence lacking.
Season	Prevalence of epistaxis in most countries is greatest in autumn and winter.
Race type/ conditions	Greater risk of epistaxis with steeplechase/hurdle (approximately 3–5/1,000 starts; 0.34–0.54%) races than with flat racing (approximately 1/1000 starts; 0.13%).
	Flat racing: epistaxis more prevalent over sprinting distances in the UK (conflicting evidence between countries).
	In the UK: increased risk of epistaxis with faster (harder) ground.

- At microscopic level all racehorses in fast exercise have some evidence of bleeding ('all horses bleed'); however, at a practical level this is clinically insignificant in most cases.
- Around half of all horses examined endoscopically post race have visible tracheal blood.
- Majority of these bleeds are minor.
- Approximately 15% of horses have grade 3 or 4 EIPH (see *Table 3.4*) and less than 0.5% of race starts are associated with blood from nose (epistaxis).
- Epistaxis affects approximately 2–3% of the racing population.

History
- Frequently an incidental finding at routine endoscopy.
- May be associated with poor performance or coughing following exercise.

Signs
- Most episodes of EIPH are subclinical: no coughing/epistaxis/poor performance.
- More severe grades of EIPH may be accompanied by coughing after exercise.
- Epistaxis following exercise does not invariably imply EIPH: may be from nasal passages.

Diagnosis
- Tracheal endoscopy is most practical method of determining severity (visual grading, *Table 3.4*).
- Laboratory analysis of tracheal lavage sample: provides little additional information of practical use. Presence of red blood cells (RBCs) (or macrophages containing their breakdown product haemosiderin) is specific and sensitive; however, all horses in fast work have microscopic evidence of EIPH (and this may persist for days/weeks beyond episode).
- Bronchoalveolar lavage is the most sensitive method for diagnosing EIPH; however, requires sedation and laboratory analysis and therefore rarely employed.
- Radiography: rarely employed but may be indicated in chronic/severe cases. Most horses with EIPH have few radiological changes; chronic 'bleeders' have bronchointerstitial pattern of density in dorsocaudal lung fields.

Effects on performance
- Bleeding into lung during exercise has potential to affect gas exchange and therefore performance.
- Dependent on severity of episode: can tolerate up to 100 ml of blood in lungs without affecting performance.
- Strong association between severe bleeding episodes (epistaxis) and poor performance.
- Lower odds of winning/placing with episode ≥grade 2.
- Despite this, many instances of horses performing well at highest level in spite of moderate–severe EIPH.

Management
- Background information important when determining significance of single episode of EIPH (previous endoscopy findings/exercise intensity/recent lower airway disease). Without sufficient information it is difficult to advise on management, and further endoscopic examinations following fast exercise may be useful.
- Uncharacteristic or single severe episode may warrant rest +/− anti-inflammatory/antibiotic medication. There are no validated recommendations for optimal period of rest from fast exercise and this should be determined by individual circumstances.

- Recurrent 'bleeders': address any concurrent respiratory disease (lower airway inflammation/upper airway obstruction), minimize severity of bleeding at fast exercise during training (*Table 3.7*) and maximize recovery times between severe episodes.
- Race day treatment/management restricted in most jurisdictions. No research support for efficacy of pre-race dehydration.

Prognosis

- Not invariably progressive and performance of horses displaying mild forms of condition may be unaffected throughout career.
- Prognosis for horses suffering an episode of epistaxis is guarded: recurrence of epistaxis is common (>30%) and does not appear to be influenced by treatment or rest.
- More severely affected horses may display continued or worsening EIPH over time and when associated with poor performance may justify retirement.
- Career longevity can be jeopardized by progressive nature of condition and penalties for epistaxis in some jurisdictions.

Table 3.7 Management aids for EIPH

TREATMENT	ACTION	RESEARCH SUPPORT FOR EFFICACY
Frusemide	Diuretic with short half-life that increases urine production (starting 15–30 minutes after administration and lasting for 2–3 hours). Reduces pulmonary capillary blood pressure and additionally is a potent bronchodilator. Dosage: 0.5–1.0 mg/kg BWT IV 2–4 hours pre-exercise (restrict water from time of administration); no apparent difference in efficacy between administration 2 or 4 hours pre-exercise. Poor/variable absorption of oral formulation.	Strong. Reduces incidence and severity of EIPH (by at least one grade in >60% of horses). Enhanced race-track performance thought to be due at least in part to weight loss arising from diuresis.
Herbal diuretics	Herbal extracts used in traditional human medicine as purported diuretics include *Sambucus* spp., *Zea mays* and *Orthosiphon stamineus*.	None/weak.
FLAIR nasal strip	Acts to reduce upper airway resistance to inspiratory airflow caused by collapse of the highly moveable nasal valve region.	Strong. Clinical effect on severity of EIPH less than that seen with frusemide.
Haemostatic/anti-fibrinolytic drugs	Drugs that have an effect on blood coagulation cascade: include aminocaproic acid, carbazochrome and tranexamic acid. Rationale for use is tenuous, as no indication that EIPH is linked to defective coagulation or fibrinolysis.	None/weak.
Vasodilatory drugs	Some theoretical rationale for use of drugs that selectively address pulmonary hypertension (e.g. the nitric oxide donor sildenafil).	None/weak.
Bioflavinoids, vitamin C	Proposed to improve integrity of capillary wall, thereby potentially limiting EIPH.	None/weak.
Omega-3 fatty acids	When supplemented over months may reduce lower airway inflammation.	Uncertain.

Research support definitions: strong (studies generally support effectiveness); uncertain (some positive findings are available, but confirming research needed); none/weak (little or no positive data available).

Pleuropneumonia

Sporadic but serious condition in which infection of the lungs spreads to the pleural space. Potentially life-threatening. Typically encountered as isolated cases (non-contagious) but clusters of disease in racing yard/training centre occasionally occur and may follow respiratory disease in wider population.

Cause
- Breakdown in normal defence mechanisms of lung leading to colonization of lower airways by oropharyngeal bacteria.
- Aerobic bacteria (beta-haemolytic streptococci, *Pasteurella* spp., *E. coli* and *Enterobacter* spp.) most commonly involved; however, mixed anaerobic infections (*Bacteroides*, *Clostridium* spp.) are responsible for up to a quarter of cases.

Risk factors
- Rare condition.
- Any age/stage of training.
- Recent (within past week) long-distance travel, exposure to viral respiratory disease or confinement with head elevated (during travel or due to injury) are recognized risk factors.
- Inability to lower head impairs normal postural drainage of respiratory secretions and leads to bacterial contamination of lower airways.

History
- Development of signs usually acute.
- Recent history of coughing and/or recurrent fever is typical.

Signs
- Fever/depression/lethargy, sometimes profound.
- +/– coughing.
- Increased respiration and heart rates, with increased respiratory effort.
- Pleural pain may mimic low-grade colic or cause horse to appear stiff/laminitic.
- +/– sternal oedema.
- +/– nasal discharge.

Diagnosis
- Blood analysis: marked acute inflammatory profile.
- Auscultation of chest: increased lung sounds in dorsal fields +/– absent/muffled lung sounds in ventral fields.
- Ultrasonography: fluid in lung parenchyma or pleural space +/– consolidated lung tissue (**Figure 3.24**); gas echoes are indicative of anaerobic infection. Assessment of deep lung tissue not possible.
- Tracheal endoscopy: tracheal mucopus not invariably present.

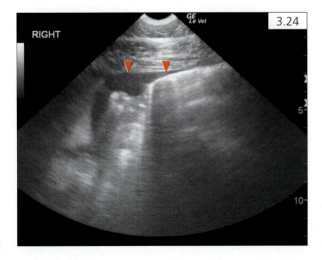

Fig. 3.24 Pleuropneumonia. Transcutaneous ultrasonographic image showing pleural fluid (arrowheads) and consolidated lung.

Management
- Require intensive management and hospitalization recommended.
- Ultrasound-guided drainage of any substantial pockets of fluid (+/– indwelling catheter) as required.
- Aggressive broad-spectrum antibiotic and anti-inflammatory medication guided by culture/sensitivity of sampled fluid. Duration of treatment 4–6 weeks.
- Supportive/intensive care (IV fluids/anti-endotoxic therapy) as required.

Prognosis
- Reasonable prognosis for survival (60–90%) with appropriate management.
- Anaerobic infections tend to be associated with poorer outcomes.
- Horses that survive have a good prognosis for return to racing (60%) regardless of duration of hospitalization.
- Complications (pulmonary abscess/thoracic mass/thrombophlebitis) associated with poorer prognosis for racing.

CHAPTER 4
CARDIOVASCULAR CONDITIONS

HEART MURMURS (Table 4.1)

Heart murmurs are abnormal sounds, generated in or around the heart, that are detectable during auscultation of the chest. They arise from turbulence of blood flow and may be physiological or the result of structural or functional defects such as heart valve insufficiency. Murmurs are defined by their timing during the heart cycle (systolic or diastolic), their intensity and quality of sound, and their location as determined by point

Table 4.1 **Types of cardiac murmur**

CLASSIFICATION	DESCRIPTION	CAUSE	PREVALENCE	SIGNIFICANCE FOR RACING
Atrioventricular (AV) regurgitation	Systolic murmur, loudest on affected side of heart.	Backflow through left or right AV valve.	Incidence and intensity increase with training and age, largely due to adaptation of cardiovascular system to training (eccentric hypertrophy of heart muscle/increased blood volume).	Valve leakage implies reduced cardiac efficiency, but generally no link between presence/severity of AV murmurs and racing performance.
Tricuspid	Right-sided (heart base) holo- or pansystolic murmur.	Backflow through right AV valve during systole.	Common in large/mature trained racehorses (>50% of mature steeplechasers); up to 25% of trained 2 YOs.	Usually low/none.
Mitral	Left-sided holo- or pansystolic murmur, loudest over apex.	Backflow through left AV valve during systole.	Uncommon in yearlings but prevalence increases with training (up to 20% of racehorses in training).	May be associated with poor performance if loud +/− increased resting HR (particularly in untrained horse): requires echocardiography.
Aortic regurgitation	Diastolic murmur, audible from both sides of chest but usually loudest on right side.	Backflow through aortic valve during diastole.	Rare in yearlings/young racehorses (<2%) but prevalence increases with age.	Potential to be associated with poor performance but determine on individual basis.
Systolic ejection	Early systolic murmur; intensity can increase with higher HRs such as during/after exercise.	Turbulence in region of aortic or pulmonary valves.	Very common in normal racehorses.	Low/none.
Ventricular septal defect	Right-sided (often audible left side) loud harsh pansystolic murmur.	Congenital defect of ventricular wall permitting left-to-right shunt.	Rare	Potentially highly significant, although can be found in effective athletes. Doppler echocardiography to determine severity/risk of poor performance.

of maximal intensity over the left or right chest walls. Auscultation is reasonably specific and sensitive for detection of valve regurgitation. Significance varies greatly and is dependent on type of murmur, age of horse, stage of training and racing form. Loud murmurs or those of uncertain origin require dynamic imaging of the heart (Doppler echocardiography) before a judgement on effect on performance can be made. Imaging of heart valves, quantifying severity and direction of any valvular backflow and measuring cardiac dimensions allows objective assessment of risk of deterioration.

ARRHYTHMIAS (*Table 4.2*)

The pacemaker of the heart, the sinoatrial (SA) node, is located in the right atrium and drives normal heart rhythm. It generates regular electrical signals that travel through the atria, down to the AV node and eventually to the ventricles. This sequential depolarization enables contraction of first the atria then the ventricles, with coordinated filling and ejection phases required for each effective heartbeat. Interruption to normal rhythm can occur at several points in the circuit and

Table 4.2 Types of cardiac arrhythmia

CLASSIFICATION	DESCRIPTION	CAUSE	PREVALENCE	SIGNIFICANCE FOR RACING
Second-degree AV block	Regular 'dropped beats' in 'regularly irregular' rhythm; abolished by exercise or excitement.	Inherent blood pressure regulatory mechanism in horse: blocked conduction of impulses generated by the pacemaker.	Entirely normal feature, occurs in most horses at rest.	None.
Ventricular premature complexes (VPCs)	Early extra beat, followed by long compensatory pause.	Depolarizations arise from ventricular muscle.	Relatively common during/after exercise in normal horses.	In general are not associated with poor performance. May warrant further investigation if frequent (particularly at rest). Several VPCs in succession (ventricular tachycardia) may indicate underlying disease.
Atrial premature complexes (APCs)	Extra early beat, followed by normal beat interval (resetting of sinoatrial node).	Depolarizations arise from outside the SA node.	Relatively common in normal horses, particularly before/during/after exercise.	In general are not associated with poor performance. May warrant further investigation if frequent (particularly at rest).
Atrial fibrillation (AF)	Chaotic ('irregularly irregular') heartbeat and high resting HR.	Pacemaker impulses from disorganized waves of depolarization in atrial muscle: loss of coordination between atrial and ventricular contraction. Sometimes caused by underlying heart disease but in most racehorses is purely an electrical disturbance.	Rare.	Always significant. Cardiac output compromised (ineffective filling of ventricles); not usually evident at rest but can cause severe exercise intolerance.

may be physiological or pathological. Auscultation of the heart often permits detection (and differentiation) of arrhythmia, but electrocardiogram (ECG) examination is typically required for definitive diagnosis. Undertaking ECG at exercise or over a long time period (24+ hours) may be necessary for detection of transient arrhythmias or to establish a relationship with poor performance.

Atrial fibrillation

In racehorses AF is usually transient or 'paroxysmal', arising without warning during exercise and causing a sudden loss of performance, pulling-up or even collapse. This may be accompanied by epistaxis (EIPH; Chapter 3, p. 229). Return to normal sinus rhythm may occur within minutes or hours. Less commonly (but more typical in older horses), sustained AF may occur.

Paroxysmal AF requires no treatment, as horses return to normal rhythm within a short time. If recurrent paroxysmal AF is suspected as a cause of poor performance, an exercising ECG should be performed.

Cases of sustained AF require conversion to normal sinus rhythm; this may be achieved through medical therapy (oral quinidine sulphate) or transvenous electrical cardioversion; in both cases hospitalization is necessary. Prognosis following return to sinus rhythm is good. Recurrence is rare.

JUGULAR THROMBOSIS/THROMBOPHLEBITIS

Partial or total blockage of a jugular vein by a blood clot (thrombus) most frequently occurs following catheterization for fluid or drug administration during hospitalization. It is usually unilateral and, once formed, the obstruction is permanent, although partial re-canalization may occur over time.

Cause
- Inflammatory cascade leads to clot formation within vein.
- Usually caused by irritation/inflammation of venous endothelium (perivascular injection of irritant drugs/long-term catheterization).

Risk factors
- Hospitalized horses with endotoxaemia (e.g. diarrhoea/colic) at greatest risk: hypercoagulable state potentiates onset.

History
- Acute onset: during or immediately following period of jugular catheterization or repeated IV injections.

Signs
- Acute phase: swelling/heat/inflammation over affected jugular vein +/– fever.
- Subcutaneous veins on affected side of face and upper neck become prominent/congested due to impeded venous return. In acute phase may be accompanied by swelling of face/lips.
- Chronic phase: non-painful but affected part of vein palpably fibrous/'corded'.
- Patency can be assessed by occluding jugular vein at base of neck and observation of venous filling.
- If bilateral (rare): initial venous congestion may be profound and cause respiratory obstruction.

Diagnosis
- Clinical findings definitive.
- Ultrasonography (aided by manual occlusion of vein) may permit assessment of extent of clot (**Figures 4.1a, b**).

Management
- Acute phase: aggressive management to limit extent of clot formation. Systemic anti-inflammatory and antibiotic medication (avoiding IV administration) +/– topical DMSO. Thrombophlebitis usually sterile but potential for bacterial colonization merits use of antibiotics
- Anticoagulant (aspirin) +/– fibrinolytic drugs may be useful in acute phase.
- Once established/chronic, medical therapy is of little use: no treatment required.
- Very rarely, unresolved septic thrombophlebitis may require surgical intervention (thrombectomy).

Prognosis
- Permanent partial/total blockage of one or both jugular veins is of little importance beyond the acute phase due to development of collateral venous return.
- No effect on racing performance.

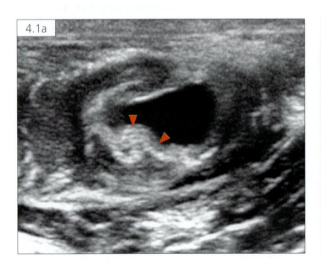 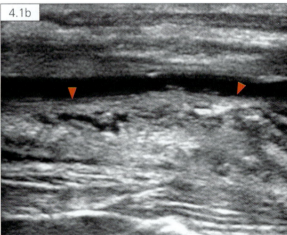

Figs. 4.1a, b Cross-sectional (a) and longitudinal (b) ultrasonographic images of a mid-cervical jugular vein with an organizing intraluminal thrombus (arrowheads).

- Main long-term consequence is inconvenience for future IV administration of drugs.
- Very rarely, septic thrombophlebitis may seed infection/clots elsewhere in body such as lungs, heart valves and synovial spaces.

EXERCISE-RELATED SUDDEN DEATH (CARDIOPULMONARY FAILURE)

Acute collapse and death of a previously apparently healthy racehorse during or immediately after exercise is rare, but accounts for 10–20% of all racetrack fatalities. The cause of death may be cardiac or pulmonary failure, pulmonary haemorrhage or blood vessel rupture, but frequently remains undetermined even after postmortem examination.

Cause
- When postmortem examination fails to reveal a definitive cause of death, it is presumed (but not possible to prove) that a fatal cardiac arrhythmia is responsible.
- Arrhythmias are electroconductive disturbances that in general do not appear to be related to pre-existing structural damage to the heart muscle.
- Arrhythmias (VPCs, p. 236) are common in the immediate post-race period in normal horses; the circumstances that lead to fatal arrhythmias are unknown but electrolyte or metabolic derangements that can occur during/after exercise are postulated to potentiate the heart to risk of ventricular fibrillation. Fatigue may contribute.
- Uncertainty over whether cases of acute fatal pulmonary haemorrhage are a severe form of EIPH (Chapter 3, p. 229).
- Aortic rupture is rare.

Risk factors
- Rare condition.
- Occurs in approximately 0.07–0.08/1,000 starts in flat turf races.
- Greater incidence in jump racing (0.3–1/1,000 starts).
- Risk factors include increasing age, greater race distance and season (greater risk in summer).

History
- Usually no history of pre-existing illness or exercise intolerance.

Signs
- Collapse and sudden death, most commonly during latter stages of a race, but also in the immediate post-race period.

Diagnosis
- Postmortem examination does not furnish a definitive cause of death in all cases.
- Cardiac failure generally considered to arise from fatal arrhythmia and typically no evidence of structural damage to heart.
- Pulmonary congestion/oedema/haemorrhage can be associated with both pulmonary and acute cardiac failure.
- Significance of pulmonary haemorrhage as a cause of sudden death in an individual is a subjective assessment based on severity.

Prevention
- At present there are no screening tests available for identification of at-risk horses.

CHAPTER 5
THE HEAD

DENTISTRY

Routine rasping ('floating')

The equine dentition is equipped to cope with grazing low-energy forage over lengthy periods. Cheek teeth constantly erupt and are composed of three materials (enamel, dentine and cementum) that differ in strength/rates of wear. This ensures a rough occlusal surface to assist breakdown of fibrous food.

Stabled horses fed concentrates spend little time chewing and may consequently develop dental overgrowths because of inappropriate wear. The upper (maxillary) arcades are broader and set further apart than the lower (mandibular) arcades. Therefore, common sites for development of sharp enamel points are the outer edges of the upper and the inner edges of the lower cheek teeth. These may impinge on adjacent cheeks/tongue causing ulceration (**Figure 5.1**) and oral discomfort. The distribution of sharp edges differs between horses and over time; they may extend along an entire arcade or be present on only a few teeth.

Routine rasping ('floating') is the process of removing sharp enamel edges using manual or motorized rasps. Most horses will accept the procedure without sedation. The occlusal (grinding) surface is not rasped, as this may cause oral pain or affect ability to chew. Routine dental examinations also afford the opportunity to detect/monitor other oral pathology and remove loose premolar 'caps' (see below). It is advisable to perform routine dentistry at 6-monthly intervals in young horses in training.

Premolar 'caps'

- First three cheek teeth in each arcade (12 teeth in total) have deciduous precursors (**Figure 5.2**).

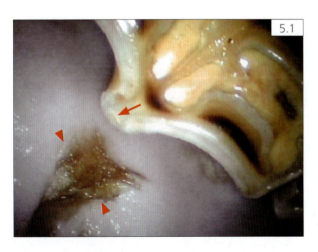

Fig. 5.1 Sharp enamel point on a caudal cheek tooth (arrow) with associated soft-tissue ulceration (arrowheads).

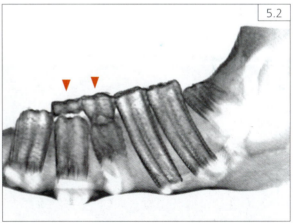

Fig. 5.2 CT image (volume rendered) of the dentition of a 2.5-YO horse. Note the deciduous premolars ('caps') on the 2nd and 3rd lower cheek teeth (arrowheads), with emerging permanent dentition (1st and 6th cheek teeth).

- Shed naturally in chronological order as underlying permanent tooth erupts and through attrition of the remaining deciduous crown (**Figure 5.3**).
- Timing of shedding of these 'caps' varies between individuals.
- Usually shed in 3–5-month cycles from late 2 YO until 4 YO.
- Shed entire or as fragments.
- Many horses show transient reduction in feed intake during cap shedding. Loose/broken caps also occasionally lacerate adjacent cheek/tongue and can cause more severe inappetence and excessive salivation.
- Removal of loose caps is readily performed in unsedated horse; however, forced premature extraction is inadvisable as may damage underlying permanent tooth.

'Wolf' teeth

- Small evolutionary remnant tooth found adjacent to first cheek tooth; not present in all individuals.
- Usually only in upper arcades (**Figure 5.4a**); unilateral or bilateral and shape/size variable.
- May remain unerupted ('blind') beneath gum.
- Never associated with inappetence.
- Link with bitting problems often assumed but difficult to prove.
- Most likely to cause bitting problems if 'blind', large/sharp or prominent following shedding of first premolar 'cap' (**Figure 5.4b**).
- Removal: routine procedure undertaken +/− standing sedation +/− local anaesthetic block; time out of ridden work not required.
- 'Blind' wolf teeth: removed under standing sedation but require small surgical incision through gum.

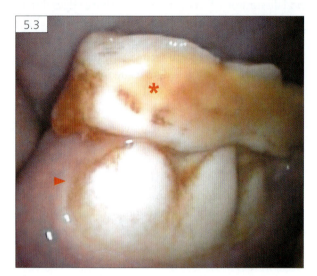

Fig. 5.3 Mandibular 'cap' (asterix) close to shedding, with underlying permanent premolar visible (arrowhead).

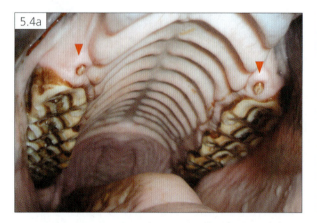

Fig. 5.4a Wolf teeth (arrowheads) in the normal position immediately forward of the first maxillary cheek teeth

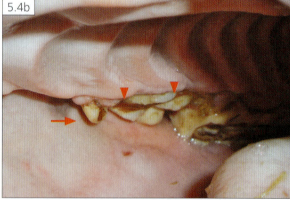

Fig. 5.4b Wolf tooth (arrow) in the right maxillary arcade; adjacent emerging 1st cheek tooth (arrowheads) following loss of premolar 'cap'.

Dental malalignment

- Although each cheek tooth arcade is composed of six teeth, they are closely apposed and act as single grinding unit.
- Teeth may occasionally erupt out of line/position, resulting in loss of continuity of dental arcade (**Figure 5.5**).
- Mid-arcade (3/4/5th cheek teeth) most commonly affected.
- Gaps between teeth can trap food and cause gum disease and oral pain/inappetence.
- Tend to be of clinical significance only when secondary gum disease worsens later in life; rare cause of oral pain in young horses in training.
- Removal of deciduous premolar 'caps' (prior to normal shedding) around the affected site may alleviate in medium term, but not curative.

'Parrot' mouth

- Congenital/developmental defect in which upper incisor arcade overshoots lower jaw (**Figure 5.6**).
- Severity ranges from mild to marked.
- Heritability plays a role but other factors probably involved.
- Surgical correction possible at early age (3–6 months) but rarely employed.
- By yearling stage unalterable and non-progressive.
- No special management required: eating/bitting unaffected and considered a cosmetic or re-sale blemish only.

Tooth root abscess

Tooth root (dento-alveolar) infection is rare. In young racehorses usually affects a single cheek tooth in mid-lower arcade (mandible), but can also affect maxillary arcade. Infection involves one or more vital pulp horns with subsequent devitalization of tooth. External signs of disease variable; purulent discharge exits through path of least resistance (lower jaw, mouth or sinus), determined primarily by location of diseased tooth.

Cause

- Mandibular cheek tooth infection: may follow inhibited eruption of permanent tooth (and subsequent vascular disruption).
- Maxillary cheek tooth infection (rare in young horses): may be secondary to dental fracture or vital pulp compromise.

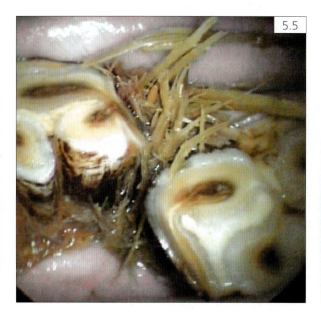

Fig. 5.5 Dental malalignment with food trapping between teeth and secondary gingival disease.

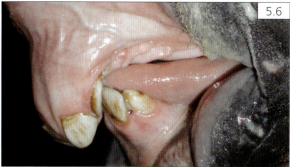

Fig. 5.6 'Parrot' mouth.

Signs
- Mandibular: unilateral firm, painful focal swelling (of variable size) of lower aspect of mandible (distinguish from normal dental 'eruption cysts', which are typically symmetrically enlarged with minimal pain).
- More advanced disease may be associated with purulent draining tract.
- Usually no oral pain.
- Maxillary infections: unilateral facial swelling or unilateral purulent nasal discharge (arising from secondary sinusitis).

Diagnosis
- Clinical findings strongly indicative.
- Oral examination (oroscopy): useful to determine tooth involvement/vitality and plan treatment.
- Radiography: useful for definitive diagnosis but can be reserved for cases non-responsive to initial therapy.

Management
- 'Best practice' involves thorough diagnostic work-up including radiography (or CT) +/− oroscopy; not always required for satisfactory outcome.
- In horses in training initial treatment is usually systemic antibiotic medication (4–6 weeks); can be fed/trained as normal.
- Poor/short-lived response to antibiotic medication should prompt further investigation.
- Surgical extraction of tooth required in small proportion of cases (including some fractured teeth).

Prognosis
- Most cases respond favourably to antibiotic treatment providing dental fracture/fragmentation not present.
- Remission of swelling may take months.
- Rarely interferes with training.

WOUNDS

Wounds to tongue
Wounds to the rostral tongue are usually the result of direct trauma from a bit or chifney. Typically a transverse cut on the dorsal surface of the tongue of variable length and depth; contamination with food is common. Lacerations to side of tongue may occasionally be caused by fractured mandibular 'cap' or cheek tooth.

Signs
- Acute oral discomfort/inappetence.
- Excessive salivation or bleeding from mouth.

Management
- Determined by severity and location.
- Most cases require antibiotic/anti-inflammatory medication and only minimal wound care (lavage) in acute phase.
- Deep/extensive dorsal injuries may benefit from sutured repair.
- Blood and nerve supply is located in underside of tongue; only the most severe injuries (with obvious signs of devitalization) should be considered for partial amputation.
- Amputation of tongue back to the level of frenulum possible without significant loss of function.
- Injuries to side of tongue require medical treatment only; inciting cause should be removed if still present.

Prognosis
- Most injuries heal well without primary closure.
- Permanent groove/defect/scar may result but tongue function unaffected.

Wounds to nostril
Sustained from interaction with stable fittings. Typically a full-thickness tear through the lateral or rostral margin of one nostril of varying length.

Signs
- Severity and configuration of wound varies between individuals.
- Initial bleeding may be profuse.

Management
- Goal is to minimize scarring/stricture of nostril, as may have negative effect on future airway function at exercise.
- Primary repair (2- or 3-layer sutured closure) should be undertaken unless injury is old/grossly contaminated/obviously devitalized.
- Wounds often break down regardless of management and may have to be repaired by delayed closure.

Prognosis
- Excellent, with appropriate management.

Fractured mandible: rostral

Fracture of incisive portion of lower jaw is most common in young colts and arises from oral play with stable fittings. Usually consists of an avulsion of one or more lower deciduous incisor teeth with variable involvement of associated bone plate (**Figure 5.7**). Invariably partially displaced and usually contaminated with food material at time of diagnosis.

Signs
- Oral discomfort is rare; eating and ridden behaviour usually unaffected and frequently only detected due to blood on stable fittings/feed manger.

Management
- Choice of treatment determined by severity and quality of remaining attachment to jaw.
- Loose single teeth with minimal gingival/bone attachments may be simply removed; no wound aftercare is required.
- Most fractures require surgical repair for best outcome. Standing surgical procedure: cerclage wire to realign fractured fragment, removal of wire 4–6 weeks later.
- May be fed/exercised as normal following surgical repair.

Prognosis
- Excellent; no interruption to training.
- Some disruption to eruption of adult teeth can be expected; however, overall cosmetic outcome usually good.

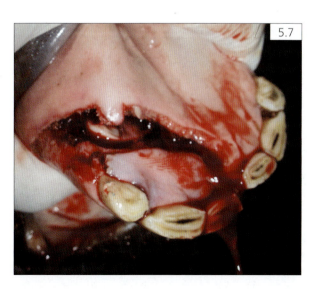

Fig. 5.7 Typical rostral mandibular fracture.

Fractured mandible: horizontal/vertical ramus

Rare injury that arises from direct trauma such as kick or as a result of being cast in stable. Unilateral and most commonly involves the horizontal ramus. Fractures are usually incomplete or non-displaced. Fracture line may exit orally and some dental involvement is inevitable.

Signs
- Non-focal thickening of lower or lateral jaw on one side.
- Pain on palpation.
- +/– excessive salivation.
- Usually no evidence of external/skin wound.
- Oral examination may reveal generalized thickening of affected mandible +/– malodour +/– focal gingival bruising.
- May resemble cheek tooth infection in initial stages.

Diagnosis
- Clinical findings usually strongly indicative.
- Radiography may assist diagnosis; however, fracture line often indistinct (especially in acute phase).

Management
- Unilateral fracture of mandible heals well without treatment, as the fragments are stabilized by muscles of mastication and remainder of jaw.
- Secondary infection (of mandible or adjacent cheek teeth) may arise if there is oral involvement: prophylactic antibiotic medication (4–6 weeks) may be warranted.
- Deterioration in appearance of jaw (or development of discharging tract) should prompt further investigation; occasionally, surgical debridement or removal of affected cheek tooth may be required, although latter is typically delayed (months) until fracture line has stabilized.

Prognosis
- Good. Minimal interruption to training.

EYES

Conjunctivitis

The conjunctiva of the eye is very sensitive to inflammatory insult due to its vascular structure and large amount of lymphoid tissue. Conjunctivitis is usually a mild and transient condition of little concern for training. May be unilateral or bilateral, depending on underlying cause.

Cause
- Most commonly arises as a primary condition (bacterial/viral/trauma/foreign body).
- May be secondary to other eye disease such as corneal ulcer (below), blocked nasolacrimal duct (p. 252) or uveitis.

Signs
- Reddening +/– swelling of conjunctival tissue.
- Usually with ocular discharge.
- Not usually associated with significant ocular pain; closed eye indicates presence of a more serious problem than conjunctivitis.

Diagnosis
- Examination of eye (+/– fluorescein staining) to rule out presence of corneal ulcer or foreign body.

Management
- Primary conjunctivitis: topical broad-spectrum antibiotic medication (triple antibiotic combinations: neomycin/polymyxin B/bacitracin; tetracyclines) 2–3×/day until resolution.
- Poor or short-lived response should prompt further investigation.

Prognosis
- Excellent. No interruption to training.

Corneal ulceration

Ulceration of the cornea is usually the result of trauma. A break in continuity of the corneal surface permits bacterial (less commonly fungal) colonization by either microbes normally resident on the cornea or primary pathogens, and the combination of infection and inflammatory products at the site may cause progressive stromal degradation. Depth of ulcer ranges from superficial to full thickness.

Cause
- Typically arises from direct trauma (e.g. from stable incident or accidental whip contact) or foreign body (seed/dirt).

Signs
- Painful eye (closed eyelids, excessive tear production, photophobia, conjunctivitis).
- Most ulcers are evident on close examination and appear as a focal defect in corneal surface +/− associated corneal oedema (opacity).

Diagnosis
- Fluorescein staining: retention of dye on exposed corneal stroma is definitive.
- Sedation +/− nerve blocking may be needed for full assessment.

Management
- Management guided by severity of stromal degradation/inflammation/ocular pain.
- Simple ulcers: topical broad-spectrum antibiotic medication (triple antibiotic combinations: neomycin/polymyxin B/bacitracin; tetracyclines) used prophylactically 2–3×/day until resolution.
- +/− pain management for secondary ocular reflexes in acute phase: topical atropine sulphate (pupil dilation) and systemic (flunixin meglumine) +/− topical NSAID (pain/inflammation relief).
- Removal from ridden exercise (to minimize exposure to dust/sunlight) until pain free.
- Eye should be monitored for healing.
- Complicated/infected ulcers (rare) are those that are deep, of large diameter or deteriorating rapidly ('melting'): require aggressive management to avoid long-term loss of vision. Treatment includes the above and topical antiproteases (EDTA); insertion of subpalpebral lavage catheter may facilitate frequent (up to every 2–4 hours) administration of topical drugs. Hospitalization may be warranted to permit intensive management.
- Poor response to initial antibiotic therapy should prompt diagnostic cytology and culture to isolate underlying pathogen and direct specific antimicrobial treatment.
- Fungal keratitis: topical (natamycin/miconazole/fluconazole/voriconazole) +/− systemic antifungal therapy.
- Surgery (conjunctival graft) may be considered if medical therapy fails.

Prognosis
- Overwhelming majority heal rapidly with simple treatment and generally display sore eye for <3 days. Interruption to training is minimal.
- Small proportion are troublesome to treat or require hospitalization.

Corneal stromal abscess

Rare but serious condition that carries high risk of unilateral blindness or restricted vision. Abscessation within the cornea may arise from direct trauma or follow the healing of an ulcerated cornea when pathogens remain trapped below the superficial corneal layers. Superficial stromal abscesses may be primarily bacterial (*Pseudomonas* spp./beta-haemolytic *Streptococcus*/*Staphylococcus* spp.) or fungal; deeper abscesses are typically fungal (*Aspergillus* spp./*Fusarium* spp.). Fungal pathogens appear to have a propensity for deeper layers of the cornea and associated disruption to normal function of corneal endothelium can result in secondary corneal oedema or hydrops (bulging).

Cause
- Cause usually not determined in individual cases but may arise from direct trauma to cornea +/− foreign body penetration; haematogenous spread of pathogens also possible.

Signs
- Painful eye (closed eyelids, excessive tear production, photophobia, conjunctivitis) is typical in acute phase.
- Single or multiple focal areas of intracorneal infiltrate, usually discoloured and often with change of external contour of cornea.
- +/− associated corneal oedema (opacity); sometimes profound.
- +/− corneal vascularization.
- +/− anterior uveitis.

Diagnosis
- Clinical findings and slit-lamp observation of corneal stromal infiltrate usually definitive.
- Fluorescein staining: usually no (or weak) uptake of stain.
- Diagnostic cytology/culture warranted but does not always result in fungal isolation.

Management
- Requires aggressive management to salvage vision and prevent recurrence.
- Topical +/− systemic antifungal therapy is cornerstone of treatment: 4–6 week treatment course is typical. Concurrent topical antibiotic medication warranted if bacterial pathogens considered to be implicated.
- Topical medication administered through subpalpebral lavage catheter: voriconazole (or miconazole/natamycin) 4–6×/day or continuous pump lavage.
- +/− pain management for secondary ocular reflexes in acute phase: topical atropine sulphate (pupil dilation) and systemic (flunixin meglumine) +/− topical NSAID (pain/inflammation relief).
- Catheterization necessitates removal from ridden exercise for duration of treatment.
- If good response to medical therapy does not result within 1–2 weeks, surgery should be considered.
- Depth of abscess determines surgical option of choice: superficial keratectomy may assist drug penetration; deep abscesses may require deep lamellar endothelial keratoplasty.

Prognosis
- Guarded to good prognosis for retention of vision in affected eye with appropriate management.
- Superficial abscesses usually respond to medical management alone; deeper abscesses frequently require surgery.
- Some degree of permanent corneal scarring inevitable.
- Loss of vision or enucleation in some cases.

AIRWAYS

Sinusitis
Air-filled sinus cavities comprise a large proportion of the skull. These communicate indirectly with the nasal passages, through which drainage of sinus secretions occurs. Infection of a sinus cavity may be primary or secondary and is usually unilateral.

Cause
- Usually primary bacterial infection.
- Less commonly: secondary to tooth root infection (p. 243), sinus masses or head trauma.
- Rarely may have fungal component.

Signs
- Unilateral purulent nasal discharge.
- +/− unilateral malodour.
- +/− deformation of facial bones/ocular discharge on affected side in advanced cases.

Diagnosis
- Nasal endoscopy: usually possible to establish that discharge is entering nasal passage from nasomaxillary drainage angle.
- Radiography: increased opacity +/− fluid line/s in affected sinus on LM projection (**Figure 5.8**).
- Further diagnostic imaging (oroscopy/sinoscopy/CT) as required.

Management
- Presumptive medical treatment (without definitive diagnosis) often favoured in first instance.
- Broad-spectrum antibiotic medication (2–4 weeks).
- Continued training plus feeding from floor (to assist drainage) recommended.
- Poor response to initial therapy: diagnostic investigation/treatment. Some cases require daily large-volume sinus lavage (small- or large-bore trephination +/− in-dwelling catheter: standing surgical procedure) until resolution (typically <1 week), or facial flap surgery (rare).

Prognosis
- Most cases of primary sinusitis resolve with prompt antibiotic therapy; training rarely interrupted and little/no effect on performance

Fungal (mycotic) rhinitis

Fungal growth may occur on any mucosal surface in the nasal passages or ethmoturbinate regions and is an uncommon cause of persistent nasal discharge. Typically unilateral.

Cause
- Inciting cause unknown but probably due to opportunistic colonization by fungal species (frequently *Aspergillus* spp.) from the stable environment.

Signs
- Persistent unilateral nasal discharge +/− malodour.
- Partially or non-responsive to antibiotic therapy.

Diagnosis
- Endoscopy: yellow/green plaque on affected mucosal surface +/− erosion/necrosis of underlying concha. Thorough examination of all nasal passages with narrow endoscope may be necessary.
- Transendoscopic capture of plaque material for laboratory analysis.
- Very rarely, advanced imaging (CT) may be required to localize lesion and differentiate from other causes of persistent nasal discharge (**Figure 5.9**).

Management
- Transendoscopic debulking of lesion and periodic lavage (usually more than three treatments required) with antifungal medication (enilconazole).
- Training may continue as normal.

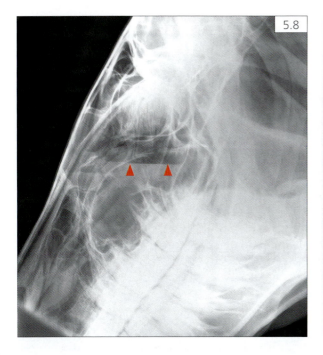

Fig. 5.8 Radiograph (LM) showing sinusitis. Note the fluid lines in the maxillary sinus (arrowheads).

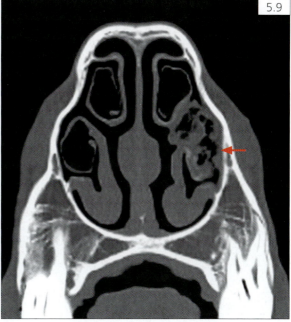

Fig. 5.9 CT image (bone algorithm/transverse) showing nasal conchal destruction caused by fungal rhinitis (arrow).

Prognosis
- Excellent; most cases resolve with treatment and do not recur.
- Rarely interferes with training.

Ethmoidal haematoma
Rare non-neoplastic, slowly progressive mass originating in the ethmoidal turbinates (or less commonly in maxillary sinuses). Ulceration of surface of mass may result in nasal bleeding. Unilateral or bilateral; additionally, some unilateral masses may extend behind the nasal septum to encroach upon other side. Typically in older (≥3 YO) horses.

Cause
- Underlying cause unknown.
- Thought to arise from recurrent submucosal haemorrhage and subsequent distension of submucosal lining to become haematoma capsule.
- Gradual expansion of mass into air spaces of nasal passages or sinuses.

Signs
- Clinical signs dependent on location and size of lesion.
- Recurrent low-grade unilateral nosebleed (epistaxis), usually unrelated to exercise.
- +/– respiratory noise.

Diagnosis
- Endoscopy: smooth-walled mass may be visible extending from ethmoid turbinate labyrinth into nasal passage. Visualization of mass is only partial and does not permit full assessment of extent.
- Radiography: smooth-margined opacity in region of ethmoid turbinates +/– sinus fluid lines usually visible on LM projection.
- CT: permits full assessment of extent of lesion and allows accurate surgical planning (**Figures 5.10a, b**).
- Definitive diagnosis only through histology of mass lining (obtained at surgery).

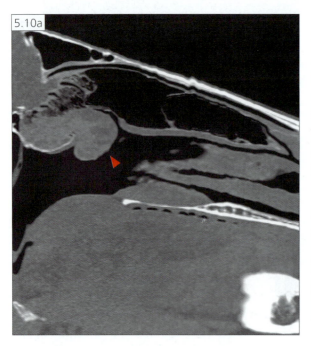
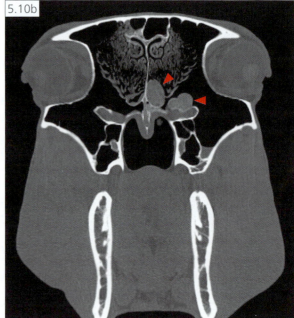

Figs. 5.10a, b CT images (bone algorithm; a, sagittal; b, transverse) of an ethmoid haematoma. Note the smooth-margined mass (arrowheads).

Management
- Without treatment mass continues to slowly expand and clinical signs will worsen.
- Choice of treatment determined by size and location of lesion.
- Small/moderate-sized nasal lesions can be treated successfully under standing sedation with laser ablation or formalin injection. Repeated treatments usually necessary.
- Lesions with sinus involvement usually require surgical ablation (facial flap).

Prognosis
- Moderate recurrence rate following treatment.
- Good medium-term remission of nasal lesions usually possible with laser ablation.
- Surgery and formalin injection associated with mortality risk (small) due to potential exposure of the central nervous system (CNS) to infection or caustic agent.

OTHER

Submandibular lymphadenopathy
Enlargement (+/– abscessation) of one or more submandibular lymph nodes. The sublingual and submandibular lymph nodes are a normal part of the lymphatic system and lie in a chain under the throat. Enlarged lymph nodes are of concern primarily because they may signal the presence of infectious disease.

Generalized mild enlargement in response to viral/bacterial challenge is common in yearlings and rarely of concern. Enlargement and recurrent abscessation of a single lymph node is also common and usually not associated with systemic illness. Differentiation from the more profound/multiple abscesses seen with *Streptococcus equi* ('strangles') infection (Chapter 11, p. 294) is important.

Signs
- Solitary lymph node enlargement: may be large, sore to palpate and intermittently discharge purulent material between periods of relative quiescence (**Figures 5.11a, b**).
- Usually without fever/systemic illness/nasal discharge.

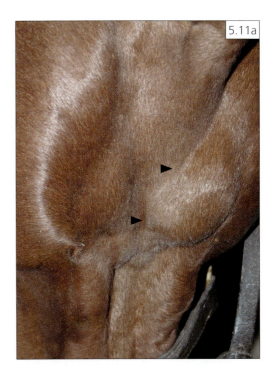

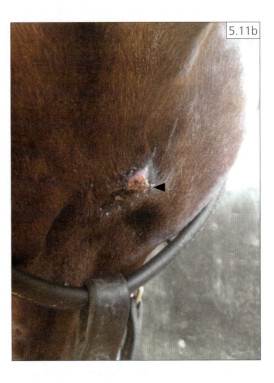

Figs. 5.11a, b Submandibular lymphadenopathy (arrowheads).

Diagnosis
- Clinical presentation and history are good indicators of risk of strangles.
- If multiple lymph node enlargement plus systemically ill +/− nasal discharge, +/− recent arrival on premises (days/weeks), precautions should be taken.
- Diagnostic tests: direct swabbing/culture of exudate +/− *Streptococcus equi* serology +/− guttural pouch/nasopharyngeal swabbing (culture and PCR).

Management
- If strangles considered unlikely: daily warm fomentation; once draining, lavage +/− antibiotic medication into cavity reduces likelihood of recurrence.
- Systemic antibiotic medication should be avoided as generally delays maturation of abscess.

Prognosis
- Occasionally may recur or persist as low-grade chronic condition with intermittent drainage for many weeks/months.
- Does not interfere with training.

Blocked nasolacrimal (tear) duct
The nasolacrimal (tear) duct is formed from the convergence of two canaliculi in the medial canthus of eye and courses through first the lacrimal then the maxillary bones to emerge in the nasal cavity. The duct serves to carry tears from the eye to the nose and varies in diameter along its course. Direct or indirect obstruction may occur, resulting in overflow of tears from eye onto face. Unilateral or bilateral.

Cause
- Most commonly from direct blockage with inflammatory debris arising from eye (following conjunctivitis).
- Pinching of duct by the bony structures that surround it (tooth root abscess/sinusitis/suture exostosis) may also cause obstruction.
- Congenital atresia of duct is rare; typically with history of long-standing ocular discharge and absence of distal nasal punctum when examined.

Diagnosis
- Fluorescein dye placed in eye should emerge at nostril within 20 minutes if unobstructed.
- Imaging of duct necessitates contrast radiography/CT or specialized endoscopy and is rarely necessary.

Management
- Catheterization of nasal punctum and retrograde (nostril to eye) irrigation of duct with saline solution; readily performed in unsedated horse and can be used for combined diagnosis/treatment. Excessive pressure should be avoided.
- If unsuccessful: topical antibiotic/anti-inflammatory eye medication and further attempt in 1–2 weeks.
- Normograde (eye to nostril) irrigation may be attempted under standing sedation.
- Congenital atresia: surgical correction (rarely undertaken).

Prognosis
- Does not interfere with training.

Cheek/lip abscess
Acute, focal infection/abscess of cheek or lip at/near corner of mouth is encountered frequently. Unilateral.

Cause
- Usually follows small penetrating injury on inside of mouth (such as from a seed/grain).
- Less commonly may arise from bit trauma.

Signs
- Pain/guarding of cheek/lip; frequently with acute, severe headshyness (usually one-sided).
- May resent fitting of bridle/headcollar.
- +/− external swelling of cheek/lip (**Figure 5.12**).
- Palpable thickening, intensely painful to light pressure.
- Gingival wound usually very small or inapparent.
- +/− malodour.

Diagnosis
- Clinical findings definitive.

Management
- Usually self-resolving.
- Daily warm fomentation.
- Systemic antibiotic medication should be avoided as generally delays maturation of abscess.
- Systemic anti-inflammatory medication in acute phase may assist with continued training.

Prognosis
- Excellent; interruption to training generally brief (days).

Nasal atheroma (dermal inclusion cyst)
Uncommon developmental epidermal cyst at back of 'false nostril' and usually visible externally. Unilateral or bilateral. Generally remains static in size but may be very slow growing.

Signs
- Typically grape-sized fluid-filled swelling at top of flexible margin of nostril.
- Painless.

Diagnosis
- Clinical findings definitive.

Management
- Does not cause problems and treatment rarely indicated.

Prognosis
- Does not interfere with training and nostril/airway function considered to be unaffected unless very large.
- View as cosmetic blemish only.

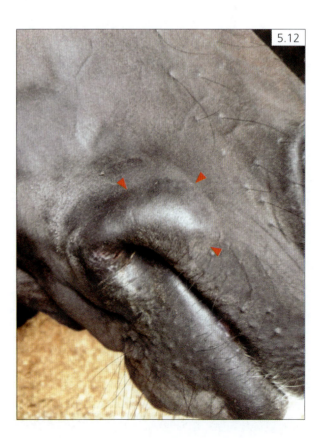

Fig. 5.12 Lip abscess (arrowheads).

CHAPTER 6
GASTROINTESTINAL CONDITIONS

Gastric ulcers

Gastric ulcers occur commonly in horses in training. Severity varies between horses and over time. Ulcers may be clinically silent or be associated with a variety of signs including inappetence, light condition and poor performance.

The horse has evolved to graze through the majority of the day; in nature the relatively small (10–15 litres) stomach is rarely empty and a constant flow of saliva serves to buffer acidity. Only half of the stomach is lined by acid-producing glandular mucosa, and because of this (and the constant inflow of acid-buffering saliva) there are marked regional differences in acidity within the stomach. Ulcers generally occur in non-glandular mucosa and are usually more severe on the lesser curvature of stomach. Gastric ulceration is a multifactorial condition that essentially represents a mismatch between the acidic environment within the stomach and the protective features of the stomach lining.

Cause
- Nutritional factors are the primary cause: concentrated meals, high-starch diets and reduced roughage of horses in training create more acidic stomach environment than in free-living horses.
- Exercise also plays a role: reduced mucosal blood flow; also increased intra-abdominal pressure leads to greater bathing of the non-glandular lining with acidic stomach contents.
- Unlike in people, 'stress' and specific microorganisms (*Helicobacter* spp.) are not thought to be contributing factors.

Risk factors
- Occurs in majority of racehorses in training (up to 90% of horses in full work).
- Horses out of work (including broodmares) can also have ulcers.
- Prevalence of ulcers, and likelihood of more severe ulcers, increases with exercise intensity.
- Up to 10–15% of horses in race training have moderate to severe gastric ulceration.
- Frequent use of concentrated electrolyte pastes may contribute.
- Drugs such as phenylbutazone or suxibuzone do not cause ulcers when used at recommended dose rates.

Signs
- Most horses with ulcers exhibit no sign of the condition.
- Clinical signs (when present) are non-specific: include poor appetite, failure to thrive, weight loss, colic around mealtimes, poor performance or behavioural changes such as irritability or sourness.
- Onset of signs usually insidious and may coincide with increase in workload.

Diagnosis
- Clinical findings non-specific and cannot be relied on for diagnosis.
- Gastroscopy: required for definitive diagnosis and grading of severity. Restriction of food (8–16 hours) and water (2–4 hours) required to

empty stomach prior to examination. Severity graded on following scale:
- Normal (**Figure 6.1a**).
- Grade 1: mucosa intact but areas of reddening +/or hyperkeratosis (**Figure 6.1b**).
- Grade 2: small single or multifocal lesions (**Figure 6.1c**).
- Grade 3: large, single or multifocal, or extensive superficial lesions (**Figure 6.1d**).
- Grade 4: extensive lesions with areas of deep ulceration (**Figure 6.1e**).

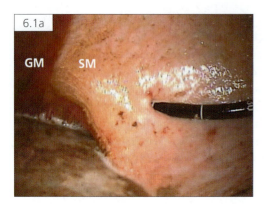

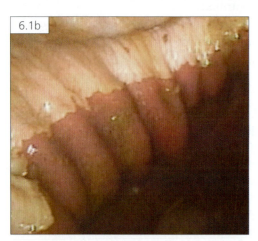

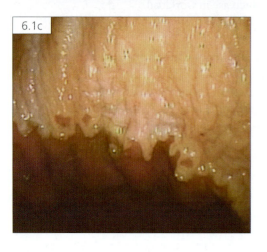

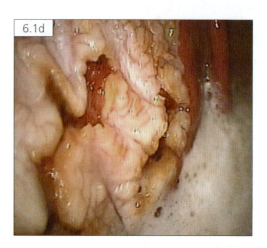

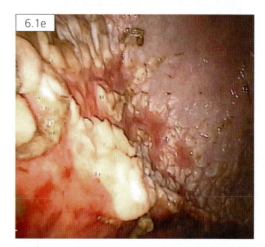

Fig. 6.1a–e (a) Normal appearance of gastric mucosa. Note the non-glandular/squamous (SM) and glandular (GM) mucosa. The endoscope is visible entering the stomach. (b) Gastric ulceration: grade 1. (c) Gastric ulceration: grade 2. (d) Gastric ulceration: grade 3. (e) Gastric ulceration: grade 4.

- Gastroscopy findings should be interpreted with caution and in context of clinical presentation. Poor correlation between clinical signs and severity; however, ulceration of grade 3 or 4 is generally considered significant.
- Blood profile is unaffected.
- Faecal occult blood detection of little/no use.

Management
- Some alteration of dietary management (provision of more hay; turnout/grazing) may be beneficial but is not curative, and return to low-starch/high-fibre diet is incompatible with intensive training.
- Alfalfa hay may be protective: high in calcium and protein and may buffer stomach acid.
- Medical treatment usually reserved for horses with both clinical signs and gastroscopic evidence of moderate–severe ulcers.
- Medical treatments/preventives need to be administered for duration of time that horse is in full training, with lapses only to permit racing free from metabolites (ulcers begin to recur within a few days off treatment).
- Treatment categories are shown in *Table 6.1*.

Prognosis
- Clinically significant ulcers, if untreated, can affect training by limiting frequency/intensity of fast work or racing (failure to maintain body condition).
- With appropriate treatment, body condition/other clinical features can be managed satisfactorily in majority of affected horses.

Table 6.1 **Gastric ulcer treatments**

TYPE	ACTION	DRUGS	EFFICACY
Inhibitors of acid production	Lower acidity of stomach by blocking production.	Omeprazole (proton pump inhibitor): the most potent licensed anti-ulcer drug. Once-daily oral dosing. Initial healing dose (4 mg/kg/BWT) for 2–4 weeks followed by maintenance dose of 2 mg/kg.	Good efficacy. Healing of ulcers occurs in 2–4 weeks (clinical effect usually more rapid).
		Ranitidine/cimetidine (histamine receptor antagonists). Require 2–3×/day oral dosing. Lengthy detection times in some jurisdictions restrict its usefulness.	Efficacy lower than omeprazole.
Antacids	Neutralize acid within the stomach.	Magnesium hydroxide/aluminium hydroxide are most common constituents.	Difficult to feed sufficient quantities to produce clinical effect; small amounts are non-therapeutic.
Mucosal protectants	Bond to exposed ulcer cavities and assist healing.	Sucralfate.	Assists healing but does not prevent ulcer formation.
		Lecithin/pectin.	Limited evidence to support use.

Colic

Colic is a general term for abdominal discomfort or pain (*Table 6.2*). There are many different causes of colic ranging from transient motility disorders ('spasmodic' colic) to strangulating torsions that lead to rupture or fatal shock unless corrected surgically. Most colic episodes are self-resolving or require only simple medical management; however, when part of the bowel becomes twisted and blood supply is compromised, deterioration can be swift. Infection, parasites and gastric ulceration can also cause abdominal pain. General points concerning the main forms of colic encountered in racehorses are as follows:

Risk factors
- Risk of colic is relatively low in well-managed racing yards (typical incidence of 5% per year).
- Main risk factors are abrupt changes in diet or management.
- Microbial population of hindgut plays a major role in digestion; sudden alterations in diet can cause shifts in bacterial population with resulting changes in acidity, gas production and gut motility.
- Racehorses on high-concentrate/low-forage diet and little access to grazing are to some degree already on a metabolic knife-edge.
- Windsuckers/crib biters at greater risk (association with altered gut transit time rather than swallowing of air).
- Tapeworm burdens associated with increased risk of spasmodic colic.
- Sudden restriction of exercise (stable rest), such as following injury, is associated with increased risk of colonic impaction colic.

Signs
- See *Table 6.2*.
- Typical signs: pawing ground, flank-watching, inappetence, recumbency +/– rolling, kicking belly, stretching to urinate, sweating.
- Severity highly variable, ranging from mild/intermittent discomfort to severe uncontrollable pain.
- Clinical parameters (pulse rate, demeanour, pain level, abdominal distension and gum colour/refill, gut sounds) are good indicators of severity.
- Should be differentiated from conditions that can present with similar signs: exertional rhabdomyolysis/pleuropneumonia/peritonitis.

Diagnosis
- Relevant history may assist diagnosis: recent management changes/current level of exercise/presence of normal faeces/previous episodes of colic.
- Typical pulse rate for mild/spasmodic colic 40–60 bpm; >60 bpm for colic possibly requiring hospitalization; and >80 bpm for horses with severe cardiovascular compromise requiring immediate hospitalization and supportive care or surgery.
- Rectal palpation (displacement/distension of abdominal organs) and nasogastric intubation (for gastric reflux) assist diagnosis. Transcutaneous abdominal ultrasound and peritoneal tap also useful.

Management
- (See *Table 6.2*).
- Pain is single most important factor in determining whether a colicking horse requires referral to a surgical facility.
- Short-acting pain control may be needed to conduct initial examination: alpha-2 agonists (xylazine/detomidine) potent and fast acting.
- Initial response to analgesics (typically phenylbutazone) +/– motility modifying medication (hyoscine butylbromide) determines management. Flunixin is used in some circumstances to differentiate need for surgical intervention, but it is a powerful and potentially masking analgesic and should be used with caution.
- Majority of cases (>90%) resolve with initial analgesic therapy +/– walking/lunging. Failure to manage pain with initial treatment indicates need for further investigation/treatment.
- High heart rate (>60 bpm) or severe/unremitting pain and deteriorating clinical signs warrants immediate transport to surgical facility; prognosis for survival declines considerably with elapsed time.

Table 6.2 **Classification of common types of racehorse colic**

TYPE	DESCRIPTION	TREATMENT	PROGNOSIS
'Spasmodic' colic	Most common form of colic; often at feeding times. Usually transient. Mild–moderate pain and gut sounds usually increased.	Spasmolytic and anti-inflammatory medication followed by short period of walking/lunging. May be fed/managed as normal following episode. Failure of initial medication/exercise to resolve pain warrants further investigation or referral.	Majority of episodes resolve with medical treatment/exercise.
Colonic (pelvic flexure) impaction	Natural hairpin bend in large colon is most common site of blockage; predisposed by narrowing of intestine at bend and local 'motility pacemaker' at pelvic flexure. Most common in horses recently confined to stable (e.g. following injury); may reflect change in intestinal motility or feed intake. Low-grade intermittent discomfort (scraping, lying quietly) over several hours few/hard faeces. Diagnosis simple with rectal palpation: impaction readily palpable (but not accessible with enemas).	Nasogastric tubing with water mineral oil (2–4 litres) magnesium sulphate (0.5–1 g/kg) to hydrate and lubricate gut contents. Restrict feed and hay until impaction cleared. Resume light exercise if feasible. Frequency of nasogastric tubing determined by size/severity of impaction: most simple cases resolve with one or two treatments.	Average clearance time 2 days; small proportion require hospitalization for intensive management or surgical intervention.
Surgical colic	Continuing signs of pain deteriorating clinical parameters (high pulse rate) in the face of initial medication warrant referral to surgical facility. Types of colic requiring hospitalization include large colon displacements (some may be managed medically), large colon volvulus/torsion and small intestinal strangulations or impactions.	Treatment determined by lesion type.	Prognosis best with early intervention. Short-term survival (to hospital discharge) 70–85%. Survival rates lower for strangulating lesions than for simple obstructions and lower for small intestinal or caecal involvement than for large or small colon involvement. Once through immediate post-surgery period, prognosis for long-term survival (1 year) is good: around 85%. Approximately 10% of horses require second colic surgery during hospitalization, and long-term survival for these horses is low (around 20%). Most (80%) horses that survive surgery return to full use; typically require 2–3 months out of ridden exercise following surgery.
Recurrent colic	Repeated episodes of colic (over weeks/months) warrant further investigation. Determine whether pattern exists (i.e. at times of increased stress or anticipation of feeding). Medical investigations include determining parasite burden (worm egg count/tapeworm serology), presence of gastric ulcers and haematology/biochemistry. High incidence of colic within a yard may indicate nutrition/feeding problem.	Identify cause/risk factor: modification of management may resolve problem. Specific medical treatment as required.	Prognosis dependent on diagnosis.

Prognosis
- See *Table 6.2*.

Parasites
Although horses in training generally have limited access to pasture, intestinal parasite burdens occur and in some circumstances can cause weight loss, colic or intestinal upsets. The major types of parasites are detailed in *Table 6.3*.

Diagnosis
- Adult parasites (roundworms and strongyles) are occasionally noted in faeces but this is a poor method of detection of worm burden.
- Diagnosis of strongyle or roundworm burden requires faecal analysis for presence of eggs.
- Positive faecal egg count (FEC) confirms presence of laying adult females, but of no value in detecting presence of larval stages (encysted or otherwise).
- Tapeworms: faecal analysis of little use due to intermittent shedding of eggs; diagnosis through serum antibody levels. Antibody levels remain detectable for up to 5 months post deworming and false positives occur.
- Blood sampling (haematology/biochemistry): poor method of detection of worm burden; larval cyathostomes sometimes associated with low plasma protein; relevance of eosinophil count unknown.

Management
- Widespread use of dewormers has resulted in genetic selection for parasites resistant to certain drug classes. No evidence that rotation of dewormer drug class prevents development of resistance.
- Most dewormers are broad spectrum but none have 100% efficacy.
- Majority of adult horses in training have only small parasite burdens; a small proportion of horses are responsible for the majority of worm egg shedding.
- Larger worm burdens more likely to be associated with clinical disease.
- Goal of parasite control programme is to identify and selectively treat horses with significant burdens to minimize shedding, while reducing reliance on dewormers.
- FECs to identify 'shedders': categorize into low (<200 eggs per gram [epg]), moderate and high FECs.
- General rule: strategic treatment of all horses in autumn and/or spring with broad-spectrum dewormer effective against strongyles and tapeworms. Additional treatments through spring/summer as required based on faecal sampling (and only for horses with FEC >200 epg).
- Avoiding unnecessary treatment of horses with a low (<200 epg) FEC helps maintain a 'drug susceptible' population of worms and limits development of dewormer resistance.
- Treatment intervals: usually based on 'egg re-appearance period' of each drug class: benzimidazoles (fenbendazole) 4 weeks; macrocyclic lactones (ivermectin/moxidectin) 6–12 weeks; tetrahydropyrimidines (pyrantel) 4 weeks.
- If treatment of encysted small strongyles desired: fenbendazole (10 mg/kg for 5 days) or moxidectin.
- Regular (twice weekly) removal of faeces from communal grazing areas to prevent contamination of pasture.

Diarrhoea
Diarrhoea is usually the result of colonic dysfunction and may arise from several different causative agents. Mild, self-limiting diarrhoea without systemic illness is common in racing yards and generally requires no intervention. Much rarer is severe diarrhoea associated with systemic illness or chronic diarrhoea associated with weight loss; infectious or parasitic disease may be responsible and hospitalization is sometimes necessary.

Diarrhoea is usually associated with abnormally rapid transit of food through the large intestine; this limits reabsorption of water/electrolytes and digestion of fibre. Large fluid losses can occur, leading rapidly to dehydration unless replenished.

Table 6.3 **Major types of gastrointestinal parasites in horses**

TYPE	SOURCE OF INFECTION	LIFE CYCLE	EFFECTS
Small strongyles (cyathostomes)	Grazing	Adults live in large intestine and eggs passed in faeces. Larvae develop on pasture; when ingested, burrow into large intestine wall ('encysted' larvae); emerge later into large intestine as adults. Common.	Seasonal emergence of large numbers of dormant larvae from intestinal wall can cause severe diarrhoea and weight loss, particularly in young horses.
Large strongyles	Grazing	2–5 cm long red worm. Adults live in large intestine and eggs passed in faeces. Larvae develop on pasture; when ingested penetrate intestine wall and migrate through blood vessels or to liver, returning to large intestine to become adults. Rare.	Feeding and migration of larvae can cause damage to small intestinal mucosa (anaemia, weight loss), blood vessels (thrombosis/colic) or other organs (liver damage/peritonitis).
Roundworms (ascarids)	Grazing	Large white worm. Adults live in small intestine and eggs passed in faeces. When ingested, larvae penetrate intestinal wall then migrate to liver and lungs. Larvae coughed up, swallowed and develop into adults in small intestine. Common.	Large numbers of worms may cause obstructions and poor growth in foals, which have low resistance. Mature horses show few signs.
Tapeworms	Ingestion of forage mites in hay/bedding/grazing	Adults live near caecum (ileocaecal valve) or small intestine/stomach. Segments full of eggs shed and ingested by intermediate host (forage mite), in which development to larvae occurs. Ingestion of forage mites (and larvae) by horse. Common.	May cause colic (spasmodic and ileal impaction).
Pinworms	Ingestion of faecal-contaminated feed/water	Adults live in colon/rectum and emerge to lay eggs around anus. Eggs stimulate irritation/tail-rubbing and larvae are ingested directly or through contaminated feed/water. Common.	Tail-rubbing.

Cause
- Transient loose faeces/mild diarrhoea: may arise from altered fermentation in large intestine due to change in diet (or poor adaptation to high-carbohydrate/low-fibre ration).
- Antibiotic-associated diarrhoea: normal balance of microflora in hindgut may be disrupted by antibiotic therapy, leading to superinfection with pathogens. Antibiotics associated with greatest risk vary with geographical region: penicillin/gentamicin, enrofloxacin, doxycycline and ceftiofur implicated on occasion. Risk greatest in horses under stress or with change of antibiotic class during treatment. Occurs in approximately 0.6% of horses in general population treated with antibiotics.
- Acute severe diarrhoea +/− systemic illness: may arise from infectious microbes (*Salmonella, Clostridium difficile/perfringens, Neorickettsia*).
- Chronic persistent diarrhoea (with weight loss): may arise from parasitic (small strongyles) or infiltrative (inflammatory or neoplastic) disease.

Signs
- Diarrhoea: severity varies from loose faeces to projectile diarrhoea.
- +/− depression/inappetence.
- +/− fever.
- Rarely, may exhibit mild colic at onset or just prior to breaking with diarrhoea.
- Clinical assessment can be reasonable guide to dehydration and the need for fluid replacement: raised pulse rate/delayed capillary refill time/dullness/reduced urine output indicate >5% dehydration.

Diagnosis
- Clinical severity and history guide diagnostic efforts.
- Mild diarrhoea/no systemic illness: further investigation generally not required.
- Moderate diarrhoea +/– mild–illness (inappetence/colic): blood analysis to determine well-being and hydration status.
- Severe diarrhoea/suspected infectious cause: multiple (3–5) faecal cultures or PCR for attempted detection of infectious microbes +/– immunoassay for clostridial toxins.
- Chronic/wasting diarrhoea: hospital-based investigation for parasitic/infiltrative disease.

Management
- Usually necessary to make treatment decisions without benefit of knowing underlying cause.
- Fluid/electrolyte imbalances (dehydration) and absorption of bacterial toxins can occur rapidly.
- Goals of treatment: replace fluid and electrolyte losses, reduce systemic and intestinal inflammation, re-establish normal intestinal function.
- Probiotics: efficacy doubtful, and considerable variability in quality between products.
- Mild diarrhoea in otherwise healthy horse: usually self-limiting and requires no treatment; address nutrition if thought to be a contributing factor.
- Moderate diarrhoea without dehydration: anti-diarrhoeal treatment warranted: clay/smectite (mucosal protectant) +/– bismuth subsalicylate by nasogastric tube (as required but up to 4×/day).
- Mild–moderate dehydration: replacement with isotonic fluids (by nasogastric intubation providing small intestine is motile).
- Severe diarrhoea +/– systemic illness: life-threatening condition requiring hospitalization and immediate supportive care (large-volume intravenous fluids/anti-endotoxic therapy/gastrointestinal protectants).
- Antibiotic therapy generally contraindicated other than in severe cases with suspected/confirmed clostridial/*Salmonella* infections; choice of drug dependent on diagnostic findings.
- Biosecurity measures if infectious disease suspected.

Prognosis
- Mild diarrhoea is usually transient and does not interfere with training.
- Severe acute diarrhoea requiring hospitalization associated with high cost of treatment and guarded prognosis for life.
- Antimicrobial-associated diarrhoea: high (approximately 20%) mortality rate due to systemic endotoxaemia or laminitis.
- Survivors have good chance of returning to training but often require lengthy convalescence due to debilitation.
- Chronic/wasting diarrhoea: prognosis dependent on underlying disease. Parasitic disease usually responds to therapy; neoplastic infiltrative disease has poor prognosis.

Oesophageal obstruction ('choke')
Acute obstruction of the oesophagus with food. Breathing is not affected. Potential for backing up of food/saliva with spillover into windpipe. Potential complications include secondary pneumonia and (rarely) oesophageal perforation or stricture.

Cause
- Usually caused by a food bolus that has been incompletely chewed or bolted quickly.

Risk factors
- Any age/stage of training.
- Most commonly occurs after post-race feed.
- Dental abnormalities (oral pain due to loose premolar cap/fractured tooth/sharp overgrowth) may inhibit normal mastication.

Signs
- Obstruction noted during/immediately after feeding.
- Typically present with acute discomfort, coughing, stretching of neck and presence of food-flecked saliva at one or both nostrils.
- Intermittent reflexive spasm/stiffening of neck.

Diagnosis
- Clinical findings definitive.

Management
- May resolve without treatment.
- Potential for development of pneumonia if food material enters lungs; warrants immediate veterinary attention.
- Withhold food and water until obstruction cleared.
- Nasogastric tubing and gentle/repeated lavage of obstruction by stomach pump while under heavy sedation (to lower head).
- Antispasmodic medication (hyoscine butylbromide) frequently used to assist clearance, but efficacy doubtful. Oxytocin may reduce oesophageal muscle tone.
- If choke has been present for some hours, prophylactic antibiotic medication should be considered and horse monitored in following days for signs of pneumonia (fever/coughing).

Prognosis
- Good; once obstruction cleared can be managed as normal.
- If horse suffers from repeated episodes, investigation of underlying cause (feeding/management/dental pathology) warranted.
- Rarely, damage to mucosa may result in oesophageal stricture.

CHAPTER 7
UROGENITAL CONDITIONS

URINARY TRACT PROBLEMS

Urinary tract problems are rare in horses in training.

Polyuria/polydipsia
- Normal maintenance water requirements for a horse in training vary according to workload, diet and climate but typically 60–70 ml/kg BWT/day (around 30 litres/day).
- Detailed history and measurement of daily water intake may assist investigation of excessive drinking/urination.
- Blood analysis, including biochemistry (blood urea nitrogen, creatinine and glucose concentrations), and urinalysis (specific gravity and presence of glucose/protein) generally permit differentiation of urinary tract disease from non-renal causes (psychogenic polydipsia).
- Excessive drinking +/– urination in healthy racehorses most commonly due to 'psychogenic polydipsia', a form of stable vice. Can also arise from high dietary protein or salt, or administration of corticosteroids or diuretics.
- Psychogenic polydipsia: only abnormality is low urine specific gravity (<1.005).
- Water deprivation testing can also be undertaken to determine whether horse is capable of concentrating urine; should not be used if evidence of renal insufficiency on blood analysis.
- Treatment of psychogenic polydipsia: restriction of water to maintenance requirements and improving level of stimulation in the stable environment.

Urinary tract infections
- Urinary tract infections very rare in young racehorses.
- May occur secondary to urinary obstruction (bladder stones/sediment).
- Can affect lower (urethra/bladder) or upper (kidney) urinary tract.
- Lower urinary tract signs: include straining to urinate, frequent small-volume urination, urine scalding.
- Upper urinary tract signs: include weight loss, fever, mild colic.
- Diagnosis: mid-stream urine sample (cytology/culture), ultrasonography, endoscopy.
- Treatment: antibiotic medication, guided by bacteriological results.

FEMALE REPRODUCTIVE SYSTEM

The oestrous cycle
Overview
- Fillies and mares are seasonally polyoestrus, with reproductive inactivity through winter and regular oestrous cycles through summer (largely brought about by increasing day length).
- Cycle length (ovulation to ovulation) is typically 21–22 days.
- 'Oestrus' ('heat'/'season'; period of sexually receptive behaviour): typically lasts 5–7 days and coincides with development of an ovarian follicle, which produces oestrogen.
- Ovulation (release of a mature egg from the follicle) occurs in the last 24–48 hours of the heat period.
- By day 6 after ovulation the follicular remnant becomes the corpus luteum.
- 'Dioestrus': progesterone produced by the corpus luteum dominates for the next 14–15 days: 'heat' behaviour is absent.

- If not pregnant, corpus luteum lysed by prostaglandin and cycle repeats.
- Progesterone level in luteal phase >1.0 ng/ml and during oestrus <1.0 ng/ml.

Transitional cycles
- 'Transitional' phases occur between dormant winter phase (anoestrus) and active summer cycling.
- Irregular pattern of heat periods during transitional phase is common.
- Spring transitional phase: several non-ovulatory waves of follicular development.
- Onset of transitional phase is stimulated by increasing day length.
- Failure to commence regular heat period may warrant further investigation.

Managing oestrus

Signs of being in season (oestrus) vary widely between individuals. In most fillies some degree of receptive behaviour is noted but daily management is not affected. A small proportion may be so dominated by the hormonal effects of the heat period that receptive behaviour overrides other activity, thereby interfering with training or racing. It may be desirable to manage oestrus in these circumstances. There is little evidence that the fluctuations of reproductive hormones that occur over the oestrous cycle have any effect on athletic performance (other than behavioural).

Transitional oestrus
- Self-limiting condition (see Transitional cycles, above), usually requires no intervention.
- Acceleration of transitional phase (by stimulation of the first ovulation of the year) often best achieved by daily oral administration of a synthetic progestin (altrenogest) for 8–15 days +/– single administration of a prostaglandin at end of treatment. Ovulation usually occurs within 15 days of end of treatment.
- Use of gonadotropin–releasing hormone (GnRH) analogue subcutaneous implant (deslorelin) may hasten ovulation.

Control/suppression of oestrus
Oestrus control is achieved either through timing of ovulation to ensure oestrus does not coincide with a particular race target, or suppression of oestrous behaviour altogether. Suppression is generally achieved through administration of exogenous progesterone or by extension of corpus luteum activity ('pseudopregnancy'). There is no single technique with complete efficacy and method of choice will depend on individual circumstances:
- Altrenogest: daily oral administration keeps filly in dioestrus. Oestrus occurs 5–10 days after end of treatment. Rarely used long term due to expense, although no detrimental effects on behaviour or BWT. Withdrawal of drug requires planning to ensure subsequent oestrus does not coincide with race day.
- Oxytocin: administration of exogenous oxytocin during dioestrus can interfere with luteolysis and prolong corpus luteum activity. Daily IM injections (60 IU) from days 7 to 14 after ovulation may suppress oestrus for 2–3 months. Requires reproductive assessment to determine exact day of ovulation, but good efficacy (60–70%) and reversible if desired.
- Intrauterine methods: implantation of spherical device (e.g. marble) at ovulation may result in prolonged dioestrus (average 2 months). Low success rate. Intrauterine delivery of plant oil (coconut/peanut oil) on day 10 post ovulation has similar effect but in need of further validation.
- Immunocontraceptive vaccine: long-term (3 to >6 months) suppression of oestrus possible following two-dose protocol of GnRH analogue vaccine (antibody response to GnRH). Safe and efficacious but rarely used as not recommended for use in fillies with breeding future.

Pregnancy and racing

Racing is generally permissible up to 120 days of pregnancy. The primary consideration regarding pregnancy is the effect of intense exercise on fetal health; however, the effect of pregnancy on athletic performance is also of interest:

- Effects of exercise on fetal health have been little researched in horses; however, in people, high levels of fitness to late term are possible with no adverse effect on maternal/fetal well-being.
- Training/racing the pregnant filly is safe; however, attention should be paid to administration of any drugs that may have effects on pregnancy/fetus. Risk of intra-articular corticosteroids unquantified but likely to be negligible with appropriate dosing.
- Effects of pregnancy on performance have not been investigated in horses.
- Considerable physiological changes occur during pregnancy but these are poorly understood in racehorses: include increased blood volume and cardiac output.
- Evidence from human athletes is ambiguous; however, aerobic power appears to be maintained well in pregnancy and may even be enhanced; some evidence that anaerobic work capacity diminishes in late term.

Mastitis

Infection of the mammary gland. Usually affects only one side of the udder; each teat is fed by a pair of mammary glands.

Cause
- Increased mammary serum production caused by high oestrogen levels may predispose to infection.
- Cyclical or seasonal factors usually responsible; however, high levels of exogenous (plant or fungal) oestrogens sometimes found in hay/haylage.
- Serum leaking may permit secondary bacterial colonization: aerobic bacteria (usually *Streptococcus zooepidemicus*) generally responsible.

Risk factors
- Rare condition.
- Occurs in fillies in and out of training.
- Risk factors not known.

Signs
- Onset usually acute.
- Painful enlargement of affected gland/s +/– oedematous filling running forward from udder along belly (**Figure 7.1**).
- +/– hindlimb stiffness/lameness.
- +/– fever.

Management
- Systemic antibiotic medication (oxytetracycline/penicillin).
- Stripping out affected teat on one or more occasions may assist resolution.
- Continued ridden exercise usually possible.

Prognosis
- Excellent: rapid response to antibiotic therapy is typical and interruption to training minimal.

Pneumovagina/urovagina

'Windsucking' of air (pneumovagina) and pooling of urine in the vagina (urovagina) are separate conditions that may be encountered in fillies in training and occasionally require intervention. Pneumovagina causes a vaginal sucking/gurgling noise during exercise. Both pneumovagina and urovagina may be associated with a secondary vaginitis/vaginal discharge and occasionally irritability and discomfort is observed.

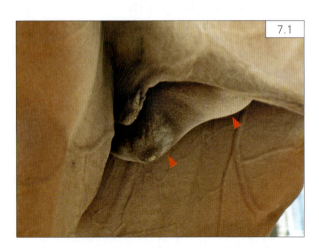

Fig. 7.1 Enlarged left teat with associated oedema (arrowheads) typical of mastitis.

Cause
- Pneumovagina: the vaginal lips and internal vestibular sphincter act as seals against aspiration of air into the reproductive tract. The vaginal seal may be compromised or more readily breached in fillies with light body condition (lack of perineal fat) or poor vulvar conformation; movement at exercise disrupts the weakened seal, allowing the vagina to fill with air.
- Urovagina: downward cranial slope of vagina or poor vestibular/vulvar conformation can lead to incomplete voiding of urine. Pooling of urine within vagina may cause inflammation and vaginal discharge.

Management
- Pneumovagina: surgical closure of the upper vaginal lips (Caslick's vulvoplasty), leaving sufficient opening for urination.
- Urovagina: if urine pooling is suspected to be secondary to a previous Caslick's, vulva should be re-opened. If due to conformation/condition, specialist surgical intervention is the only treatment: rarely warranted in fillies in training.

Prognosis
- Rarely interfere with training.
- Secondary infection associated with both conditions may have implications for fertility.

Contagious equine metritis
See Chapter 11, Infectious diseases.

MALE REPRODUCTIVE SYSTEM

Castration
Techniques
Castration may be performed as an open (non-sterile) surgical procedure under standing sedation, or under GA using either the same surgical approach or an aseptic sutured technique. The benefits of standing castration are lower cost and lower risk of serious complications, while aseptic sutured castration under GA offers lower risk of interruption to training due to post-surgical infection.

Management
- Standing castration: large surgical incisions, prophylactic antibiotic/anti-inflammatory medication and early return to ridden exercise (trotting/light cantering resuming within 2–5 days) reduce risk of postoperative swelling/infection. Daily cleansing of scrotum +/− greasing of hindlimbs to prevent scalding.
- Sutured (GA) castration: 1 week of walking prior to resumption of ridden exercise. No/little wound care required.
- Fertility may persist for up to 6 weeks post castration.
- Behavioural changes may not be observed for weeks/months depending on prior temperament and age at castration.

Complications (Table 7.1)
- Standing castration: approximately 20% of horses require some treatment for postoperative swelling or infection. Risk of serious complication (death/eventration of intestine) very low regardless of age.
- GA castration: risk of minor complications (infection, swelling) much lower than standing castration; however, risk of death (arising from GA) is 0.05–1%.

Cryptorchids ('rigs')
Cryptorchidism is a failure (partial or total) of one or both testicles to descend into the scrotum. The retained testicle is typically much smaller than the external testicle. Usually only one testicle is affected. Affected testicle is more likely to be intra-abdominal if left-sided than if right-sided. Bilateral cryptorchids and monorchids (one testicle completely absent) are very rare.

Cause
- Testes develop within abdomen of fetus and are programmed to migrate from their origin near each kidney through the internal and external vaginal rings of the abdominal wall to the scrotal sac.
- Migration guided by structure known as the gubernaculum and subject to hormonal control.

Table 7.1 **Complications associated with castration**

COMPLICATION	DESCRIPTION	TREATMENT	PROGNOSIS
Post-castration haemorrhage	Minor bleeding is common in hours following open castration. Persistent and profuse bleeding is rare and is usually result of incomplete crushing of testicular artery.	Bleeding usually minor and of no concern. If drips/small stream, no treatment required but restrict exercise until stabilized. Profuse bleeding: administration of acepromazine may decrease severity. Persistent profuse bleeding: clamp cord leaving forceps in place for 24–36 hours; if unsuccessful, exploration under GA or standing laparoscopy may be required (very rare).	Good. Intervention rarely required.
Post-castration swelling	Minor swelling around scrotum/sheath common in days following standing castration.	Swelling of sheath (prepuce) indicative of insufficient daily exercise.	Resolves with exercise.
Eventration	Abdominal cavity and scrotum communicate; creates potential for intra-abdominal contents to herniate through surgical wound. Very rare. May involve small intestine or omentum. Usually within 4 hours of surgery.	Prolapsed omentum: transect under standing sedation. Eventration of small intestine: surgical emergency, requires cleaning/protection of exposed intestine and immediate surgical referral.	Excellent survival rates (>85%) for small intestinal eventration with appropriate management.
Infection	Swelling of one/both sides of scrotum at 1–2 weeks following open castration is common; usually coincides with incision healing and subsequent lack of drainage. Painful scrotal/inguinal thickening +/– fever +/– hindlimb lameness or stiffness.	Systemic antibiotic +/– anti-inflammatory therapy (to effect). Re-establish drainage +/– flushing scrotal wound (antiseptic solution) as required.	Most cases resolve within 1–2 weeks of treatment. Very rarely, infection of spermatic cord non-responsive to medical therapy (funiculitis) can develop over months and necessitate surgical removal of infected stump.
Infection (peritonitis)	Self-limiting (5–7 days) non-septic peritonitis is common after open castration and requires no treatment. Septic peritonitis is rare: recurrent pyrexia/colic/weight loss/diarrhoea in weeks following castration.	Broad-spectrum antibiotic +/– anti-inflammatory therapy +/– hospitalization.	Good with appropriate management.

- Final descent of testes into scrotum occurs either just prior to, or in days after, birth.
- Failure of descent can result in testicle being retained anywhere along migratory path, from fully intra-abdominal (usually near body wall) to within inguinal canal.
- Cryptorchids ('rigs') classified as abdominal, incomplete abdominal or inguinal.

Risk factors
- Genetic factors thought to play a role, but direct heritability unlikely in most cases.

Effects
- Abdominal testicles are generally sterile but produce testosterone.
- Cryptorchids display normal colt behaviour.

- Retained testicle almost never responsible for lameness/gait abnormality (although frequently blamed).

Diagnosis
- Diagnosis based on clinical evaluation and history is usually sufficient.
- Thorough examination may require sedation; if inguinal, the high testicle may be partially palpable.
- Further confirmation may be required for surgical planning (or when possibility of previous hemicastration exists); passport should be checked for declaration of previous surgery.
- Transabdominal ultrasonography: high sensitivity and specificity for detection of both abdominal and inguinal testes.
- Blood hormonal assays: serum oestrone sulphate (high sensitivity for retained testicular tissue in horses >3 YO); stimulation of testosterone production by administration of human chorionic gonadotropin (hCG) (blood samples before and 1 and 24 hours after IV injection of 6,000 IU hCG) highly sensitive for the detection of testicular tissue but not in young horses (<18 months of age) or during winter.

Management
- Of little concern for training aside from planning for appropriate castration technique.
- Full descent of testicles occurs within weeks of birth in most normal horses; however, descent of an inguinally located cryptorchid testicle may occasionally occur in young adult life (yearling to 2 YO).
- Determining likelihood of full descent of retained testicle is not possible.
- Hormonal treatment (hCG) to assist descent of inguinal testes has low efficacy.
- Castration technique determined by location of retained testicle: inguinal or scrotal surgical approaches under GA, or standing laparoscopic removal (if abdominal).

INTERSEX DISORDERS

Disorders of sexual development are very rare but may be encountered during investigations into infertility or aberrant testosterone levels. Sex differentiation is a complex process that begins with chromosomal make-up (determined at fertilization). Gonadal development and subsequent hormonal production then contribute to the external characteristics of sex such as body type, bone mass and behaviour. Genital development has a natural tendency towards female differentiation in the absence of testosterone, with masculinization being an active process requiring both testosterone production and tissue sensitivity to it.

Developmental abnormalities can occur at any stage of this process, therefore a great variety of intersex conditions exist. Affected horses may be outwardly normal but sterile/subfertile, have ambiguous or under-developed internal sexual organs or external genitalia, or display inappropriate behaviour. Diagnosis may sometimes be presumptive based on clinical findings and blood levels of reproductive hormones, but definitive diagnosis often requires exhaustive genetic analysis. The heritability of various forms of the intersex condition has been poorly investigated; however, both recessive and sex-limited dominant transmission are recognized.

The key considerations regarding intersex disorders are gender assignment to satisfy the concerns of racing regulatory bodies and determination of fertility status in the case of horses intended for breeding. Once racing authorities have been made aware of the ambiguous sex status of a racehorse, restrictions may be imposed on the type of races the horse in question is permitted to enter. This is usually done on an individual basis and approach may vary between jurisdictions. Classification as male or female in many affected animals is far from simple; human sporting bodies have moved away from arbitrary categorization based on chromosome analysis to a system that takes into account hormonal effects and external phenotype.

CHAPTER 8
NEUROLOGICAL CONDITIONS

VERTEBRAL COLUMN CONDITIONS

'Wobbler' syndrome (cervical stenotic myelopathy, cervical vertebral malformation)

'Wobbler' syndrome is a syndrome in which malformation or instability of the cervical vertebral column leads to compression of the spinal cord, causing neurological gait deficits of varying severity.

Impingement on the cord may be constant (static) or may worsen with changes in head/neck position (dynamic). Sites most commonly affected are C3–C5 for dynamic compression and C5–C7 for static compression, although generalized narrowing of the canal is usually present regardless of the actual lesion location.

The peripheral location of nerve tracts involved in voluntary control of skeletal muscle means that upper motor neuron signs (incoordination, weakness +/− spasticity) define the syndrome. Because of the more superficial location of nerve tracts servicing the hindlimbs they are usually more severely affected than the forelimbs.

Cause
- Developmental condition.
- Probably result of both genetic and nutritional factors, with rapid growth, high energy intake and micronutrient imbalances leading to disease in some genetically susceptible horses.
- Patterns of heritability thought to be complex.
- Compression of spinal cord can occur through generalized narrowing of spinal canal or malformation/malalignment of certain vertebrae.
- In older horses, static compression may arise from arthritis of APJs in neck base, with bony impingement through the intervertebral space.

Risk factors
- Prevalence in young Thoroughbred population estimated at 0.5–2%.
- More common in males than females (3:1).
- Large, rapidly growing individuals appear at greatest risk; growth plate enlargement and developmental orthopaedic disease implicated.

History
- Onset of signs usually occurs between 6 months and 3 YO and is typically insidious.
- Acute-onset disease; signs that fluctuate in severity are also encountered.
- Riders may raise concern about stumbling, poor action or lack of hindlimb propulsion.

Signs
- Incoordination (ataxia, *Table 8.1*) and postural muscle weakness (paresis) are main presenting signs: may walk as though sedated ('truncal sway').
- Cranial nerve function and mental status are normal.

Table 8.1 **Grading of ataxia**

GRADE	SIGNS
0	Normal
1	Minimal neurological deficits noted with normal gaits; requires manipulative tests for detection
2	Mild deficits noted at walk; obvious response to manipulative tests
3	Readily apparent at walk
4	Very ataxic; may fall if turned tightly or backed
5	Recumbent

- Ataxia is usually of greater severity in hindlimbs than forelimbs.
- When turned in tight circles: exaggerated circumduction of outer hindlimb +/− interference or crossing over of hindlimbs.
- When backed up: dragging of hindlimbs and weakness.
- When walked forward with head elevated (particularly downhill): spasticity in all limbs +/− dragging of forelimbs.
- When walked forward and tail pulled each side: lateral weakness and overcorrection on release.
- +/− loss of tail tone.

Diagnosis
- Presumptive diagnosis usually based on clinical findings and radiography.
- Definitive diagnosis may require advanced imaging (contrast myelogram/MRI/CT) under GA and is sometimes only possible post mortem.
- Radiography: flare of caudal physis ('ski jump')/caudal extension of dorsal lamina/vertebral malalignment most useful for diagnosis (**Figures 8.1, 8.2**). Caution when interpreting neckbase arthropathy, as common in normal horses.
- Radiography: measurement of intravertebral sagittal ratio (ratio of minimum sagittal diameter of canal to width of corresponding vertebral body) allows assessment of vertebral canal stenosis (**Figure 8.3**). Ratio ≤50% of any vertebra from C4–C6 (≤56% at C7) is strongly linked to disease, although operator variation is in the order of 5–10%.

Management
- Horses with ataxia graded ≥2 are generally considered to be unsafe to ride and may require care in handling, especially when sedated.
- Euthanasia may be considered in moderately/severely affected horses; insurance status may necessitate interim period of conservative management prior to final assessment.
- Conservative management may stabilize condition: stable rest (4–8 weeks), dietary changes and anti-inflammatory (corticosteroid) medication. Improvement in neurological signs may result but complete recovery sufficient to resume training is uncommon.

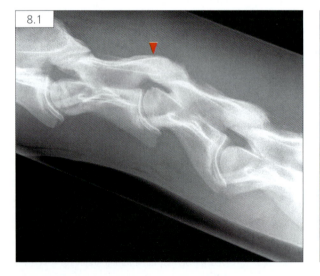

Fig. 8.1 Radiograph (laterolateral) showing vertebral malalignment (arrowhead) at C3/C4.

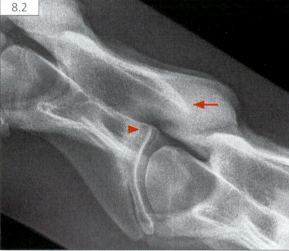

Fig. 8.2 Radiograph (laterolateral) showing caudal extension of dorsal lamina (arrow) and flare of caudal physis (arrowhead) at C4/C5.

- Dietary management aimed at slowing growth while maintaining balance of key nutrients: restriction of energy and protein intakes to 75% of National Research Council (U.S.) Committee on Animal Nutrition recommendations (+/− supplementation with vitamins A, E); low carbohydrate (CHO) diet.
- Surgery (fusion of adjacent vertebrae at affected sites) may be considered for valuable individuals and can result in return to athletic use. Lengthy recuperation (6–12 months), frequently incomplete recovery (by 1–2 neurological grades) and concerns over ethical aspects of breeding from affected horses mean that surgical intervention is rare in racehorses.

Prognosis
- Prognosis for racing generally considered to be poor.
- Up to 30% of horses with milder grades (1–2) of ataxia may race following conservative/medical management.
- Surgery: majority of horses improve by 1–2 grades; return to athletic use is more likely in horses with dynamic compression and those in which clinical signs were only present for <1 month.

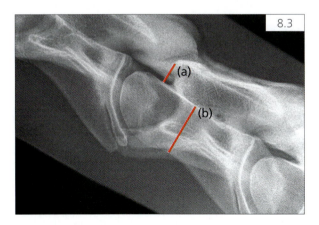

Fig. 8.3 Measurements used for intravertebral sagittal diameter ratio: minimum intravertebral diameter (a) and vertebral body width (b).

VIRAL INFECTIONS

Equine herpesvirus-1 myeloencephalopathy

Equine herpesvirus (EHV)-1 is endemic throughout horse populations worldwide and most horses are exposed at some point early in life and become latent carriers. The virus most frequently causes respiratory disease but occasionally is associated with neurological signs. Outbreaks of ataxia and weakness caused by the neurological form of EHV-1 are rare but occur sporadically in racing yards. Severely affected horses may become recumbent and require euthanasia, and disruption to yard operations is inevitable due to movement restrictions until spread of disease has been controlled.

Cause
- Neurotropic strain of EHV-1 causes vasculitis in the CNS with resulting widespread ischaemic necrosis of neural tissue.
- Non-neurotropic strains can also cause myeloencephalopathy (less common).
- Patient factors, including immune status and stress, may play a role in development of disease but poorly understood.

Risk factors
- Usually adult horses; any stage of training.
- Previous vaccination for EHV-1/4 does not currently preclude development of neurological disease.

History
- Acute-onset ataxia.
- Recent respiratory disease (within past 1–2 weeks) in affected individual or yard is frequently reported.

Signs
- +/− initial fever, followed within 7 days by neurological signs in some horses.
- Ataxia +/− paresis; usually symmetrical and affects hindlimbs to greater extent (may 'dog-sit').
- +/− urinary incontinence (bladder paralysis).
- Ataxia may be transient or progress to recumbency.

- Respiratory disease and limb oedema may be noted in larger population at time of outbreak.

Diagnosis
- Virus isolation (nasopharyngeal swabs/blood sample); also PCR and seroconversion (≥4-fold increase in titre in samples 10–20 days apart).

Management
- In case of neurological EHV: strict adherence to statutory requirements and current recommendations from regulatory bodies including isolation of premises.
- Monitoring rectal temperature twice daily in all in-contact horses, with further testing for horses that develop fever.
- Avoid stress/strenuous exercise in at-risk horses until disease status known.
- Movement restrictions for 1 month; lifting of restrictions only when either serological monitoring determines no further activity within at-risk group or >14 days from onset of signs in last clinical case.
- Initial 1–3 days: dexamethasone +/− NSAID +/− antiviral (nucleoside analogues [e.g. valacyclovir]) medication.
- Vaccination of at-risk horses in the face of an outbreak carries risk of potentiating neurological form of disease and should be avoided.
- No current vaccines prevent the neurological form of the disease; however, some evidence that virus shedding (and therefore severity of outbreak) may be lower in vaccinated yards.

Prognosis
- Ataxic horses that remain ambulatory have good prognosis for return to full function but may take months.
- Recumbency >24 hours is poor prognostic indicator but intensive supportive care of recumbent horses generally rewarded with partial recovery (guarded prognosis for return to athletic use).
- Mortality 5–30%.
- Horses recovered from neurological EHV do not appear to pose any greater risk of future infection to susceptible populations.

Equine protozoal myeloencephalitis

Equine protozoal myeloencephalitis (EPM) is a neurological disease caused by a protozoal parasite (primarily *Sarcocystis neurona*; less commonly *Neospora hughesi*). Disease is currently restricted to horses living in or originating from the Americas (geographical limit of parasite).

Cause
- Parasitic life cycle and means of transmission not completely understood.
- Definitive host of *Sarcocystis neurona* is the opossum.
- Oocysts are passed in opossum faeces and the infective stage may contaminate feed or water.
- Birds, insects and other vectors may act to disseminate the parasite.
- Horse (along with other mammals) is a 'dead-end' host in which the parasite does not replicate but rather may cause disease during its colonization.
- Following ingestion, parasite passes from gastrointestinal tract to bloodstream then eventually localizes in CNS.
- Many factors involved in development of clinical disease including stress at/after infection, number of parasites ingested and location within CNS (spinal cord, brainstem or brain) of protozoal activity.
- Most horses mount an effective and long-lasting immune response against parasite and never develop clinical disease.

Risk factors
- Majority of horses (approximately 30–80% depending on location) within the USA have serological evidence of exposure to *Sarcocystis neurona*; however, clinical disease only develops in a small proportion (approximately 0.14%).
- Likely that some horses are more susceptible than others to disease; risk factors unknown.
- Risk greatest in young (<5 YO) horses.
- Transmission between horses does not occur (horses do not produce any infective stages).
- Thought that transplacental transmission also does not occur.

History
- Onset of clinical disease usually insidious, but can occasionally be acute.
- Disease is predominantly limited to the Americas.
- Occasional clinical case encountered in Europe/Australasia in horses originating from the Americas; clinical signs may arise many months or even years after original exposure to parasite.

Signs
- Neurological signs vary widely and determined by location and extent of lesions within CNS.
- Most commonly involves spinal cord (rather than brain).
- May mimic other diseases such as wobbler syndrome (p. 271).
- Primary characteristic that differentiates it in many cases is asymmetry: of neurological dysfunction or muscle wastage.
- Ataxia, weakness, abnormal gait.
- Selective loss of muscle of face, limbs or topline.
- Less commonly, brain signs: head tilt, seizures.

Diagnosis
- Definitive diagnosis currently difficult due to lack of specificity of tests.
- Blood serology does not differentiate exposure to parasite (common) from clinical disease (rare).
- Combination of blood and cerebrospinal fluid testing currently used to determine likelihood of disease.
- More reliable serological testing likely to be available in future.

Management
- Affected horses pose no risk of infection to other horses.
- Due to difficulties associated with definitive diagnosis, presumptive treatment may be appropriate.
- Early treatment is important for successful outcome.
- Anti-protozoal medication (ponazuril or nitazoxanide): duration of course dependent on manufacturer's advice but typically 4–6 weeks.
- Anti-inflammatory medication may be used to manage some clinical signs in short term.

Prevention
- Minimizing exposure to infective protozoal stages: securing feed from possible contamination by opossums and rodents.
- Gene sequencing likely to lead to effective vaccines.

Prognosis
- Clinical cases if not treated will deteriorate, although may take months/years.
- Better prognosis for cases treated early in course of disease.
- Majority (60–70%) of cases treated promptly show significant clinical improvement, with up to one-third of these recovering completely.
- Best chance of complete recovery for less severely affected horses.
- Relapse in small proportion of cases.

Arboviral encephalitis

Arboviral encephalitis is a broad term for a group of viral diseases (West Nile virus [WNV], Eastern [EEE], Western [WEE] and Venezuelan [VEE] equine encephalomyelitis, Murray Valley encephalitis [MVE], Japanese encephalitis [JE]) spread by mosquitoes (and less commonly other biting insects) and causing predominantly neurological signs. The natural reservoir for disease is primarily the wild bird population (also rodents for some diseases), with horses being a 'dead-end' host for the virus. Horse-to-horse and horse-to-human transmission is highly unlikely because of the low levels of virus circulating in infected animals (although can occur with VEE). Seasonal appearance of clinical cases is typical.

The geographical distribution of the main equine arboviruses within and between countries varies seasonally with climatic conditions and spread of natural hosts and insect vectors. Currently:
- WNV: Americas, parts of Europe, Africa, Middle East, Australasia.
- EEE and WEE: Americas.
- VEE: Central and South America.
- MVE: Australia.
- JE: Australasia.

Cause
- Reservoir of infection in natural host (predominantly wild birds), with transmission of virus to horse by mosquito bite.
- Inflammation of CNS may ensue after initial viraemia, resulting in neurological signs.
- Proportion of infected horses that develop clinical disease and severity of disease varies between viruses and virus strains.
- Incubation period 3–15 days.
- Horses that recover from infection generally develop long-term immunity.

Signs
- Vary in type, severity and progression between both causative viruses and individual horses.
- May include combinations of: fever, depression, weakness, ataxia, cranial nerve deficits, altered mental state (depression, aggression or hyperexcitability), head pressing, blindness, convulsions.
- Severe cases may progress to recumbency +/− death within 2–3 days.
- Neurological signs not always symmetrical.
- WNV: neurological morbidity approximately 10%.

Diagnosis
- Presumptive diagnosis often based on clinical presentation and knowledge of disease status of locality.
- Should be differentiated from other diseases with similar signs: EPM/EHV/wobbler syndrome/rabies/botulism/bacterial meningitis.
- Serology (≥4-fold change in antibody titre in paired samples 10–14 days apart) often strongly indicative.
- IgM ELISA.
- Definitive diagnosis may require postmortem sampling; care in handling tissues of horses suspected of having the disease, as human infection possible.

Management
- No specific therapies exist.
- Supportive care: hospitalization/fluids/anti-inflammatory medication.
- WNV: hyperimmune plasma early in disease may improve outcome.
- Severe clinical signs or rapid deterioration may warrant euthanasia.

Prevention
- Vaccination (WNV/EEE/WEE) for animals living in, or travelling to, endemic areas.
- Primary vaccinations/annual boosters should be completed before onset of risk period for mosquitoes.
- Minimize exposure to mosquitoes: stabling and lighting management/use of insect deterrents and insecticides/elimination of standing water.

Prognosis
- WNV: around 30% of horses with clinical disease die or require euthanasia.
- Recumbent horses have poor prognosis for survival.
- Mortality rate of EEE, VEE and WEE can be high (50–90% for EEE, the most pathogenic).
- Many horses that recover from clinical disease (up to 30% for WNV) have residual neurological deficits (e.g. gait abnormalities) that can persist for months/years.
- MVE: low morbidity and mortality (approximately 10%) rates.

CHAPTER 9

SKIN CONDITIONS

INJURIES

Interference injuries
See Chapter 1, pp. 11–13.

Girth 'gall' ('girth sore')
Acute bruising/myositis of girth region. Usually most severe within 12 hours of incident and diminishes over subsequent days.

Cause
- Overtight/pinching girth.

Signs
- Swelling/oedema just behind girth (on lower midline or one/both sides) (**Figure 9.1**).
- +/– mild palpable tenderness.
- Hair loss unusual, and usually no break in skin.
- Occasionally a firm, painful enlargement of underlying pectoral muscle/s.

Diagnosis
- Clinical findings definitive.

Management
- Topical +/– systemic NSAID or corticosteroid medication in acute phase to reduce swelling.
- Severe swelling (rare): may benefit from 1–2 days out of ridden exercise.

Prognosis
- Resolves rapidly and rarely interferes with training.

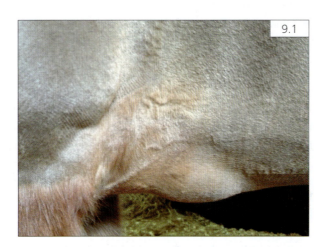

Fig. 9.1 Girth 'gall'.

INFECTIONS

Cellulitis/lymphangitis

Ascending generalized infection of (usually) single limb with resulting inflammation/swelling. Most frequently affects cannon region. Severity and progression varies.

Cause
- Typically but not invariably associated with small entry point for infection (puncture, cut or focal dermatitis).

Signs
- Filling/oedema of limb.
- Severity varies and in worst cases may extend to upper limb.
- Generalized pain response to palpation.
- Mild (most commonly) to severe lameness; typically warms up with forced exercise.

Diagnosis
- Clinical findings usually definitive.
- Diagnostic procedures rarely required.
- If lameness severe and/or unremitting: consider investigation to rule out synovial sepsis (see Chapter 1, p. 15).

Management
- Broad-spectrum antibiotic and anti-inflammatory medication.
- Exercise assists resolution and disperses filling: appropriate level of exercise determined by severity, but in general forced walking during acute phase and return to ridden exercise as soon as possible.

Prognosis
- Most cases respond favourably to treatment, with little interruption to training.

Pastern dermatitis ('cracked heels'/'mud fever')

Inflammation/infection of heel/low pastern region of one or more limbs; characterized by dry or wet dermatitis, crusting and variable localized filling. Severity and response to treatment varies. Often involves white limbs. Some horses appear more prone to condition than others.

Cause
- Multifactorial.
- Generally an opportunistic infection by bacterial pathogen/s due to breakdown in local skin defences.
- Factors that contribute to development: excessive wetting or wet–dry cycles; poor cleaning following exercise; inappropriate skin dressing; skin trauma from interference or boot rubs.
- Frequently a seasonal problem (winter/wet conditions).
- Bacterial species generally free-living in environment: most commonly involves mixed bacterial population; may include *Staphylococcus* spp.

Signs
- Patch of dry or wet crusting/matted hair (**Figures 9.2a, b**).
- +/− cellulitis/inflammation of pastern.
- +/− localized pain on palpation.
- +/− lameness (only with secondary cellulitis).
- May crack/bleed during exercise.

Diagnosis
- Clinical findings definitive.
- Bacteriological investigation (culture) rarely useful.

Management
- Management guided by recent history of previous treatment.
- Variety of approaches to treatment: most incorporate cleaning/debridement and topical medication.
- Initial topical application of debriding/keratolytic cream useful to lift crusts, followed by daily/twice-daily application of antibiotic cream until resolution.
- Daily management: light barrier cream (paraffin) for exercise; gentle cleansing (chlorhexidine solution) and drying post exercise, followed by application of topical antibiotic cream.

- Choice of topical antibiotic cream determined by local experiences and efficacy.
- Clipping of any long hair around site may assist treatment.
- Avoid aggressive cleaning/irritation of site.
- +/– systemic antibiotic medication if cellulitis present.

Prognosis
- Rarely interferes with training but significant daily care often needed.
- May persist for weeks/months in troublesome cases.
- Susceptible horses require careful management/vigilance to prevent recurrence; generally a favourable response to prompt treatment.

Boils and 'runners'

Acute, localized skin infection characterized by raised papule (usually solitary) and intense pain. Most commonly found in areas of tack contact/pressure, particularly withers or flank.

Cause
- Bacterial (usually staphylococcal) infection.
- Usually an opportunistic infection caused by breakdown of local skin barrier.
- Sweating, failure to dry properly, contact pressure and dirty tack may be risk factors

Signs
- Raised oedematous papule often with small central 'head'.
- +/– single or multiple raised lymphatic 'runners' (**Figure 9.3**).
- Usually intensely painful to palpate and may interfere with tack.

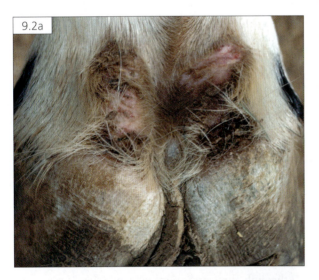

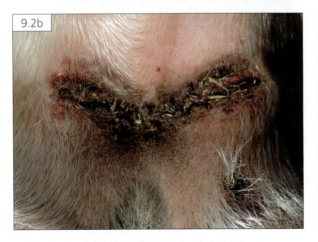

Figs. 9.2a, b Examples of pastern dermatitis.

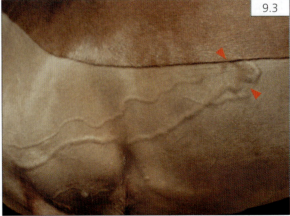

Fig. 9.3 Bacterial 'boil' (arrowheads) with lymphatic 'runners' on flank.

Diagnosis
- Clinical findings definitive.

Management
- Systemic antibiotic (3–5 days) medication +/– topical antibiotic ointment.
- Fomentation may encourage rupture and early resolution.

Prognosis
- Resolves rapidly with treatment.
- Interruption to training depends on lesion location/severity and potential interference with tack (but usually short term, <2 days).

Bacterial folliculitis
Bacterial infection of hair follicle/s, most commonly at sites prone to sweating +/– pressure from tack (back/flanks/neck).

Signs
- Multiple small firm dermal papules, which usually develop 'heads' and focal secondary hair loss (**Figure 9.4**).
- May resemble fungal infection (dermatophytosis/'ringworm'/'girth itch').

Diagnosis
- Clinical findings usually definitive.
- Monitoring progression of disease over initial days usually permits differentiation from fungal infection (easy loss of hair with latter).

Management
- Topical medicated/antibacterial shampoos or chlorhexidine solution, taking care to gently raise scabs/heads.

Prognosis
- Good. Rarely interferes with training.

Dermatophytosis ('ringworm'/'girth itch')
Contagious fungal skin infection causing crusting and hair loss. Most commonly occurs at girth, flank, neck or face (areas in contact with tack). Infections most common in young horses, as previous exposure leads to reasonable (but not complete) resistance to reinfection in older horses.

Cause
- *Trichophyton* spp. most commonly implicated but *Microsporum* spp. also encountered.
- Fungal spores are resistant to environmental conditions and may persist for years.
- Contagious through direct or indirect contact (environment, tack, grooming equipment).
- Usually also requires lowered local skin defences through abrasion, sweating or pressure.

Signs
- Time period from exposure to development of skin lesions approximately 10–14 days.
- Initial appearance is of clusters of raised hairs, progressing rapidly to crusting and hair loss (**Figures 9.5a–c**).
- Lesions may be solitary/focal or extensive.
- Crusting/scaling is usually 'dry'; less commonly manifested as wet dermatitis.
- May resemble other types of dermatitis (Bacterial folliculitis), particularly on neck; can usually be differentiated by ready plucking of hair from lesion edges and rapid progression over few days.

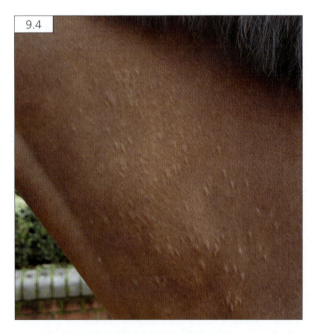

Fig. 9.4 Bacterial folliculitis on neck.

Diagnosis
- Clinical findings usually sufficient.
- If definitive diagnosis required: hair/crust plucks from lesion edges reveal fungal hyphae and spores on microscopic examination.
- Fungal culture rarely warranted.

Management
- Lesions eventually resolve spontaneously but treatment is undertaken to minimize spread.
- Presumptive treatment warranted if justified by clinical signs: better to treat as precaution than risk spread.
- Topical fungicidal medication (enilconazole/miconazole/lime sulphur): focal or entire coat depending on signs.
- 2–3 treatments at 3–4-day intervals recommended for common topical medications.
- Application of keratolytic/debriding cream useful to lift crusts prior to antifungal treatment.
- Lesions in close proximity to sensitive sites (eyes, muzzle, ears, girth) best treated with topical fungicidal cream.
- During infectious period care should be taken to disinfect tack/rugs/grooming kit (sporicidal disinfectants/fumigation) to prevent spread between horses.
- May infect stable staff/riders: caution with handling of active lesions and vigilance for skin lesions.
- Efficacy of in-feed oral antifungal medication (griseofulvin) has not been demonstrated.

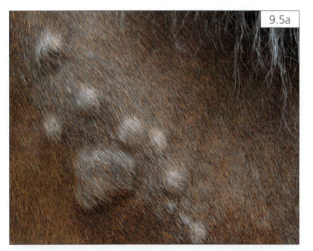
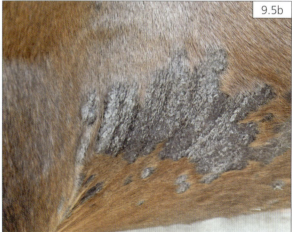
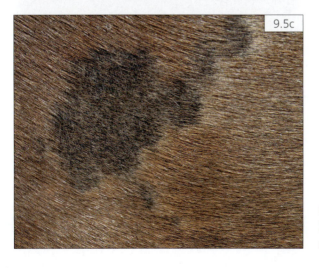

Figs. 9.5a–c Dermatophytosis: (a) raised hairs of early lesions; (b) active lesions; (c) healing lesions (hair growth returning).

Prognosis
- Most cases resolve over 1–2 weeks with treatment; rarely interferes with training.
- New lesions may continue to appear for some time after treatment: due to time delay between infection and resulting hair loss rather than ineffectual medication.
- May interfere with racing and international travel while lesions are visibly active.

Dermatophilosis ('rain scald'/ 'rain rot')

Skin infection characterized by crusting/wet dermatitis that occurs most commonly over areas of the body subject to wetting/sweating such as quarters or back; less frequently on front of hind cannons. Usually in horses at pasture or with winter coats; uncommon in stabled horses.

Cause
- Opportunistic colonization of wet/damaged skin by microbe present in environment (*Dermatophilus congolensis*).

Signs
- Wet dermatitis in which exudate causes hard matting of hair.
- Crusts may come away leaving painful moist/raw lesions.

Diagnosis
- Clinical findings usually definitive.
- Laboratory work (cytology) can be undertaken if necessary but rarely required.

Management
- Medicated (keratolytic) washes/creams or chlorhexidine cleansing to remove matted hair/crusts, followed by topical antiseptic/antibiotic creams until resolution of dermatitis.
- Systemic antibiotics (oral potentiated sulphonamides) may assist healing if lesions widespread.

Prognosis
- Good. Rarely interferes with training.
- If treatment delayed or inappropriate, permanent alopecia/white hairs may ensue.

OTHER CONDITIONS

Urticaria ('hives')

Common clinical manifestation of allergy (rather than single disease entity). Allergic response to inhaled/ingested/injected/contact allergen/s. Typically acute onset. Severity varies and duration ranges from transient (few days) to many weeks/months (rare).

Cause
- Inflammatory response causes increased vascular permeability and leakage of protein and fluid into skin, resulting in skin oedema or 'wheals'.
- May be associated with change in feed/bedding/management; however, inciting cause rarely determined with confidence.

Signs
- Multiple raised patches of hair/flat oedematous wheals throughout coat (**Figure 9.6**). Generally circular but sometimes ring-shaped.
- Most prominent over face/neck/flank, usually affects both sides of body; pressure from blanket may keep lesions away from trunk.

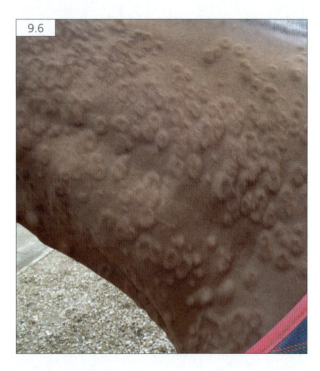

Fig. 9.6 Urticaria.

- Transient improvement (hours) may be noted following exercise.
- Small proportion of cases develop severe exudative wheals, with resulting secondary crusting/hair loss.

Management
- Remove inciting cause, if identified.
- Corticosteroid medication: dexamethasone (0.01–0.02 mg/kg BWT IV) will usually resolve the clinical signs for 3–4 days and transient cases may require no further treatment.
- Recurrent cases: may require low-dose oral prednisolone (1 mg/kg BWT/day given early morning until lesions resolve, then every other day) over days/weeks; alternatively, repeated dexamethasone dosing as required.
- Rarely, lesions of variable severity may persist for many months: may be manageable by minimizing time spent in stable environment and determining whether dietary factors are involved.
- Allergen-specific immunotherapy (based on intradermal testing) may reduce need for corticosteroid use, but is rarely employed due to cost and duration of treatment.

Prognosis
- Good.
- Rarely interferes with training, although drug administration needs to be planned around racing engagements.

Papillomatosis ('warts')

Common viral (papillomavirus) skin disease. Moderately contagious; incubation period approximately 2 months. Seen predominantly in young (yearling/2 YO) horses, as older horses develop good immunity. May bleed if traumatized but generally benign and of no importance.

Signs
- Single or (more commonly) multiple grey/pink vegetative lesions (**Figures 9.7a, b**).
- Most common sites are lips and muzzle, lower limb and groin/sheath.

Diagnosis
- Clinical findings definitive.

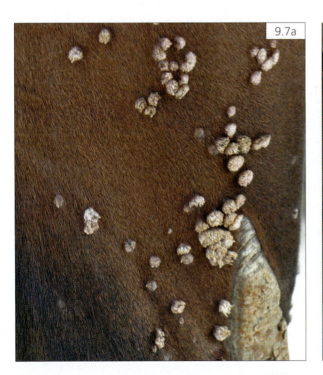
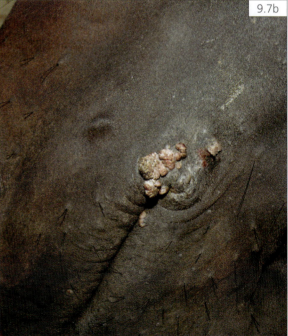

Figs. 9.7a, b Papillomatosis ('warts') (a) on the forearm and (b) at the corner of the mouth.

Management
- Usually no treatment required.
- Spontaneous regression in 2–4 months.
- Troublesome warts suffering from repeated trauma (corners of mouth, pastern) may warrant removal (sharp dissection/cautery/topical caustic ointment).
- Good efficacy reported with autogenous vaccines but rarely used.

Prognosis
- Good. Rarely interfere with training and resolve (with no recurrence) within months.

Sarcoids
Fibroblastic skin tumours that can take several forms and often behave unpredictably. Do not metastasize but may spread locally. Spontaneous resolution can occur but highly unusual; most lesions are slowly progressive.

Cause
- Multifactorial disease process.
- Considered to arise from exposure to bovine papillomavirus with predilection sites being those most prone to fly-bite (belly/sheath/face).
- Risk factors for individual horses (such as genetic susceptibility) poorly defined.

Signs
- Lesions may be solitary or multiple. Classified into the following recognizable forms depending on appearance:
  - Occult: affected sites (most usually around mouth/eye/groin) appear as poorly defined areas of thick/hard skin, sometimes with change in overlying hair.
  - Verrucous: classic 'warty' appearance; anywhere on body (**Figure 9.8a**).
  - Nodular: firm, non-painful nodules frequently with normal overlying skin. Most commonly around eye, sheath and groin (**Figure 9.8b**).
  - Fibroblastic: similar appearance to proud tissue with areas of ulceration/haemorrhage and often extensive local spread.
  - Mixed: lesions with features of any of above.

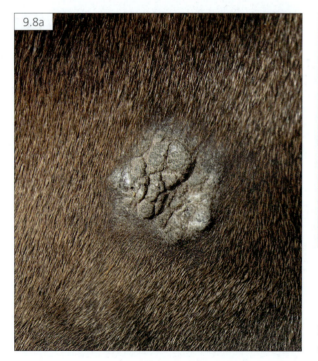

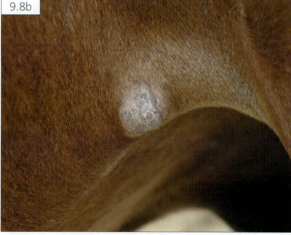

Figs. 9.8a, b Common sarcoids: (a) verrucous; (b) nodular.

Diagnosis
- Can generally be distinguished from other common skin conditions (warts, proud flesh) on clinical appearance, although solitary nodules (+/− ulcerated margin) may resemble other nodular disease (mast cell/basal cell tumours).
- Undertaking biopsy to confirm diagnosis is inadvisable: aggressive re-growth/spread is common following partial excision.

Management
- If appearance is suggestive of sarcoid, should be managed as such.
- Most sarcoids do not interfere with training during racehorse career; treatment usually reserved for lesions that interfere with tack or are growing rapidly.
- Unless a sarcoid is to be removed in its entirety, it should be left alone.
- Because of the considerable risk of aggressive re-growth, important that initial therapy (if undertaken) is appropriate.
- Choice of treatment is determined by location of lesions and economic factors.
- Solitary, well-defined sarcoids with relatively small skin 'pedicle' are readily ligated (rubber elastrator/thread ligature) and generally do not recur.
- Several treatment options available for more serious lesions: good efficacy with laser excision, topical cytotoxic (5-fluorouracil/aciclovir) ointments and intralesional chemotherapy and radiotherapy.
- Periocular lesions: iridium-192 interstitial brachytherapy (90% success rate; time to maximum resolution up to 2 years) or topical 5% imiquimod cream.

Prognosis
- Sarcoids rarely interfere with training but can have implications for resale.

Eosinophilic collagen necrosis/granuloma
Common, non-painful focal nodular skin lesion/s. Typically over back and flank. Usually do not progress or enlarge and may remain unchanged permanently or resolve spontaneously over months.

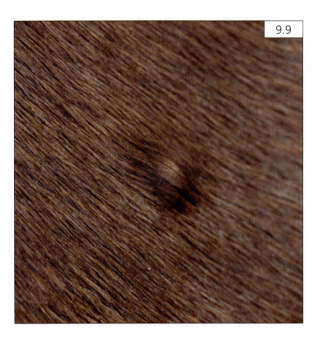

Fig. 9.9 Eosinophilic collagen necrosis nodule.

Cause
- Cause unknown but risk factors include pressure of tack and insect bites.

Signs
- Small, firm and non-painful dermal nodules (**Figure 9.9**).
- Solitary or multiple.
- Hair loss not a feature unless rubbed by tack.

Diagnosis
- Clinical findings definitive.

Management
- Usually not treated, as cosmetic blemish only.
- Perilesional or systemic administration of corticosteroids may result in improvement/resolution but rarely warranted.

Prognosis
- Usually remain a long-term minor skin blemish but do not interfere with training.

Tail rubbing/pruritus

Pruritus over quarters or tail base may result in persistent irritation and traumatic dermatitis of tail. Severity varies between individuals; can affect horses of all ages. Usually of cosmetic importance only.

Cause
- Frequently undetermined as typically a cycle of trauma/infection/irritation.
- Often part of a more generalized pruritus.
- Uncommonly initiated by tail rub/dermatitis sustained during transport.
- Other causes of pruritus include worms (*Oxyuris equi* resides in lower bowel and deposits eggs on perianal skin) and *Culicoides* allergy (p. 288); however, these are rare in racehorses.
- Presence of skin lesions elsewhere on body may indicate parasitic or allergic origin.

Signs
- Broken and lost hairs at tail base with some crusting dermatitis.
- +/− pruritus when quarters/tail base stimulated.

Diagnosis
- Diagnostic work usually not undertaken as more practical to treat than diagnose.
- Care should be taken to determine whether horse is truly pruritic, as this will direct management.

Management
- Deworming (unless recently treated).
- Initial treatment should be directed at breaking the dermatitis/irritation cycle.
- Repeated washes with keratinolytic/antibacterial medicated shampoo (selenium sulphide products also have antipruritic/antifungal action) +/− daily topical emollient +/− tail bandaging resolves most cases.
- Systemic corticosteroid (prednisolone) medication may be warranted in acute phase.

Prognosis
- May persist for weeks/months but does not interfere with training.

Linear keratosis

Rare dermatitis characterized by linear bands of crusting (hyperkeratosis), generally on neck, shoulder or flank.

Cause
- Unknown; likely to be an autoimmune disorder.

Signs
- Vertical (continuous or broken) line of hair loss or crusting that resembles a 'run-off scald' (**Figure 9.10**).
- Usually unilateral.
- Pruritus and pain are not features.

Diagnosis
- Clinical findings definitive.

Management
- Treatment not usually needed (or effective).
- Steroid or keratolytic creams may reduce severity of some lesions temporarily (if desired).

Prognosis
- Life-long condition, although spontaneous resolution may occur.
- Does not interfere with training.

Harvest mite dermatitis

Seasonal pruritic dermatitis caused by the biting larvae of the harvest mite (*Trombicula autumnalis*). Primarily in horses with access to pasture (chalky soil) in late summer/autumn; however, mites can also be found in hay and stabled horses may therefore be affected at any season in mild climates. Not contagious but more than one animal may be affected.

Signs
- Areas of crusting/hair loss on face or lower legs, with characteristic orange 'droplets' of dried serum.
- Pruritus (rubbing face, stamping legs) is a key feature.
- Larvae rarely seen as only on horse for brief periods to feed.

Diagnosis
- Clinical findings strongly indicative.
- Confirmation by microscopic examination of crust/debris for mites.

Management
- Topical insecticidal washes.

Prognosis
- Responds well to treatment.

Lice

Infestation with biting (*Damalinia equi*) or sucking (*Haematopinus asini*) lice causes irritation/itching and is most common in winter and spring. Contagious through direct or indirect (rugs/grooming kit/environment) contact. Horses free from clinical signs may be carriers of lice.

Signs
- +/− pruritus and resulting dermatitis.
- Rubs, hair loss and scurf typically along base of mane/tail or over quarters.
- Close examination may reveal eggs (small/pale/oval 'nits') attached to hairs of mane (**Figure 9.11**) or lice in coat.

Diagnosis
- Clinical findings usually definitive.
- Coat groomings can be placed on a dark surface and examined for movement of lice.

Management
- Insecticidal powders/washes/topline treatments; treatment on 2 occasions 7–10 days apart usually recommended.
- In-contact horses should be treated if feasible.

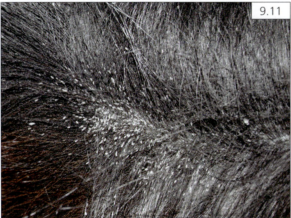

Fig. 9.11 Lice eggs ('nits'): small white eggs adhering to hairs of mane.

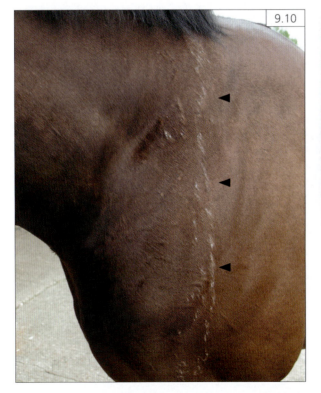

Fig. 9.10 Linear keratosis (arrowheads).

Prognosis
- Good. Resolves rapidly with appropriate treatment.

Culicoides hypersensitivity ('sweet itch')
Allergic dermatitis caused by biting midges (*Culicoides* spp.). Seasonal (summer). Rarely seen in racehorses.

Signs
- Thickened scaly skin at base of mane/tail with broken hairs.
- Pruritus.

Diagnosis
- Clinical findings usually definitive.

Management
- Topical insecticidal washes/topline treatments.
- Insect repellents applied to belly (most common site for the midge bites that initiate inflammatory cascade).
- Systemic corticosteroid therapy may be useful to manage initial pruritus.

Prognosis
- Most cases can be managed satisfactorily.
- Rarely interferes with training.

Dermoid cysts
Congenital cysts within the skin. Thought to arise from aberrant placement of tissue during embryonic development. Presence noted early in life. Generally remain unchanged in appearance throughout training.

Signs
- Small, non-painful skin nodules of similar size and appearance to eosinophilic collagen necrosis (p. 285) but differentiated by being found invariably on dorsal midline of back.
- Not associated with hair loss but few white hairs may be observed over each nodule.
- Single or multiple.

Diagnosis
- Clinical findings definitive.

Management
- Generally no treatment required.
- Exceptionally, may interfere with tack and in these cases surgical excision is curative.

Prognosis
- Remain present throughout life but do not interfere with training.

Intertrigo
Rare exudative dermatitis of contact areas of skin in high groin (or, rarely, axilla). May arise secondary to 'chafing' and seen on occasion in colts with large testicles or following open castration.

Signs
- Areas of shallow ulceration, focal in early stages but often coalescing to involve extensive regions of in-contact skin (**Figure 9.12**).
- May be associated with considerable local inflammation/soreness and wide-based hindlimb gait.

Diagnosis
- Clinical findings definitive.
- Progression of dermatitis can be rapid; swabbing (for bacteriological analysis) may be warranted prior to commencement of any treatment to guide choice of antimicrobial.

Management
- Frequently a troublesome condition that requires meticulous management to optimize healing.
- Topical antiseptic/antibiotic/antifungal ointment +/− systemic NSAID indicated in initial stages and may be guided by laboratory findings.
- Daily cleansing with dilute antiseptic solution and careful drying of affected site followed by application of barrier (zinc oxide) cream; often painful and may require sedation.

Prognosis
- Full resolution may take weeks and some interference with training can be expected in initial stages.

Calcinosis circumscripta

Rare, benign subcutaneous calcified growth typically found overlying a joint, most commonly the stifle. Cause is unknown. Unilateral or bilateral. Detection of mass typically occurs during yearling/early training phase or at routine pre-purchase radiography.

Signs
- Firm, non-painful subcutaneous mass over lateral aspect of stifle.
- Size of mass varies but can be extensive.
- Overlying skin not involved, of normal appearance and can be moved freely over lesion.
- Rarely associated with lameness.

Diagnosis
- Clinical presentation definitive.
- Radiography: heterogeneous/granular radiopaque body lateral aspect of stifle (**Figure 9.13**).

Management
- No treatment required in most cases.
- If considered to be causing lameness, or large and growing (rare): surgery. Close association with stifle joint capsule means surgical excision is not without risk of complication including wound breakdown.

Prognosis
- Rarely interferes with training.
- Life-long condition; however, growth of mass, if it occurs, is very slow and of little concern.

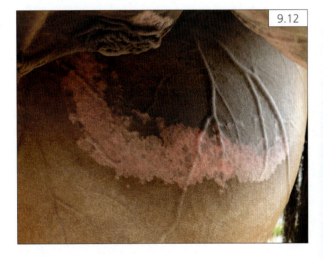

Fig. 9.12 Intertrigo.

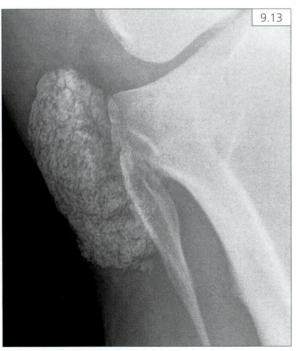

Fig. 9.13 Radiograph (CdCr) showng a calcinosis circumscripta lesion overlying the stifle.

CHAPTER 10
MISCELLANEOUS CONDITIONS

Stable vices (stereotypic behaviours)

Stable vices or stereotypic behaviours are habitual and repetitive behavioural patterns that serve no apparent function. They include the following:
- Crib-biting: grasping of fixed object with incisor teeth, contraction of ventral strap muscles of neck and production of a 'grunt'.
- Windsucking: as for crib biting (+/− grasping of fixed object) with swallowing/gulping of air.
- Weaving: habitual swinging of head/neck from side-to-side with associated shifting of weight.
- Boxwalking: habitual pacing/walking in or around stable.
- Other variations of tongue/lip play, wood-chewing, stall-kicking and hole-digging.

Causes
- Horses in free-range conditions move and forage for a large proportion of the day and have continual social interactions; stable vices are thought to result largely from absence of this natural behaviour.
- Some evidence that gastrointestinal (gastric ulcers, intestinal transit times) and dietary (low forage, high concentrate) factors are important.
- Management at weaning can have a strong influence: feeding of concentrates and housed (as opposed to pasture) weaning both associated with greater risk of development of stable vices. Stress, gastrointestinal factors and frustrated sucking behaviour may play a role.
- May be copied from other horses, although learned behaviour likely to be less of an influence than other risk factors.
- Certain behaviours may be precipitated by stress (e.g. change of yard).

Effect
- Main stable vices are generally considered to be an unsoundness: negative impact on saleability/value.
- Racetrack performance is unaffected.
- Horses that crib-bite or windsuck are at increased risk of developing colic.
- Air swallowed while windsucking does not transit the gastrointestinal tract and in itself does not cause colic; more likely to relate to undefined factors such as intestinal transit times/gastric ulceration.
- Stall-kicking and door-banging may cause injuries or cosmetic blemishes such as acquired bursae over front of carpus.

Management
- Once a horse has developed a stable vice, management changes frequently have little or no effect.
- Stabling that permits some social contact or visual interaction with other horses may be useful in minimizing/preventing behaviour.
- Large mirror placed on stable wall or obstacles (tyres) on floor may limit weaving/boxwalking behaviour.
- Provision of salt/mineral lick or interactive feeding devices/toys may reduce crib-biting.
- Investigation/treatment of gastric ulceration if thought to be implicated.
- Forced prevention of stereotypical behaviour (e.g. crib strap) rather than addressing underlying causes may actually increase stress levels.
- Surgery (neurectomy of ventral branch of spinal accessory nerve plus myectomy of omohyoideus/sternothyrohyoideus muscles): reasonable (not total) efficacy for preventing crib-biting but rarely undertaken.

CHAPTER 11

INFECTIOUS DISEASES

Equine influenza

Equine influenza (EI) is the most important viral respiratory disease in the racehorse population worldwide. Similar in many respects to human influenza A; antigenic drift and strain mutation ensure outbreaks occur periodically even in vaccinated populations.

Signs
- Fever (often high), nasal discharge and coughing.
- Severity of signs depends on immune status of individual: in a naïve population signs may be dramatic.

Transmission
- Incubation period 1–5 days.
- May shed virus for 7–10 days after infection.
- Direct and indirect spread through respiratory route.
- Young or inadequately vaccinated horses at greatest risk.
- Survival of virus in environment for hours/days.
- Dry, cool conditions appear to favour spread.
- Wind-borne spread (kilometres) possible and has been recorded when windspeed >30 km/hour.

Diagnosis
- Laboratory diagnosis.
- Nasopharyngeal swabs: PCR detection of virus from day 1–10 of infection.
- Blood sampling: seroconversion by day 8.

Management
- Supportive care includes rest +/– antibiotic medication for horses with persistent respiratory disease.

Prevention
- Vaccination is a requirement of most racing jurisdictions.
- International surveillance panel monitors epidemiological shifts in active strains and makes recommendations to vaccine manufacturers for vaccine updates.
- Current vaccines provide reasonable but not total protection against emerging strains and boosting 2–3 times/year is recommended.

Equine herpesvirus

There are several types of herpesvirus that affect horses. Types 1 and 4 are of greatest importance. EHV is endemic and is notable for its ability to remain dormant in previously infected individuals (latency in lymph nodes and the trigeminal ganglia), with stressors prompting periodic reactivation and shedding of virus. Variable strains of EHV-1 and EHV-4 are involved in outbreaks of disease; virulence (and clinical signs that develop) differs depending on strain characteristics and individual horse immune factors.

Signs
- EHV-4: primarily associated with signs of respiratory disease (coughing, nasal discharge, fever). Can occasionally cause individual abortions.
- EHV-1: can cause respiratory disease (as above) as well as neurological disease and contagious abortions.
- Neurological form (usually caused by neurotropic strains): may be preceded by respiratory disease +/– fever. Progressive ataxia (usually hindlimb but may progress to forelimb or complete recumbency) +/– urinary overflow incontinence (Chapter 8, p. 273).

Transmission
- Most horses are exposed early in life.
- Main reservoir of infection is reactivation of latent virus in outwardly healthy 'carrier' horses.
- Reactivation episodes may be prompted by stressors such as travel, sales or racing.
- Incubation period 2–10 days.
- Virus spread by direct or indirect contact with respiratory secretions; shedding of virus occurs from initial fever for up to 2 weeks depending on immunity.
- Virus may survive in environment for weeks.

Diagnosis
- Laboratory diagnosis: virus isolation is gold standard (nasopharyngeal swabs/blood sample); also PCR and seroconversion (≥4-fold increase in titre in samples 10–20 days apart).

Management
- Neurological/paralytic EHV: strict adherence to statutory requirements including isolation of premises. Movement restrictions for 1 month, with lifting of restrictions only when serological monitoring determines no further activity within at-risk group. (See also Chapter 8, p. 274)
- Respiratory EHV: generally no treatment required (antibiotic medication may be needed for persistent respiratory disease/secondary bacterial infections). Biosecurity measures as for neurological/paralytic EHV recommended, but rarely implemented as less serious outcomes of respiratory EHV rarely prompt diagnosis/management.

Prevention
- EHV is endemic and all horses are potentially carriers.
- Routine vaccination with current vaccines may limit susceptibility of a yard to outbreak of infection (reduced virus shedding) but does not prevent either respiratory or neurological disease from occurring.
- Routine disinfection of stables and transport advisable.

Strangles
Strangles is a highly infectious bacterial respiratory disease caused by *Streptococcus equi*. Endemic in wider equine population. Up to 10% of horses that have recovered from infection may become clinically silent carriers, with infection reservoir in guttural pouches and intermittent shedding of bacteria for months/years.

Signs
- +/– initial fever.
- +/– inappetence.
- Nasal discharge.
- Swollen submandibular and pharyngeal lymph nodes, with eventual abscessation and discharge of purulent material.

Transmission
- Direct transmission between horses through respiratory secretions and open abscesses.
- Shedding does not begin until 1–2 days after initial fever.
- Incubation period 1–3 weeks.
- Indirect transmission via equipment, tack, staff and shared water sources.
- In ideal conditions may survive in environment for weeks; likely to be much shorter in sunlight or on soil.

Diagnosis
- Clinical presentation of enlarged/abscessed pharyngeal lymph nodes +/– nasal discharge is strong indicator of possible infection.
- Laboratory detection of bacteria (culture or PCR) needed for confirmation: from abscess discharge/nasopharyngeal swabs/guttural pouch sampling.
- Repeated nasopharyngeal swabbing (three swabs at weekly intervals) or a single endoscope-guided guttural pouch wash submitted for culture and PCR is recommended. False-negative PCR tests possible. Sensitivity of three nasopharyngeal swabs (PCR) is around 90%.

- Blood ELISA test: good sensitivity and specificity for previous exposure (positive from 2 weeks to around 6 months following exposure), although false positives and negatives occur. Blood test best used as screening tool; only minority of seropositives are carriers. Weak positives may represent recent infection or residual antibody response and should be re-sampled in 7–14 days.

Management
- Suspicion of clinical strangles should prompt strict isolation of premises and adherence to statutory requirements and current recommendations from regulatory bodies.
- See Chapter 17 (Herd health) for general quarantine principles.
- Division of all horses on premises into risk groups: clinical disease/direct or indirect contact/no contact. Blood ELISA testing of latter two groups. Testing of clinical cases (three nasopharyngeal swabs or single guttural pouch PCR) following resolution of disease and before release into wider population. Testing best performed >30 days after last clinical signs.
- Treatment of clinical cases not necessary and is dependent on stage/severity of disease and determined on individual basis. Possible to halt disease in early cases (pyrexia) with 3–5 days antibiotic medication (antibiotic of choice is penicillin). Cases with lymph node abscessation best managed with NSAIDs rather than antibiotics.
- Treatment of guttural pouch carriers: large volume/repeated lavage of guttural pouches with benzylpenicillin/gelatin solution.
- Following outbreak: rest contact pastures for 4 weeks, disinfection of wooden surfaces and water troughs.

Prevention
- Vaccines for *S. equi* have shown variable efficacy in the past and are not available in all countries.
- Good biosecurity practices such as isolation and/or blood sampling of all arrivals considered to be high risk should minimize likelihood of disease entering yard.

Equine viral arteritis
Equine viral arteritis (EVA) is a viral disease causing respiratory signs, abortion and vasculitis. Primarily a disease of concern to breeding establishments, with shedding by carrier stallions and transmission at mating leading to abortion.

Signs
- Infection not always accompanied by clinical signs.
- Fever/depression.
- Filling of lower legs.
- Conjunctivitis and puffiness around eyes.
- Nasal discharge.
- Swelling of scrotum or mammary glands.

Transmission
- Main route of transmission is venereal at mating.
- Respiratory spread through direct or indirect contact also occurs.
- Incubation period 2–14 days.
- Infected stallions remain long-term carriers, while mares show transient disease (respiratory signs +/– abortion).

Diagnosis
- Laboratory diagnosis: virus isolation/PCR/seroconversion.

Management
- Strict adherence to statutory requirements and current recommendations from regulatory bodies.
- Isolation of clinical cases and contacts.
- No treatment available.
- Castration of infected stallions may be considered.

Prevention
- Blood sampling prior to breeding.
- Vaccination of breeding stallions.
- Certification of seronegativity prior to vaccination is important to facilitate international travel.

Equine infectious anaemia ('swamp fever')
Equine infectious anaemia (EIA) is a viral infection with worldwide distribution that can cause severe anaemia and death. Recovered horses remain infected for life and act as a reservoir of infection.

Signs
- Highly variable (may be subclinical).
- Acute disease: fever/weight loss/diarrhoea/depression/ataxia/jaundice.
- Chronic disease: recurrent fever/anaemia/weight loss.

Transmission
- Transmission is through infected blood/plasma.
- Insect vectors may play a large role: predominantly biting flies.
- Insects involved in transmission do not normally travel large distances.
- Other possible routes of transmission include contaminated veterinary or dental equipment, contaminated blood products (plasma) and transplacental transmission.
- Incubation period variable but typically 1–3 weeks; can be ≥90 days.

Diagnosis
- Laboratory diagnosis.
- Coggins blood test (agar gel immunodiffusion test): detection of antibodies possible from 7–14 days post infection. Is the official test for EIA for international movements.
- ELISA blood test: rapid screening but associated with false positives/negatives.

Management
- Strict adherence to statutory requirements and current recommendations from regulatory bodies including isolation of premises.
- No treatment available.
- Compulsory slaughter of affected horses and quarantine of direct contacts is requirement in most jurisdictions.

Prevention
- No vaccine available.
- Routine serological monitoring of breeding stock and blood donors.
- Caution when travelling to countries with endemic disease.

Contagious equine metritis

Contagious equine metritis (CEM) is a bacterial infection of the reproductive tract caused by *Taylorella equigenitalis*. Main Thoroughbred populations largely free of the disease apart from sporadic outbreaks; endemic in non-Thoroughbred breeding populations in mainland Europe (sporadically in USA). Economically important disease, although causes only mild clinical signs (endometritis/vaginitis/cervicitis).

Signs
- Fillies in training: very low risk group but infections can occur through indirect transmission; usually no external sign of infection.
- Mares: mucopurulent vaginal discharge +/– temporary infertility (early return to oestrus) following covering.
- Stallions: no external signs of infection.

Transmission
- Direct venereal contact at mating or teasing.
- Indirect spread through handlers/equipment.
- Some mares become long-term carriers without showing further signs: pathogen resides in clitoral tissues (rarely in uterus).
- Stallions can become long-term (months/years) carriers without showing signs of disease: pathogen resides in the urethral sinus/fossa and sheath.
- Foals of carrier mares may be infected at birth and remain carriers.

Diagnosis
- Genital swabbing to isolate pathogen.
- Swabbing protocol determined by breeding/import requirements and risk status of horse/country.
- Fillies/mares: clitoral sinuses and fossa +/– endometrial/cervical swab during oestrus.
- Colts/stallions: distal urethra, urethral fossa and sinus, penile sheath.
- *Taylorella equigenitalis* is difficult to culture: use of antibiotics in week prior to swabbing or delay in processing of swabs >48 hours can reduce reliability of testing. Culture time: 3 days for growth, 7 days for negative.

- PCR highly specific and sensitive and more rapid than culture but currently not widely accepted as pre-export test.
- Testing usually combined with screening for other bacterial causes of endometritis (*Klebsiella pneumoniae/Pseudomonas aeruginosa*).
- Serological testing currently not reliable for detection of infection in all circumstances.

Management
- Notifiable in many jurisdictions: strict adherence to statutory requirements and current recommendations from regulatory bodies.
- Positive culture from filly/mare may be treated with repeated antiseptic washing (clitorectomy for intractable cases), followed by re-testing protocol to ensure clear of infection.

Prevention
- Prevention dependent on avoiding contact with infected individuals.
- Genital swabbing prior to breeding (or international travel).

Piroplasmosis

Piroplasmosis is a tick-borne disease caused by the protozoal parasites *Theileria equi* and *Babesia caballi*. *T. equi* is most common but dual infections also occur. Parasite colonizes RBCs, causing cell destruction and anaemia. Disease occurs in horses living in (or transported to) regions where parasite is endemic; however, also problematic when healthy but seropositive horses fail testing requirements for international shipping. Horses born to mares from endemic regions may be seropositive.

The disease is widespread throughout southern, central and eastern Europe, Asia, Africa and Central and South America. High seroprevalence within horse populations in endemic zones.

Signs
- Acute disease: fever/severe anaemia/jaundice/oedematous filling of legs, abdomen/depression/raised respiration and pulse rates/red urine (haemoglobinuria)/abortion.
- Chronic disease: milder signs including recurrent fever/anaemia/weight loss.
- Most infections of horses born in endemic regions are non-fatal.
- Fatality rate in other horses: 10–50%.

Transmission
- Ticks are natural means of spread between horses (several species are recognized vectors for disease).
- Incubation period: *T. equi* 12–19 days, *B. caballi* 10–30 days.
- Other possible routes of transmission: mechanical spread through contaminated veterinary equipment (e.g. needles) or blood products.
- Once recovered from infection, many horses become long-term carriers with no outward sign of infection.
- Occasionally, stress/other disease may precipitate a relapse in a carrier.
- Infected horses pose no risk of infection to other animals in the absence of appropriate tick vector.

Diagnosis
- Laboratory diagnosis to detect antibodies to parasite/s.
- Indirect fluorescent antibody test (IFAT) preferred.
- ELISA also used.

Management
- Strict adherence to statutory requirements: some countries free of disease require quarantine, export or compulsory slaughter in order to prevent parasite from becoming established in local tick population.
- Acute disease: good efficacy of antiprotozoal drugs for control of acute infection.
- 'Seropositive but healthy': some antiprotozoal drugs have shown reasonable efficacy for elimination of infection of *B. caballi*; *T. equi* is relatively resistant, with lower success rates of treatment.
- Dosage of antiprotozoal drugs (imidocarb dipropionate, diminazene aceturate) required for attempted complete elimination of infection is close to toxic threshold: severe side-effects (colic/diarrhoea) common and supportive care necessary.

- Success of elimination regime often cannot be determined for some months as antibodies remain detectable for lengthy periods.

Prevention
- No vaccine available.
- Management to minimize risk of contact with ticks in endemic regions.
- Avoid practices that might spread infected blood between horses.

African horse sickness

African horse sickness (AHS) is a viral infection spread by bite of infected midges. African horse sickness virus (AHSV) causes damage to cellular lining of blood vessels, resulting in widespread effusion and haemorrhages in body cavities/lungs.

The disease is endemic in sub-Saharan Africa. Previous outbreaks in the Middle East and southern Europe. *Culicoides* midges involved in transmission are widely distributed throughout northern Europe and the UK and spread of the related midge-borne bluetongue virus (sheep/cattle) has demonstrated risk of introduction of AHSV, facilitated by changing climatic conditions.

Signs
- Several forms of disease.
- Acute respiratory form: short incubation period/high fever/respiratory distress/frothy nasal discharge/inflamed conjunctivae/highest (>90%) mortality.
- Subacute cardiac form: swollen eyelids/oedematous shoulders/neck/chest/heart failure/moderate (>50%) mortality.
- Mixed form: mixed respiratory and cardiac signs; high (>70%) mortality.
- 'Fever' form: fever/swollen eyelids/no mortality.

Transmission
- Spread by the bite of infected *Culicoides* midges.
- Weather conditions and climate change thought to contribute to spread: warm, wet weather, wind dispersal.
- No direct horse-to-horse transmission.
- Variable incubation period.

Diagnosis
- Laboratory diagnosis: blood testing for antibodies (ELISA/PCR). Also virus isolation.

Management
- Strict adherence to statutory requirements and current recommendations from regulatory bodies including isolation of premises, compulsory slaughter and implementation of large exclusion zone.
- No treatment available.

Prevention
- At present vaccination restricted to Africa or reserved for outbreak events in disease-free countries.
- Current vaccines do not entirely prevent subclinical infection.

Dourine

Dourine is a serious venereal disease caused by the protozoan parasite *Trypanosoma equiperdum*. It is found in Asia, Africa, southern and eastern Europe and South America.

Signs
- Signs develop over weeks/months.
- Variable severity.
- Swelling/oedema of genitalia; may extend to perineum and lower abdomen.
- Purulent vaginal or urethral discharge.
- +/− conjunctivitis.
- Urticarial-type plaques over body.
- May progress to neurological signs (progressive weakness, paralysis).
- Loss of condition (despite good appetite).
- High (>50%) mortality outside of endemic areas.

Transmission
- Sexually transmitted (natural mating or artificial insemination [AI]).
- Most commonly from stallions to mares.
- Mare to foal transmission possible.
- Parasite cannot survive outside living host.

Diagnosis
- Laboratory diagnosis required.
- Blood testing for antibodies (CFT/IFAT).

Management
- No effective treatment.
- No available vaccine.
- Usually notifiable in non-endemic areas; strict adherence to statutory requirements and current recommendations from regulatory bodies including isolation of premises.
- Prevention of transmission through identification of infected animals (blood testing for antibodies).
- Horses should not leave endemic areas without certified freedom from disease.
- As no long-term cure, surviving infected horses are subject to breeding and movement restrictions indefinitely (or euthanasia).

Glanders
Glanders is a serious, potentially fatal bacterial infection (caused by *Burkholderia mallei*) that causes nodular abscessation/ulceration in the respiratory tract and lymphatic system. May infect people. It occurs in the Middle East, parts of Asia, Africa and South America.

Signs
- Development of signs may be acute or chronic.
- Three main forms of disease: nasal (nodules/ulcers in nasal passages/purulent nasal discharge/coughing); pulmonary (coughing/difficulty breathing/weight loss); and cutaneous (also known as 'farcy': abscessation/rupture of subcutaneous lymph tracts).
- All forms of disease may be associated with fever and debilitation.

Transmission
- Subclinical carrier state exists.
- Ingestion of water or feed contaminated with respiratory/cutaneous discharge from infected/carrier horses.
- Incubation period highly variable and dependent on route/dose/host factors: days to months.

Diagnosis
- Laboratory diagnosis required.
- Blood testing for antibodies (CFT): accurate, sensitive to infections of >1 week duration (including carrier state).
- Culture of organism can be difficult and may require repeat sampling of purulent discharge.

Management
- No available vaccine.
- Notifiable in non-endemic areas; strict adherence to statutory requirements. Compulsory slaughter policy is typical as antimicrobial treatments are ineffectual at eliminating carrier state.

Part 3
TRAINING AND MANAGEMENT

CHAPTER **12**   Selection of the racehorse

CHAPTER **13**   Exercise physiology and training

CHAPTER **14**   Nutrition

CHAPTER **15**   Ergogenic aids

CHAPTER **16**   Blood analysis

CHAPTER **17**   Herd health

CHAPTER **18**   Transport

CHAPTER 12
SELECTION OF THE RACEHORSE

OVERVIEW

Pre-purchase examinations vary in content with type of animal, intended purpose and client demands, and may comprise any combination of physical inspection, assessment of airway function, radiographic and ultrasonographic imaging and blood analysis. Examination of horses for private sale typically follows the recognized standard of 'five-stage' inspection encompassing pre- and post-exercise phases (+/− supplementary diagnostic imaging), while examination in the context of public auctions typically has a curtailed examination depending on type of horse and circumstances of sale.

Pass or fail?

The pre-purchase examination represents a 'risk assessment' of the potential for a horse not to fulfil the particular purpose for which it is being considered. Every purchasing client has different perceptions of risk and what is acceptable to one buyer may 'fail' for another. Criteria for horses purchased ('pinhooked') specifically for public or private resale at a future date must necessarily be more stringent than for horses bought primarily for racing. Acceptability of orthopaedic conditions that require some patience in handling or that may necessitate medication to maintain soundness is determined largely by the client's requirements. It is therefore important for the clinician to establish clearly the purpose for which the horse is being bought and the level of acceptable risk. Significance of clinical and imaging findings can vary markedly depending on the age of animal, stage of training and intended purpose.

Expectations

Purchasing an unbroken yearling is a high-risk investment when considering the likelihood of racetrack or resale earnings providing a return over and above the combined cost of purchase and training. This risk is considerably lower for the horse in training that has typically been selected for examination on the basis of demonstrable athletic ability. Expectations of athletic potential for a yearling should be considered in the context that only 40–50% of horses will race at 2 YO, and around 20% of horses will not have started a race by the end of their 3 YO season.

Conflicts of interest

Prior to undertaking a pre-purchase examination the examining clinician should attempt to establish the identities of both vendor and potential purchaser in order to avoid any possible conflict of interest. Clinicians should avoid knowingly undertaking examinations on horses that have been under their care and if such a situation is unavoidable, the examination should only proceed on the understanding that the potential purchaser is informed of this conflict and that the vendor gives permission for the clinician to declare all relevant history relating to that animal.

All information gathered during the course of the examination is solely reportable to the potential purchaser. While the vendor has no right to this information, judicious sharing of pertinent findings (with permission of the purchasing agent) is courteous and usually beneficial to all parties.

Conditions of sale at public auction

Conditions of sale at public auction differ between sales companies and types of sale. Most have clauses regarding return of lots due to undeclared infirmity of wind, stable vices and use of anti-inflammatory drugs, and it is important to be familiar with the relevant conditions when undertaking pre-bid inspections. Legislation in some countries permits the return of animals with latent defects far beyond the scope of published conditions of sale; however, preventing such situations arising in the first instance through competent examination is always preferable.

THE VETTING PROCEDURE

Preliminaries
- Establish the intended purpose for which the horse is being examined; imaging requirements and relevance of findings differ between jurisdictions.
- Communication with vendor prior to examination regarding level of exercise required/recent medication.
- Verbal or written statement from vendor regarding stable vices and history of previous surgery, EIPH or any other significant veterinary intervention.
- Establish recent racing form.
- Verify identification from passport and record vaccination history.

Physical examination: summary
- Condition and conformation: apparent fitness, overall health and obvious conformational faults.
- Eyes (*Table 12.1*): horses with severely impaired vision can function seemingly normally in training with few or no behavioural irregularities. Gross assessment, direct ophthalmoscopy and evaluation of ocular reflexes. Menace reflex is reasonable test of vision (requires intact sensory and motor pathways), unlike pupillary light reflex.
- Heart: rate, rhythm and murmurs. Auscultation from both sides of chest at rest and immediately following exercise.
- Mouth: teeth (evidence of stable vices); corners of mouth (bit damage).
- Neck: throat and submandibular space (scarring/lymph nodes); jugular grooves (patency of jugular veins/recent injection); poll and wither (headshyness/injury).
- Girth, topline and belly: sarcoids (interference with tack); muscular pain/asymmetry of topline and pelvis; abdominal scars (previous surgery); tail (tone and injury).
- Genitalia: both testicles fully descended/palpably normal (colts); mammary glands and vulval conformation (fillies).
- Limbs: palpation weight-bearing and with limb in flexion.
- Feet: foot symmetry, balance, hoof quality and type of shoeing.

Action
- Examination at walk and trot in hand before exercise.
- Exercise component should ideally incorporate fast work so that dynamic respiratory obstructions and propensity for EIPH can be assessed.
- Second examination at walk and trot following cooling-off period.

Flexion tests
- Flexion tests are non-specific and response varies between horses.
- May exacerbate subclinical lameness.
- Force and duration of flexion can strongly influence results; important that a standardized approach is used and 'positive' responses (obvious lameness which persists for ≥3 strides) are compared against the opposite limb and interpreted with caution.

Table 12.1 Significance of ocular findings

	FINDING	CAUSE	SIGNIFICANCE
Globe	Small/shrunken globe.	May be congenital (+/− concurrent lens luxation and blindness) or acquired (secondary to inflammatory disease).	Vision usually severely affected.
Cornea	Oedema.	May be primary/secondary, temporary or permanent.	Effect on vision dependent on extent. Not usually progressive.
	Keratitis.	Multiple causes (viral/bacterial/fungal/immune) and variable severity.	Most respond favourably to treatment; some conditions are recurrent.
	Ulceration.	Multiple causes (trauma/infection).	Most respond favourably to treatment with little/no permanent effect on vision.
Anterior chamber	Uveitis.	Inflammation of anterior chamber/iris.	Frequently recurrent. Considered high risk for development of future episodes of vision-affecting disease.
	Synechiae (adhesions).	Indicates previous inflammation (uveitis) in eye.	Considered high risk for development of future episodes of vision-affecting disease.
Iris	Coloboma.	Congenital focal weakening/prolapse of iris.	No effect on vision.
	Corpora nigra and iris cysts.	Can reach large size and occasionally detach to cause inflammation of eye.	Generally considered benign and no risk for vision.
Lens	Cataracts.	Anterior (Y-shaped) and posterior suture opacities are common (up to 20%).	Not progressive and do not significantly affect vision. Central capsular cataracts may interfere with ophthalmoscopic examination of retina, but do not normally affect vision (some interference with vision possible when pupil constricts in bright daylight).
	Luxation.	May be anterior or posterior; always associated with cataract and inflammation.	Blindness or severely affected vision.
Fundus (retina)	Peripapillary chorioretinopathy ('butterfly' lesions).	Localized loss of retinal pigment. Very common; may arise from previous inflammation.	Not progressive and do not affect vision.
	Focal chorioretinopathy.	'Bullet hole' loss of retinal pigment.	Variable outcome but when extensive may be a risk for future vision impairment.
	Optic disc atrophy or loss of vascularization.	Loss of blood supply to optic nerve.	Usually indicates blindness.
	Retinal detachment.	Multiple causes (trauma/congenital/viral).	Severe impairment to vision.

Ancillary tests
- Blood/serum samples obtained for analysis for presence of anti-inflammatory +/– other classes of drugs.
- For horses that are intended to travel internationally, appropriate blood +/– reproductive tract samples according to the specific entry requirements of receiving country.
- Assessment of respiratory function, ultrasonography and radiography as required.

History
- While not a compulsory component of the pre-purchase examination, a full and frank disclosure of veterinary history (particularly with regard to timing/frequency of orthopaedic medications) can greatly assist the interpretation of any radiological abnormality or lameness that is encountered during the examination.

PRE-PURCHASE RADIOGRAPHY

Pre-purchase radiography is a standard procedure for yearlings at premier public auctions and many horses in training. Pre-purchase radiography should be considered a survey of the common radiographic lesion predilection sites, rather than a comprehensive warranty of future soundness. Several important orthopaedic conditions encountered in racehorses are either radiologically silent or occur at sites not routinely surveyed during a pre-purchase examination.

The radiographic protocol (minimum specified views) varies with the age of the horse and the requirements of the sales company/purchaser, and reflects the relative importance of certain pathological conditions at various stages of training. The proximity of image acquisition to sale date is usually stipulated by the conditions of sale (typically 3–6 weeks) and examining clinicians should still be alert to pathology that may arise in the intervening period. The standard protocols are listed in *Table 12.2*.

Supplementary projections
The need for additional radiographic projections is dictated by clinical findings. Bony enlargements/splints not adequately covered on standard projections may warrant lesion-oriented obliques to assess activity. The importance of fetlock condylar pathology in horses in training makes a strong case for inclusion of flexed dorsopalmar/plantarodorsal projections into any comprehensive protocol. Multiple DLPaMO projections of the carpus are beneficial for assessment of the middle carpal joint when activity at this site is suspected.

Image interpretation
Radiographic series are assessed for diagnostic quality, completeness, date of acquisition and accurate labelling and any deficiencies noted. The relevance of certain radiological lesions to future soundness may differ between individuals with similar defects, and clinical evaluation of the affected site is essential for accurate interpretation in many cases. The relative importance of radiological findings can also differ considerably depending on stage of career. As a general rule, developmental orthopaedic disease (osteochondrosis: OCD/bone cyst) and abnormalities associated with the PSBs (sesamoiditis, foal sesamoid fractures) are viewed more critically in the yearling because any influence on trainability remains untested. When these same faults are detected in a horse that has been trained to 'breeze-up' stage (p. 312) and the horse remains clinically unaffected, they can be interpreted more leniently, and when detected in a horse-in-training with recent racing form they can often be disregarded (or at least considered low risk for future interruption). Radiological signs of active arthritic change in important high-motion joints (fetlock/middle carpal joint) should be interpreted in the context of physical findings but may be significant at any age.

Table 12.2 **Standard protocols for pre-purchase radiography**

SITE	PROJECTION	YEARLING	HORSE IN TRAINING
Front fetlock	Dorsopalmar (DPa) elevated 20°	*	*
	Dorsolateral oblique (DLPaMO)	*	*
	Dorsomedial oblique (DMPaLO)	*	*
	Standing lateromedial (LM)	*	*
	Flexed lateromedial (flexed LM)	*	
	Flexed dorsopalmar (flexed DPa)		(*)
Hind fetlock	Dorsoplantar (DPl) elevated 30°	*	*
	Dorsolateral oblique (DLPlMO)	*	*
	Dorsomedial oblique (DMPlLO)	*	*
	Standing lateromedial (LM)	*	*
	Flexed plantarodorsal (flexed PlD)		(*)
Knee (carpus)	Dorsopalmar (DPa)	*	*
	Dorsolateral oblique (DLPaMO)	*	*
	Dorsomedial oblique (DMPaLO)	*	*
	Standing lateromedial (LM)	*	*
	Flexed lateromedial (flexed LM)		*
	Skyline distal row (flexed D35°PrDDiO)		*
Hock (tarsus)	Dorsoplantar (DPl) slightly (10°) lateral	*	*
	Dorsolateral oblique (DLPlMO)	*	*
	Dorsomedial oblique (DMPlLO)	*	*
	Standing lateromedial (LM)	*	*
Stifle	Lateromedial (LM)	(*)	(*)
	Caudolateral oblique (CdLCrMO)	*	*
	Caudocranial (CdCr)	*	*
Front foot	Lateromedial (LM)		*
	Upright pedal (D60°Pr-PaDiO)		*

(*) Non-compulsory projections; inclusion dependent on specific requirements/clinical judgement.

The prevalence of radiological abnormalities in yearlings presented for sale at public auction (*Table 12.3*), and their impact on future performance, has been investigated in a small number of studies (USA, Australia, New Zealand, South Africa). There are only a few consistent or strong relationships between radiological findings and key measures of performance that include likelihood to start, time to first start and career placings/prize-money (although it should be noted that these studies do not take into account previous or subsequent surgical intervention). Regardless of this general lack of direct 'risk association', risk may still be attached to some abnormalities on an individual basis because of the consequences for that individual should lameness arise.

Digital images

Due to the large file size of acquired images, image compression is used both to facilitate data archiving and to permit transmission of images to remote servers. Image compression can either be reversible ('lossless') or irreversible ('lossy'). The type and level of compression that is diagnostically (or legally) acceptable varies with application and current guidelines are neither definitive nor universal to all situations. The often low range of contrast in equine skeletal imaging calls for a conservative approach to image compression; the quality of the viewed image is also frequently limited by the resolution of the viewing screen as much as by file size.

It is recommended that the DICOM (Digital Imaging and Communications in Medicine) format is used where possible for diagnostic, pre-purchase and teleradiology applications of radiographic and ultrasonographic images, as this involves no image degradation and permits full adjustment of window levels and other post-processing. By contrast, the window level of JPEG and TIFF formats is set at the time of creation of the image and cannot be altered by the viewer; additionally, it is possible for JPEG images to be manipulated such that lesions are obscured. JPEG images should only be used as part of a pre-purchase examination if there is no visual loss of image quality due to compression.

Table 12.3 **Prevalence and significance of radiological abnormalities in public auction yearlings**

SITE	FINDING	PREVALENCE	RISK FOR TRAINABILITY	RISK FOR RESALE (AS HORSE IN TRAINING)
Carpus	Dorsal medial carpal disease	2.7%[$]	Medium; dependent on severity. Less likely to start a race. May require medication in training.	High; dependent on severity.
	Chip/fragment/spur	2.5[$]–4%	Medium. May require medication in training.	High.
	Distal radial cyst	0.09%[$]	Medium.	Medium.
	Radial carpal bone cyst	?	Medium. Most remain clinically silent but those that develop lameness can be problematic to manage.	Medium.
	Ulnar carpal lucency/cyst	8.33[†]–22.2%	Low/negligible.	Negligible.
	Accessory carpal bone fracture	0.08–0.4%[$]	Low (if clinically silent); however, significance is untested prior to training.	Medium–high depending on intended market.

Table 12.3 (continued)

SITE	FINDING	PREVALENCE	RISK FOR TRAINABILITY	RISK FOR RESALE (AS HORSE IN TRAINING)
Hock	DIT/TMT spur	9.92†–35.4%	Low/negligible. No effect on performance.	Low/negligible.
	OCD (tibiotarsal joint)	4*–8.7% (distal intermediate ridge most common: 3%)	Low. No effect on performance.	Low.
	Wedged-shaped or collapsed T3	1.2%§	Mild severity: low. Marked/collapsed: moderate–high: less likely to start a race and may predispose to slab fracture.	Mild: negligible. Marked: medium.
Front fetlock	Sagittal ridge OCD (lucency)	17.4§–37.1%	Low/negligible No effect on performance.	Negligible.
	Chip/fragment: dorsoproximal	0.7–1.6%†§	Low. Less likely to start a race.	Low.
	Chip/fragment: palmaroproximal	0.4–2%†	Low (dependent on type/size). No effect on performance.	Low/negligible.
	Bone cyst (distal Mc3 or prox P1)	0.7%§	Medium–high.	Medium–high.
	Supracondylar lysis (moderate–severe)	0.1–2.1%§	Medium–high. Less likely to start a race (at 2 or 3 YO).	Medium.
Hind fetlock	Sagittal ridge OCD (>10 mm length)	0.7–1.6%§	Medium. Fewer starts/less likely to start/greater time to 1st start.	Low.
	Chip/fragment: dorso-proximal	1.6†–3.3%§	Medium Less likely to start a race (at 2 or 3 YO).	Low.
	Chip/fragment: plantaroproximal	5.9§–7.1%†	Low (dependent on type/size). No effect on performance.	Low.
	Bone cyst (distal Mt3 or prox P1)	0.2%§	Medium–high.	Medium–high.
Pastern joint	Lucency (P1/P2; midline/condylar); visible on multiple radiographic projections	2.4%††	Low (dependent on size/appearance). Bone cysts medium–high risk depending on size/location/appearance.	Low–high (dependent on size/appearance).
Proximal sesamoid bone: forelimb	Marked sesamoiditis (≥3 irregular vascular channels >2 mm)	2–3.6%	Medium (determine SLB involvement). May affect performance at 2 and 3 YO.	Low–medium.
	Fracture	0.9§–1.5% (medial most common)	Medium–high (dependent on severity). Less likely to start a race (at 2 or 3 YO).	Medium–high.
	Elongated/abnormal shape	5.6%§	Low. No effect on performance.	Low.
	Modelling (osteophytes/ entheseophyte/s)	1.6§–3.8%	Medium (determine SLB involvement). Less likely to start at 2 and 3 YO.	Low–medium.

(continued overleaf)

Table 12.3 *(continued)*

SITE	FINDING	PREVALENCE	RISK FOR TRAINABILITY	RISK FOR RESALE (AS HORSE IN TRAINING)
Proximal sesamoid bone: hindlimb	Marked sesamoiditis (≥3 irregular vascular channels >2 mm)	2[‡]–3%	Medium (determine SLB involvement). Fewer starts and lower earnings at 2 and 3 YO.	Low–medium.
	Fracture	1.7–2.9%[§]	Low–medium (dependent on severity). Limited effect on performance.	Low–medium.
	Elongated/abnormal shape	2.8%[§]	Low.	Low.
	Modelling (osteophytes/entheseophyte/s)	4%	Low. No effect on performance.	Low.
Stifle	OCD (defect/fragment): lateral trochlear ridge	3*–5.1%[§] **(lesion >40 mm in 0.5%)**	Horses with smaller lesions (total length <6 cm) undergoing surgery prior to 2 YO season have similar trainability to normal horses; longer time to 1st start. Horses with more extensive lesions (total length >6 cm) less likely to race.	Medium.
	OCD (defect/fragment): medial trochlear ridge	0.3[§]–0.7%	Medium.	Medium.
	Medial femoral condyle: bone cyst	2*–5.6%	Medium–high. >6 mm deep: less likely to start a race at 2 or 3 YO.	Medium–high (dependent on radiological appearance/clinical history).
	Medial femoral condyle: lucency	16%*	Low–medium (dependent on radiological/ultrasonographic appearance).	Low.
	Patellar fracture	0.1%	High.	High.
Front foot	P3 cyst	2.3%[§]	High.	High.
	P3: proliferative modelling (toe)	6.1%	Low. No effect on performance.	Low.
	P3: proliferative modelling (dorsal)	14.5%	Low/negligible.	Negligible.
	P3 fracture	0.3%	Low–medium (dependent on type).	Low–medium (dependent on type).
	Bipartite navicular bone	?	High. Usually cause lameness (untreatable) in training; small number of horses remain clinically unaffected and race.	High.

Bold Jackson M, Vizard A, Anderson G *et al.* (2009) A prospective study of presale radiographs of Thoroughbred yearlings. *RIRDC* **No 09/082**.

[§] Kane AJ, Park RD, McIlwraith CW *et al.* (2003) Radiographic changes in Thoroughbred yearlings. Part 1: Prevalence at the time of the yearling sales. *Equine Vet J* **35(4)**:354–365.

*Oliver LJ, Baird DK, Baird AN *et al.* (2008) Prevalence and distribution of radiographically evident lesions on repository films in the hock and stifle joints of yearling Thoroughbred horses in New Zealand. *NZ Vet J* **56(5)**:202–209.

[†] Furniss C, Carstens A, van den Berg (2011) Radiographic changes in Thoroughbred yearlings in South Africa. *J S Afr Vet Assoc* **82(4)**: 194–204.

[‡] Spike-Pierce D, Bramlage LR (2003) Correlation of racing performance with radiographic changes in the proximal sesamoid bones of 487 Thoroughbred yearlings. *Equine Vet J* **35(4)**:350–353.

[††] Vargas J (2011) Racing prognosis of Thoroughbred yearlings with subchondral bone lucencies in the proximal interphalangeal joint. *Proc 57th Ann Conv Am Assoc Equine Practitnrs* p. 243.

PRE-PURCHASE ULTRASONOGRAPHY

Ultrasonographic assessment of the forelimb cannon/fetlock region is commonly included in pre-purchase examinations of moderate- to high-value horses-in-training. Sensitivity for detection of previous tendon injury is high; interpretation of suspensory ligament appearance is more subjective but major lesions are usually readily apparent. Examination of other areas (e.g. pelvis) may be indicated if clinical abnormality or reported history demands it. Ultrasonography is less common in yearling inspections, but very useful to assess integrity of the SLB–sesamoid bone interface (Chapter 2, p. 86) particularly if radiological evidence of sesamoiditis is present.

Satisfactory image acquisition is usually possible without clipping the limb. Sequential cross-sectional and longitudinal images of the major structures of the palmar cannon (flexor tendons, inferior check and suspensory ligaments) and of the SLBs are obtained of both forelimbs and assessed for symmetry, size, echogenicity and fibrillar pattern. Particular care should be taken to assess the most important sites of injury: SDFT, suspensory ligament origin (proximal metacarpus) and SLB insertion.

ASSESSMENT OF AIRWAY FUNCTION

Physical examination/history
- Vendor declaration on unsoundness of wind or previous respiratory surgery should be sought.
- Palpation of throatlatch for detection of surgical scars, congenital laryngeal abnormalities and laryngeal muscle atrophy.

Resting endoscopy
- The upper airway conditions of greatest importance to the racehorse (Chapter 3, p. 201) are dynamic in nature and cannot be fully assessed at rest.
- Despite this, resting endoscopy is still the mainstay of respiratory tract assessment at public auctions and most private horse-in-training examinations. Useful for more advanced grades of RLN, congenital abnormalities and arytenoid chondritis (Chapter 3, p. 218). Not useful for palatal function.
- Laryngeal function graded according to symmetry and synchrony of movement of the arytenoid cartilages (Chapter 3, p. 205); observation of full range of cartilage movements assisted by inducing swallowing or nasal occlusion.
- Acepromazine is in common use at public sales as a behaviour-modifying drug and has potential to temporarily weaken observed laryngeal function.
- Epiglottic size/flaccidity generally not associated with potential for future dynamic obstructions; however, markedly flaccid or short epiglottis usually viewed with considerable caution in the untrained yearling.

Video endoscopy
- Availability of recorded resting endoscopy (by clinician acting for vendor) is commonplace at public auctions in some jurisdictions.
- To be considered of diagnostic quality, recordings should include identification of horse, be of sufficient length and display full range of arytenoid movements (both resting and induced by swallowing/nasal occlusion).
- Throats that are 'fixed' open may indicate use of prior exercise (high respiration rate evident) or nasal twitch to stimulate laryngeal dilation and are problematic to interpret.
- Non-diagnostic video endoscopic recordings justify endoscopic reappraisal.

Wind testing
- Presence and character of abnormal respiratory noises not necessarily specific for type of respiratory obstruction (Chapter 3, p. 203).
- Any use of tack that might affect upper airway function (noseband/tongue-tie) should be noted.

Laryngeal ultrasonography
- Objective assessment of intrinsic laryngeal muscle atrophy/degeneration.
- May be used as adjunct to resting endoscopy to determine significance of 'borderline' grades of laryngeal function.

Overground endoscopy
- Useful in situations in which concern exists over respiratory noise/previous respiratory surgery/racing form.

PUBLIC AUCTION VETTING: THE YEARLING

Pre-bid inspections of yearlings at public auction are often undertaken under challenging circumstances due to constraints of time and convention. Examinations typically consist of a brief physical inspection in the stable followed by observation at a walk (examination at a trot is not generally accepted practice and reserved for horses with radiological lesions or suspected lameness).

Physical examination
Particular attention to enlargement of PSBs (plus deep palpation of SLB insertions), distal radial growth plates and effusion of important high motion joints. Major conformational faults or physical traits that might affect trainability are noted. Opportunities to observe action are limited and importance is placed on stride length and indicators of neurological dysfunction/incoordination when turned.

Airway function
Upper airway is frequently inflamed +/− pharyngeal lymphoid hyperplasia (Chapter 3, p. 217): may obscure full visualization of abducted arytenoid cartilages; intermittent displacement of the soft palate (Chapter 3, p. 210) is common.

Radiography
Particular attention should be paid to the following:
- Developmental orthopaedic disease (osteochondrosis: OCD/bone cysts): significance varies with location and appearance.
- PSBs: fractures and sesamoiditis.
- Articular modelling of important high motion joints (middle carpal joints/fetlocks).

Ultrasonography
Useful to assess SLB–sesamoid interface for subclinical ligament injury. 'Juvenile' SDFT tendinitis (Chapter 2, p. 96) is a common finding of little relevance.

PUBLIC AUCTION VETTING: THE 'BREEZE-UP' 2 YEAR OLD

'Breeze-up' ('ready-to-run') auctions differ from other formats in that the horses being offered for purchase are unraced 2 YOs that must complete a short fast-exercise 'breeze' prior to sale. Although untested on the racetrack, these horses have undergone a training preparation and many of the unquantifiable risks attached to imaging/physical defects seen in yearlings can therefore be interpreted with greater objectivity.

Physical examination
As for yearlings. Examination of action at a trot is permissible. Dorsal metacarpal disease ('sore/bucked' shins, Chapter 2, p. 102) is common in breeze-up 2YOs: may be associated with lameness and thereby complicate interpretation of physical findings. Of little long-term significance but may interfere with training in immediate post-sale period.

Airway function
Format of breeze-up auctions permits observation at exercise and assessment of respiratory noise.

Radiography
Particular attention should be paid to the following:
- Carpus: middle carpal joint changes (if present) can be expected to progress with further training. May have implications for resale later in career and may be predictive for future carpal lameness in training.

- Fetlocks: active joint margin modelling is not uncommon; determine significance (training and resale) on individual basis. Sesamoid bone changes (sesamoiditis, old fragments/fractures) can generally be viewed more leniently than in yearling if clinically silent.

PUBLIC AUCTION VETTING: THE HORSE IN TRAINING

Level of fitness and recent racing form are of considerable importance for interpretation of findings. It is possible to be less critical of certain imaging/clinical faults in a fit horse that has run recently than in a horse unraced for some months. Many significant injuries (including SDFT tendinitis and stress fractures) can be difficult to detect clinically after even short periods of rest and/or anti-inflammatory measures.

Physical examination
Examination at a trot is permissible; action should be considered in the context of level of fitness/excitability. Recent lameness may be diminished/abolished with short periods of rest or intra-articular medication prior to sale. Particular attention should be paid to joints, tendons and ligaments, especially asymmetry of any structure.

Airway function
Particular attention should be paid to endoscopic evidence of previous surgical intervention (larynx/palate); palpation of throatlatch region for surgical scars (often subtle)/laryngeal muscle atrophy.

Radiography
Requirement for pre-purchase radiography is dictated by needs of buyer and/or intended racing jurisdiction. Particular attention should be paid to the following:
- Carpus: middle carpal joint changes are common and are considered in the context of clinical findings. Assess for possible future interruptions to training arising from chip/slab fracture rather than previous activity. Long-standing arthritic change of settled appearance may be acceptable in absence of clinical abnormality.
- Fetlocks: long-standing arthritic change of settled appearance may be acceptable. Problematic subchondral lesions or condylar fatigue cracks are usually not detectable with standard radiographic projections (require 'flexed dorsopalmar/plantarodorsal' projection).

CONFORMATION

Overview
Judging athletic potential from body type and limb conformation displayed early in life is highly subjective. Accurate measurement of conformation is difficult and current scientific knowledge is based largely on information derived from yearlings vetted at public auction, a population of animals already selected for saleability. The main conformational faults appear to be heritable to a variable extent. The importance of conformation lies primarily in its influence on limb loading (and thereby predisposition to injury) and, less quantifiably, on force generation during locomotion (particularly the hindlimb). Opinions on conformation/body types most suitable for different racing distances (sprint/middle-distance/staying) are widely held but not currently supported by any evidence base. Smaller/shorter horses are more likely to race as 2 YOs (and have more career starts) and base-narrow horses are less likely to run as 2 YOs. Taller yearlings are more likely to be elite performers.

There are some general trends of association between certain conformation types and development of specific injuries; however, exceptions to all rules exist and conformation should be viewed in the context of body type, pedigree, action and intended use. Significance for future unsoundness is greater the more severe a conformational fault is, although in general there is only a weak association between conformation and racetrack performance. Excluding severe conformational faults, pedigree is a far greater influence on racetrack performance than conformation. Conformation assessment is of greater importance at yearling examinations (prior to training) than in horses that have trained at least one season and in which any adaptive effects have become tangible either clinically or on imaging.

Changes with maturity

In general horses tend to be proportional, such that length of limb bones is related to height. Bone length changes little beyond 12 months of age, and by 18 months most yearlings are nearly (95%) full adult height.

Limb conformation may change up to the point of skeletal maturity and considerable self-correction of many carpal and fetlock conformational faults occurs in foals. From yearling stage into adulthood, limb conformation generally changes little: straightening of toe out hind fetlocks and back-at-the-knee occurs, while offset knee/toe in conformation may worsen. Consideration of body type, severity of fault and activity of growth plates, and prior experience of closely related animals may help determine the importance of limb conformation in a particular individual.

Corrective surgery

If corrective surgery for a fault has resulted in a normalization of conformation without untoward effects (such as on dynamic foot balance), then as a general rule any importance to potential trainability can simply be judged on the yearling's limb conformation as presented at time of sale.

Conformation faults
Offset ('bench') knee
- Carpus and cannon laterally offset (with varying severity) relative to radius.
- Common finding.
- May worsen from yearling to adulthood.
- Greater loading through medial splint bone: higher likelihood of developing splint enlargement or fracture.
- Association with risk of developing fetlock problems (in same limb).
- Strong anecdotal indication that moderate–marked severity is associated with carpal lameness (specifically pathological loading through dorsomedial carpus).

Carpal valgus
- Angle of radius–mid-carpus–mid-fetlock is >180^0.
- Common finding.
- Mild–moderate carpal valgus may reduce risk of carpal fracture.

Back-at-the-knee
- Proximal row of carpal bones positioned caudal to front edge of radius, resulting in 'concave' appearance to knee when viewed from side.
- Strongly heritable.
- Uncommon finding.
- Improves from yearling to adulthood.
- Anecdotally associated with greater risk of carpal fracture, particularly involving radiocarpal joint.

Over-at-the-knee
- Rare finding.
- May worsen from yearling to adulthood.
- Associated with greater risk of pastern fracture.

Fetlock–toe out
- Very common finding (small amount of outward rotation through the fetlock is normal).
- May predispose to interference injuries.

Upright forelimb pastern
- Common finding: up to 20% of yearlings.

Long/sloping pastern
- Uncommon finding.
- Greater risk of fracture in same limb (including carpal chip fracture).

Straight through the hock
- Uncommon finding.
- Greater risk of developing hindlimb lameness, particularly hind suspensory desmitis.

Sickle hocks
- Uncommon finding.
- Greater risk of developing lower hock joint osteoarthritis or curb.

Uneven feet
- Uncommon finding.
- Uneven front feet (one upright/boxy, other flat-heeled) may develop either from 'sidedness' when grazing at young age or chronic lameness or DIPJ contracture.
- Merits caution: determine significance on individual basis.
- Correction usually not possible/advisable.

HEART SIZE

Accurate measurement of cardiac dimensions in the live horse may be undertaken with echocardiography. As a general rule heart size is a poor predictor of athleticism in the racehorse. The following points are relevant:
- Heart size is strongly related to body size.
- Chamber dimensions and heart muscle mass increase considerably with training.
- Heart dimensions therefore often change markedly between yearling and mature (trained) racehorse.
- Top-performing sprinters often have hearts ≤ average size.
- Heart size is a more important predictor of endurance capacity; not relevant in yearlings/2 YOs but may be useful in National Hunt (hurdle/steeplechase) racehorses.
- 'Heart scores' derived from ECG assessment of ventricular depolarization (QRS duration) may bear some relationship to heart size but correlation with performance is weak.

GENETICS OF SELECTION

A horse's athletic potential remains largely unknown until completion of a training programme and tested against peers during fast exercise in training/racing. Even following full maturity, considerable experimentation on the racetrack may be needed before a horse's optimal racing distance is determined. Given that athletic ability is largely determined by cardiovascular and muscular capacity and that around 35% of variation in performance is heritable, it is understandable that interest in the use of gene sequencing to predict a horse's potential is increasing.

The closed Thoroughbred gene pool, intense selection for performance and the physiological features of large muscle mass and a high-capacity cardiorespiratory system has led to identification of gene variants that may contribute to performance. Genes associated with energy production and utilization at a cellular level may have a direct bearing on a horse's anaerobic and aerobic capacity and total oxygen uptake. Variants of the myostatin gene have been shown to be highly predictive of potential for sprinting/staying ability and were the first commercially available genotype test for racing ability. C:C (sprinting) and C:T (middle-distance) genotypes are in general more precocious and more successful as 2 YO than T:T (staying) genotypes. In addition to optimum racing distance, evidence is emerging that variants of genes involved in mitochondrial respiration and regulation of insulin sensitivity and glucose uptake may be predictive for elite performance.

CHAPTER 13
EXERCISE PHYSIOLOGY AND TRAINING

OVERVIEW OF EXERCISE PHYSIOLOGY

The ability to perform and sustain athletic effort is determined by energy production in skeletal muscle. During exercise, constant replenishment of muscle energy stores is required; this can occur through aerobic or anaerobic metabolic pathways. The generation of energy by aerobic means is most efficient but is limited by the many factors that make up the supply chain of oxygen to muscle, chiefly cardiorespiratory function and blood oxygen carrying capacity (haemoglobin). When the supply of blood and oxygen to muscle can no longer keep pace with energy expenditure, anaerobic metabolism begins to contribute. Anaerobic energy production is relatively inefficient and results in increased production of lactate (lactic acid). Rising levels of lactate in muscle and blood impair muscle contraction and further energy (glycolytic) production, resulting in fatigue.

Over flat racing distances, fatigue arises from the build-up of the by-products of energy production (lactate and heat), rather than depletion of energy reserves. The energy pathways used are self-regulated at a cellular level, with the relative contributions of aerobic and anaerobic metabolism primarily influenced by exercise intensity and duration. Slow paces (trot and slow canter) are purely aerobic; however, all performances at racing speeds derive energy from both pathways, regardless of distance. Energy production during races over staying distances (>3,200 metres/2 miles) is estimated to be around 80–90% aerobic, and even those run over sprint distances (<1,200 metres/6 furlongs) are predominantly (70%) aerobic. Short periods of acceleration during a race (whether at the start or in the closing stages) are anaerobic efforts and consequently cannot be sustained for long (typically <600 metres/ 3 furlongs).

THE RACEHORSE AS ATHLETE

Evolution as a fight-or-flight prey animal has resulted in the modern horse being skeletally mature at a young age and capable of tasks requiring speed or stamina. Further selective breeding has given the racehorse several intrinsic anatomical and physiological characteristics that make it an effective athlete:

- Large muscle mass relative to BWT, with muscles primarily positioned in the upper limbs/trunk allowing for great efficiency of motion.
- Large cardiovascular capacity to supply this muscle mass with oxygenated blood: main feature is ability to greatly increase heart rate in response to workload.
- Large reserve of RBCs stored in the spleen, which is released at onset of exercise to dramatically increase oxygen-carrying capacity of blood.
- Efficient cellular-level utilization of oxygen in skeletal muscle through high activity of enzymes involved in energy pathways.

Cardiovascular system

Resting heart rate is 28–36 bpm; it increases rapidly at onset of exercise, and at racing speeds the maximum heart rate is 200–240 bpm. Although high heart rates reduce the time available for the cardiac chambers to fill, the horse succeeds in also raising the amount of blood pumped with each beat (stroke volume) by about 50%. In this way up to >300 litres/minute of blood can be circulated at peak exercise, supporting the high metabolic demands of the musculoskeletal system. Total circulating blood volume in the resting racehorse is about 45 litres (9% of BWT). With exercise (or excitement), splenic contraction can effectively double the circulating RBC concentration.

Respiratory system

The primary function of the respiratory system is gas exchange: transfer of oxygen into the bloodstream and removal of carbon dioxide. The racehorse has a large respiratory capacity relative to body size, and increased demand for oxygen at exercise is met by an increase in breathing rate. At faster paces, breathing and locomotion are intrinsically coupled such that exhalation occurs when the forelimbs strike the ground. The horse is an obligate nasal breather and is therefore reliant on correct functioning of the dynamic components of the upper airway for optimum respiratory efficiency.

Muscles

The function and capacity for different types of workload vary between muscles depending on anatomical location. Muscle fibres are either 'slow twitch' (aerobic) or 'fast twitch' (greater anaerobic capacity), and the relative proportions of these are largely genetically predetermined. Central/axial muscle groups tend to have a greater postural role and therefore a higher proportion of slow twitch fibres; however, recruitment of muscles varies according to speed, gait and duration of exercise. Muscle concentrations of energy substrates (primarily glycogen) in racehorses are considerable; along with high cellular enzymatic activity this contributes to a high capacity for buffering against the acidic conditions that lead to fatigue.

ADAPTATIONS TO TRAINING

The goal of training is to stimulate adaptation of key body systems (skeletal, muscular, cardiovascular) to the demands of racing. Training serves both to condition the musculoskeletal system to withstand the forces imposed during peak exercise and to maximize efficiency of energy generation and utilization, culminating in 'fitness'. Different tissues have specific responses to the stimulus of training.

Cardiovascular system

Training results in strengthening and enlargement of the left side of the heart, with hypertrophy of left ventricular muscle permitting greater propulsion of blood to the exercising body. Unlike human athletes, neither resting heart rate or maximal heart rate at exercise (HR_{max}) are significantly affected by training.

Training causes some increase in resting RBC figures (such as haemoglobin concentration and total red cell count); however, the changes are too small to be used reliably as a measure of fitness. Resting acid–base and electrolyte status does not change with training.

Respiratory system

Training has little effect on ventilatory capacity.

Muscle

Muscle is probably the most responsive of all body tissues to training and most changes occur within 4 months of the commencement of exercise. Above an exercise threshold the majority of changes occur rapidly and relate primarily to improvements in oxidative capacity brought about by greater enzyme activity and increased network of capillaries. Trained muscles have a greater ability to utilize oxygen, thereby raising the threshold for anaerobic metabolism; combined with enhanced buffering against lactate, the result is a delay in onset of fatigue. High intensity exercise may also lead to muscle cell hypertrophy and greater potential for power generation.

Bone

Bone is a dynamic tissue that remodels continually in response to the loads placed upon it. These loads are influenced by speed, conformation, track surface and jockey weight among other factors. Architectural adaptations involving bone shape and size and trabecular orientation of cancellous bone appear to be more important to acquired strength than increases in bone density or mass.

Tendon and ligament

Adaptation of the flexor tendons to conditioning exercise occurs early in life. From the age of 2 years, no strengthening of tendons occurs, although some increase in tendon size is often noted (as a result of greater water content of tendon matrix rather than tendon hypertrophy). The suspensory ligament undergoes some strengthening into early training.

Cartilage

While training has little or no adaptive effect on articular cartilage, free exercise as a foal is important to future health of the joint. Restricted exercise early in life has the potential to hinder normal articular cartilage development, making it less able to withstand the rigours of training.

FUNDAMENTALS OF TRAINING

Training usually commences before the age of 2 years. Training strategies vary widely both geographically and between individual trainers and in large part are shaped by tradition and local conditions. Although there is no universal template for conditioning a racehorse, most programmes share elements of the following:
- Foundation low-intensity phase: low-speed, predominantly aerobic exercise (trot and slow canter). HR <160 bpm and no increase in blood lactate. Goal is to improve aerobic capacity and limb strength as well as educate the horse.
- Gradual increase in training load (cantering speed +/or distance) every 2–3 weeks ('overload principle') to improve aerobic and anaerobic fitness as well as musculoskeletal strength. Exercise intensity is more important than duration.
- Combined aerobic and anaerobic phase: periodic high-intensity exercise improves muscular strength and stamina. Causes adaptation/recruitment of the 'fast twitch' (type II) muscle fibres that assist in developing anaerobic metabolism. Typically done by closing submaximal (70–80% of race speed; 14–16 seconds/furlong) workouts with a short distance (1–3 furlongs) of top speed (95–100% of maximal speed).

The capacity for exercise (mental and physical) varies between horses. Training programmes are modified to account for this as well as stage of maturity and career goals. Training not only targets physical fitness but also mental development (stalls and race training). Rest days after fast exercise or racing days are important for recovery and frequency of high-intensity bouts (typically 1–2/week) is determined on an individual basis. Overreaching (in this context: short-term/single session excessive training load relative to fitness) may diminish performance and cause loss of appetite. Fitness is maintained well in the short term and in general it is preferable to apply short intense training loads on an intermittent basis, with allowance for rest/light exercise periods, than to maintain constant high-volume training stimulus.

The goal of achieving muscular and cardiovascular fitness must be balanced with conditioning of the musculoskeletal system. Incremental increase in workload (through manipulation of intensity, duration or frequency of exercise) stimulates conditioning; however, unless sufficient time is allowed for adaptation, stress-related injuries may result. The main musculoskeletal tissues have different 'windows of opportunity' for adaptive change. For cartilage, tendons and ligaments these are in the first year of life and there is some indication that judicious application of conditioning exercise in addition to spontaneous paddock activity might be advantageous. Bone strength is highly responsive to early training and the better overall career longevity of horses trained and raced as 2 YOs probably reflects greater potential for the musculoskeletal system to adapt during this period of relative immaturity.

Training speeds

Terminology to describe canter speeds differs worldwide. Frequently, there is also considerable variation between trainer/jockey perception of paces and measured speeds. Factors such as stage of season, time of week, track surface and flat or hillwork have been demonstrated to have an impact on actual (as opposed to described) speeds; to determine work intensity accurately, objective measurement using GPS equipment is required. Typical training speeds are shown in *Table 13.1*.

Overtraining
- Poorly defined syndrome characterized by underperformance.
- Mismatch between training load and recovery.
- Frequently suspected but difficult to prove.
- May be indicated by changes in condition and behaviour.
- Loss of condition/BWT without a drop in feed intake.
- Irritability and unwillingness to train.
- No effective test for diagnosis.

Detraining
- Short periods of restricted exercise (<1–2 weeks) do not result in great loss of fitness.
- Cardiovascular fitness may return to pre-training levels after 2–3 weeks of inactivity. This is not influenced by level of fitness immediately prior to the break.
- Loss of fitness can be significantly offset if the horse is allowed some daily walking/paddock turnout rather than being confined to the stable.
- Effects of detraining on musculoskeletal system are less certain. Some degree of limb loading and motion is required to keep articular cartilage healthy.

TRAINING AIDS

Hill work
- Inclines of 5–10% typical.
- Exercising uphill permits application of a similar training load at slower speeds than would be needed if exercised on the flat (maximal exercise intensity occurs at 10–12 metres/second on a 6% hill, but 14–16 metres/second on the flat).
- Permits increase in volume of training, which stimulates anaerobic pathways without causing fatigue and overtraining.
- Training at lower speeds reduces risk of certain musculoskeletal injuries, although greater loading of hindlimbs can lead to higher prevalence of some hindlimb problems.

Treadmills
- Adjustable for speed (up to gallop) and incline (typically 0–10%).
- Fan-cooled.
- Majority of horses readily become accustomed to treadmill exercise after a short introduction period (1–2 sessions).
- Allows great control over training loads and individual tailoring of exercise programmes.
- Useful for horses that are unwilling/difficult to train under rider; also horses recovering from musculoskeletal injury or those with sore backs preventing use of tack.
- Little information available on treadmill-specific injury patterns; however, risk of serious/catastrophic injury during use is very low.

Table 13.1 **Typical training speeds**

	TROT	CANTER (SLOW)	CANTER (1/2 PACE)	CANTER (3/4 PACE)	FAST GALLOP/BREEZE
km/h	10–16	18–29	36–47	48–54	>54
mph	6.5–10	11–18	22–29	30–34	>34
m/s	3–4.5	5–8	10–13	13–15	>15
s/furlong		>25	20–15	15–13	<13

km/h, kilometres/hour; mph, miles/hour; m/s, metres/second; s/furlong, seconds/furlong.
1 furlong = 220 yards = 201.2 metres.
1 mile = 8 furlongs = 1,609.3 metres.

Water treadmills
- Adjustable water height: encourages change in stride length/character during use (longer stride length if at knee–elbow height).
- Increased workload relative to regular horse-walker.
- Unless utilized heavily, has little demonstrable conditioning effect on cardiorespiratory or muscle function.

Swimming
- Generally considered a non-essential cross training aid, as stimulates adaptations specific to swimming rather than running.
- Has a role in rehabilitation and some training programmes.
- Exercise intensity similar to trotting/slow cantering (HR 140–180 bpm): submaximal aerobic exercise.
- Tethered (tail) swimming with short periods of encouragement may achieve efforts with HR >200 bpm.
- Markedly altered respiration pattern compared with ridden exercise: brief inspiration, breath holding and prolonged, explosive expiration.
- Greater pressure of water on chest and abdomen may necessitate more forceful breathing: possible 'training' of respiratory muscles.

GPS/ECG monitors
- GPS tracking can allow accurate monitoring of daily workload (speed and distance).
- Primary benefit is objective analysis of fast exercise performance (**Figure 13.1**).
- Poor performance in closing stage of fast exercise often found to be result of unplanned events early in exercise session (e.g. too quick too early).
- Encourages improvement in pace consistency of work riders.
- HR data from ECG monitors may be used longitudinally over period of time to document fitness/athletic potential of an individual; interpret with caution as influenced by many variables.

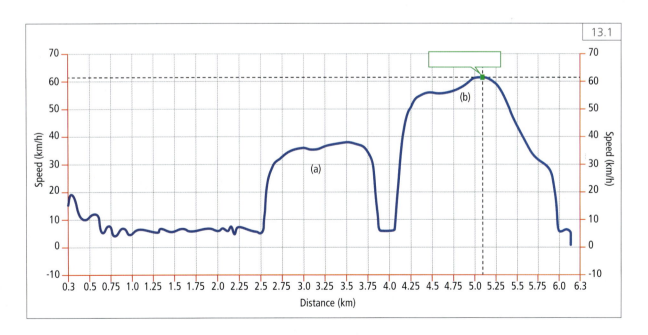

Fig. 13.1 Typical GPS speed graph from normal training gallop: (a) warm-up canter (first peak); (b) fast exercise (second peak).

Warm-up
- Has little effect on injury risk, but can enhance performance.
- 'Primes' the muscles: improves oxygen and fuel availability/utilization such that during subsequent race more energy is provided by aerobic sources and onset of fatigue is delayed.
- Splenic contraction increases circulating red cell fraction (and oxygen-carrying capacity) of blood; may also occur through anticipation/ excitement.
- Likely that high-intensity (canter) warm-up is more beneficial than low-intensity (walk/trot).
- Cantering down to start of race probably beneficial to subsequent race performance.

Cool-down
- 'Cool-down' in immediate post-gallop/race period also important.
- Most efficient cool-down exercise for optimizing clearance of blood lactate is 10 minutes fast trot (at 65–70% of maximal HR) rather than passive recovery or walking.
- Replenishment of muscle glycogen stores after high intensity exercise is usually relatively slow (3 days).
- If faster recovery is desired (e.g. because of proximity of next race), it is important to provide water, electrolytes and high-energy diet and avoid low-energy feed (hay) in post-race period. Consider IV fluid therapy (glucose).

FITNESS TESTING

Assessment of fitness (readiness to run) and individual athletic ability is the central role of the trainer. This is typically judged through appraisal of body condition and observation of an individual's performance during fast exercise or trial gallops relative to that of other horses in the work group (accounting for factors such as jockey weight and instructions). The ultimate measure of fitness is racetrack performance, where these estimations can be tested against a broader group of animals. This process is lengthy and inexact, and more objective methods of determining fitness would be desirable. Measurement of aerobic capacity (maximal oxygen uptake) is possible with treadmill studies incorporating ventilation capture, but this is a specialist procedure that is rarely practical. Some other measures that are sometimes applied are discussed below.

Blood analysis (haematology)
- Not useful for assessing fitness.
- Changes in oxygen-carrying capacity of blood occur early in training but are an unreliable guide to fitness later in preparation.
- Large splenic reserve of blood cells means assessment of circulating blood sample is often an inaccurate measure of whole-body status anyway.
- Little correlation between resting or post-exercise RBC or WBC values (or blood enzymes) and fitness.

Heart rate
- Unreliable measure of fitness.
- Maximal and resting HR vary between horses.
- Training does not alter resting HR (unlike human athletes).
- Training does not alter maximal HR at exercise. Rather, with increasing fitness a horse will achieve higher speeds at this HR_{max}: this speed is known as VHR_{max}.
- No correlation between maximal HR and racetrack performance.
- VHR_{max} can be used as measure of fitness but requires standardized conditions and GPS/ECG monitoring.
- HR recovery after standardized exercise test difficult to utilize for fitness assessment, as HR naturally drops rapidly at end of exercise.

Respiration rate
- Commonly used for subjective appraisal of fitness by training staff.
- Poor/prolonged return to normal respiration rate after fast exercise is an indicator of overexertion/ unfitness/illness.

Body condition
- Highly subjective and requires close familiarity with individual horse and knowledge of workload and appetite.
- Considerable variation in ideal condition and BWT at peak fitness between individuals.
- BWT can be used as indirect measure of race-readiness; of most use when information on previous weights in relation to performance is available.

Speed
- VHR_{max} broadly correlates to ability and fitness.
- Many variables can confound interpretation of VHR_{max}: stress/illness/rider/track.

Blood lactate (lactic acid)
- Build-up of lactate in muscle and blood occurs when intensity of exercise exceeds aerobic capacity; typically occurs during medium/fast cantering.
- 'Anaerobic threshold' is considered to be the speed at which horse has blood lactate concentration of 4 mmol/l.
- Increasing fitness allows work at faster speeds without lactate accumulation (rise in threshold).
- Blood lactate can rise from resting levels of <2 mmol/l to >20 mmol/l with intense exercise; returns to normal levels within 3 hours post exercise.
- Measurement of blood lactate immediately after (or during) exercise is a good test of aerobic (but not sprint) fitness; can also be used as guide to ability.
- Portable hand-held, whole-blood lactate analysers permit accurate measurement.
- More suited for treadmill testing: exercise variables must be tightly controlled and samples obtained within 3 minutes of cessation of cantering (or trotting).
- Treadmill field test: blood lactate obtained immediately after strenuous but submaximal exercise; speed of test can vary but typically medium-fast canter. Variables such as warm-up/distance should be kept constant.

TRACK TYPES

A variety of track types are used in training and racing worldwide and in many training centres a choice of track surfaces is available for slow and fast work. The main classes of track are discussed below.

Turf
Turf is the preferred surface for racing and training in many jurisdictions. While many turf tracks are purpose-built (with layered construction and drainage), many turf training areas have developed with no planned construction over generations of use. Turf tracks typically consist of a topsoil/root zone layer that is comparatively shallow (10–15 cm), above sand and deeper gravel layers that serve to drain water away. Shear strength of the topsoil layer is determined not only by grass root structure but by its soil content, with clay being relatively more cohesive than sand, particularly in the presence of moisture. The incorporation of polypropylene fibre, mesh or strands in the upper sand layer is common in high-rainfall climates and fortifies the shear strength of the root zone (smaller divot size). Suitability to local growing conditions determines optimum grass type, with root growth, strength and resilience to wear being more important than sward above the ground. Ideal soil temperatures for root growth differ between grass varieties: common cool-season grasses are Kentucky bluegrass and ryegrass, while kikuyu, bermudagrass and couch predominate in warmer climates. It is common for racetracks to be composed of a mix of grass varieties to cope with local weather conditions. The length of sward is typically maintained at 10–15 cm; however, while this may provide some slight cushioning effect for footfall, the interaction between horse and ground is primarily a function of the topsoil/root zone.

Maintenance of grass tracks is labour-intensive, requiring specialized management of soil, grass and water resources. Ease of management and uniformity of surface under different weather conditions varies with track design and drainage as well as local factors such as soil type and water table depth. Regular upkeep includes replacement of divots, rolling and thatch removal; heavy use or use in wet conditions can result in serious deterioration of the track. In many jurisdictions, turf racetracks are maintained to higher standards than turf training grounds, despite the latter carrying the majority of traffic.

Dirt

Dirt racing tracks typically consist of varying proportions of medium, fine and coarse sand with a smaller amount (approximately 5%) of clay, which acts to bind the sand and therefore contributes to shear strength. The main track designs in use include those with a shallow (9–12 cm) dirt cushion lying directly on a hard foundation base, and deeper dirt tracks in which selective management of different depths creates a shallow cushion over either a 'false base' hardpan layer or a partially compacted pad. The level of maintenance required depends on design and rainfall, but in general dirt tracks weather well and can support heavy use.

Sand

Sand tracks are in wide use in training centres as a relatively cheap all-weather surface. They can support heavy use and are used for both foundation and fast work. Sand tracks vary widely in construction and material, but surfaces are typically deep. Maintenance requirements (regular harrowing/rolling, occasional top-ups) are generally lower than many other surfaces. Shear strength diminishes considerably when saturated.

Synthetics

Synthetic tracks were initially developed to provide consistent footing and a lower-maintenance surface in the face of weather challenges and high-volume traffic. Synthetic surfaces vary in their composition between manufacturers, but generally consist of mixtures of sand, synthetic/natural fibres and non-compressible fillers (rubber/foam) coated with waxes, oils or polymers. Fibres provide shear resistance and act much in the same way as root structure does in turf tracks, while the waxes or oils bind the constituents together and repel water. Synthetic tracks are typically laid as a layer 15–25 cm thick (with a loose top 1/3) on a multi-layer porous foundation of aggregate rock that serves to drain water away from the track, with central perforated drainage pipes beneath. Synthetic surfaces are generally softer than dirt and generate lower peak ground reaction, acceleration and hoof vibration forces than dirt and turf tracks to the extent that they have been proposed to reduce injury rates. Track characteristics (speed) can vary markedly with ambient temperature. Maintenance protocols vary with different products but typically involve regular (daily/multiple daily) rolling/grooming and occasional top-ups. The working depth of the top surface can be altered with the depth of harrowing.

Woodchip

Woodchip surfaces are in wide use as all-weather training tracks. The construction characteristics of the foundation layers vary between sites. They are considered to provide safe, even footing if maintained (harrowed, rolled) regularly (daily/multiple daily) but replacement/resurfacing is required on a regular basis (approximately 10–25% top-up/year).

Track design

Tracks vary widely in configuration and design. Local topography and historical factors account for much of this variation. In addition to track surface, crossfall and other drainage factors contribute to a track's performance under different conditions and determine whether and how track bias may develop with weather, traffic and maintenance. The design of new tracks increasingly has to incorporate features that contribute to horse and jockey safety, that minimize disruption to race meetings from weather events and that take account of local water availability and quality.

Track condition and maintenance

The provision of a surface that is consistent in character during the course of a training session or race meet, or in the face of weather and climate variables, is challenging. In general terms, the greatest influence on the mechanical characteristics of dirt and turf tracks is moisture and on synthetic tracks is temperature. The maintenance regime required to provide a consistent surface therefore depends on geographical location and local weather variability.

Turf tracks require complex maintenance year-round that includes watering, mowing, soil aeration and thatch removal. Wear of the track can be managed by moving the inner rail to provide fresh ground. Dirt and synthetic tracks require regular light harrowing and grooming during use to prevent compaction from increasing the hardness of the track in areas of high use; dirt tracks are more susceptible to this compaction. Deeper tilling and rolling on a periodic basis is also important to freshen the track. Such maintenance does not impact significantly on shear strength, which is determined by moisture (and clay) content in dirt tracks and fibre density of synthetic tracks. The mechanical characteristics (and thereby speed) of synthetic tracks change with ambient temperature due to changes in wax viscosity; peak temperatures in the top layer usually occur mid-afternoon. They can also change in composition over time, with degradation of fibres, loss of wax/oil and contamination with organic material; the need for top-ups and re-waxes is guided by regular depth checks and quality control.

Accurate determination of racetrack firmness is essential for trainers, groundstaff and the betting public. Official pre-confirmation/declaration and race day reports of turf track conditions (ranging from 'heavy' to 'hard') have traditionally relied on subjective assessment, but increasingly the aggregated measurements of penetration and/or shear strength obtained from instruments such as the GoingStick are used to derive the 'going'. Such measurements are interpreted in the light of local track characteristics and do not necessarily permit direct comparisons between tracks; they do, however, allow detection of variability in the track and can guide maintenance and watering efforts.

CHAPTER 14
NUTRITION

PRINCIPLES OF FEEDING

The horse is a grazing animal with a gastrointestinal tract that has evolved to digest grasses that are consumed throughout the day. The large amount of 'gut fill' associated with natural grazing is, however, incompatible with the athletic demands of the racehorse. In consequence, while some forage is required for the hindgut to function properly, energy-dense concentrates form the basis of racehorse diets.

Concentrates are primarily cereal-based. The starch and fats that comprise the majority of energy in these feeds are largely absorbed in the foregut (small intestine), while the hindgut is the site for digestion of fibre, through fermentation by a large resident population of microbes. Overfeeding of concentrates may result in 'spillover' of starch into the hindgut: subsequent changes in the microbial population of the hindgut may cause diarrhoea or colic. It is therefore necessary to split the daily concentrate ration into three or four separate feeds to avoid overlarge meal size. Because a large part of the horse's digestive function relies on the hindgut microbial flora, dietary changes should be made gradually in order to allow adaptation to occur.

Feeding strategies vary widely between trainers and derive from tradition, personal preference, local availability of feed and economic factors. When a diet is grain-based, a 'balancer' is usually fed to ensure that nutritional imbalances do not arise; alternatively, complete feeds offer the advantage of being formulated to provide all major nutrients in a single, uniform product. It matters little how the ration is fed providing the diet is balanced (not over- or underfortified in key nutrients) and feed intakes and health/performance are satisfactory.

KEY NUTRIENTS

Carbohydrates
Carbohydrates utilized by the horse derive primarily from starch. Starch is broken down by enzymes in the small intestine into sugars (glucose), which are readily absorbed across the gut wall into the bloodstream.

Proteins
Proteins are made up of amino acids and form the building blocks of the body; they are needed for maintenance and growth. The horse can synthesize some but not all of its required amino acids and must source the remainder from dietary protein. Proteins are broken down by enzymes in the small intestine into their constituent amino acids. Protein quality and digestibility are important factors in the value of a protein source: higher quality protein is that which conforms closest in amino acid make-up to that required by the tissues and is digestible in the small intestine. A common measure of protein content is crude protein (CP): this is not a measure of digestibility or quality; therefore, protein source should be considered carefully.

Protein requirements increase only by a moderate amount with full work; it is rarely necessary to supplement protein as increased ration intake with workload usually covers losses. High protein does not equal high energy, and feeding too much protein may be detrimental to performance.

Fats
Although fats make up a very small proportion of the horse's 'natural' diet, their digestion is surprisingly efficient. The small intestine is the main site of fat digestion and absorption.

Fibre

Much of the horse's natural diet is made up of fibre. As with ruminants, the horse does not have enough innate enzymatic activity in the gut to break down all the fibre that passes through it into useable molecules. For this it relies on a large population of bacteria and protozoa in the hindgut to ferment dietary fibre into volatile fatty acids, which are then absorbed and used as an energy source.

Electrolytes

Electrolytes are water-soluble salts and minerals that control the fluid balance of the body and have key roles in nerve and muscle activity, energy metabolism and many cellular functions. The primary electrolytes are sodium, chloride, potassium, calcium and magnesium. Sweat contains salt and as a consequence the exercising horse loses sodium, chloride and potassium. Other than calcium, the body has little in the way of stores of electrolytes and must replenish losses on a daily basis.

Minerals

Minerals are inorganic nutrients and include the above electrolytes as well as phosphorus, sulphur and trace minerals (iron, zinc, copper, selenium, iodine, manganese, cobalt) that are needed for normal growth and development. Mineral requirements are typically small and vary with workload and age. Absorption and utilization of trace minerals is complex, with dietary source and interactions between certain minerals being as important as absolute intake. One of the key interactions relevant to the racehorse is that between calcium and phosphorus. The body's reservoir for both minerals is bone, and if the dietary ratio is insufficient, calcium can be lost from bone to maintain blood levels, resulting in reduced skeletal strength and increased injury rates. Cereals are high in phosphorus, and use of an appropriate balancer +/− forage (high in calcium) is required to ensure that the calcium:phosphorus ratio is within optimal range (1.2–2:1). Most commercial complete feeds are formulated to have a balanced calcium:phosphorus ratio.

Vitamins

Vitamins are organic compounds that are essential for many cellular processes. Vitamins are required in very small quantities for maintenance of health; however, little is known of the ideal dietary requirements of the racehorse. Many diets and supplements are fortified with vitamins based on the premise that if particular vitamin deficiencies are detrimental, then supplementation must be beneficial, without accounting for normal daily intakes. The body is able to store fat-soluble vitamins (A, D, E and K), allowing some flexibility with regard to daily intakes, but overfortification can occasionally lead to toxicity. Water-soluble vitamins by contrast are not stored but many are produced within the body (B vitamins by microbes in the hindgut, vitamin C from glucose in the liver), and overfortification simply results in excretion through the kidneys rather than toxicity. B vitamins have important roles in energy metabolism and horses in full work may have increased requirements, meriting some supplementation. The benefits of vitamin C and, to a lesser extent, vitamin E supplementation are controversial, with mixed evidence of antioxidant effects and bioavailability of nutritional sources varying considerably.

BASIC FEED TYPES

Forage
The hindgut requires a certain amount of forage to function correctly; a minimum daily intake of 1% BWT is recommended. Feeding less than this increases the risk of intestinal upsets, such as colic, or of deficiencies of nutrients found predominantly in forage (potassium deficiency: may lead to exertional rhabdomyolysis). Forage is fed as either hay or haylage.

Hay
Grasses (rye/timothy/orchardgrass/bluegrass) and legumes (alfalfa) can be cut for hay. Energy density and cleanliness (from dust and microbial spores) are largely determined by maturity and weather conditions at the time of cutting. Leaves are more nutrient-rich than stems, and forage cut at a later stage of maturity (when it has greater stem) has a lower energy and protein content and more indigestible fibre. The dry matter (DM) content of hay should be approximately 85–90%; moisture levels greater than this (<85% DM) may permit fungal spoiling. The nutritional value of most hay does not diminish significantly with storage:
- Grass hay (rye/timothy/fescue): CP levels 9–11% for average quality hay.
- Legume hay (alfalfa): CP levels 16–20% for mid-bloom; greater digestible energy and calcium content than grass hays. Leaves may shatter more readily than grass hay, causing loss of nutrient density and greater dust.

Chaff
The main purpose of feeding chaff is to slow down the intake of concentrates. Chaff made from alfalfa or good quality forage is preferable to that made from straw.

Haylage
Grasses cut for haylage are baled when wilted and have a greater moisture content than hay (55–65% DM). Haylage is dust-free and more palatable than hay. Although having a higher moisture content, the fermentation process limits mould contamination. Because of the lower DM compared with hay, more (25–50%) haylage should be fed by weight per day if fibre and potassium deficiencies are to be avoided.

Mould contamination
Mould contamination is primarily a feature of hay. It arises from inadequate drying at baling and therefore is more of a problem in countries with wet/unpredictable summers. Fungi may affect health through mycotoxins (diminished appetite/compromised immunity). Mycotoxins are resistant to high temperatures and are not destroyed by hay steamers.

Cereals
Cereals are rich in starch and contain more digestible energy than hay. They are relatively deficient in calcium. Cereal types differ in their energy and nutrient content and digestibility. One of the primary goals when feeding cereals is to optimize digestibility in the small intestine and limit potential spillover of starch into the hindgut. Processing achieves this by increasing digestibility:
- Oats: grain size, palatability, digestibility and good quality protein make oats a safe cereal to feed unprocessed.
- Naked oats: varieties that lose husk readily so therefore have higher energy and oil content than normal oats (30% higher digestible energy than oats).
- Barley: hull is more closely adhered than that of oats and therefore requires rolling/crimping.
- Wheat: requires processing. Very high starch content so less safety margin than oats.
- Maize: double the energy density of oats but less readily digestible in foregut, therefore greater fermentation in hindgut (less desirable).

Other common feed products
- Wheat bran: produced from husk of wheat grain. CP 14–16%. Rich in phosphorus and deficient in calcium. Palatability and ability to absorb water make it a common choice as mash.
- Rice bran: fat supplement. Should be heat-stabilized to prevent spoiling.
- Sugar beet pulp: highly digestible fibre. Similar protein content and quality to cereals.
- Linseed meal: protein supplement (CP 20–35%) with high omega-3 fatty acid content.
- Soybean meal: protein supplement (CP 45–50%).
- Lupins: protein supplement (CP 28–34%); digested predominantly in hindgut. Usually fed in processed form.

Oils
Digestion of oil/fats is very efficient and takes place entirely in the small intestine. Vegetable oils are energy dense, containing approximately three times the digestible energy of oats. It is therefore possible to increase the energy density of the diet without increasing the volume of feed intake; substitution of oil for starch may also be beneficial to gut function. Oils should be introduced gradually, but a total dietary content of 10% oil is usually well-tolerated. The typical quantity topdressed to racing diets is 50–150 ml/day.

Oils found in most cereals are rich in omega-6 fatty acids, while a few cereals (linseed, rapeseed and soya) and fish oils are rich in omega-3 fatty acids. There are some possible anti-inflammatory benefits from a diet relatively high in omega-3 fatty acids; linseed meals or use of linseed/soya oil is therefore preferred to other sources of fat.

Electrolytes
As electrolytes are not stored in the body, losses through sweat and urine need to be replenished on a daily basis. Most electrolyte requirements are met by feeding a balanced diet. Sodium and chloride requirements are influenced by workload and temperature/humidity, but are usually covered by addition of salt to the diet or provision of salt licks/rock salt.

SUPPLEMENTS

Biotin
Biotin is a water-soluble B vitamin. It can improve the speed and quality of hoof growth with long-term supplementation. Supplementation at 15–25 g/day is recommended for horses with poor hoof quality or foot balance; the effect is on new hoof growth and positive changes therefore take months to be noticeable.

Probiotics
Probiotics are live microbes (bacteria and yeasts) used as dietary additives to provide possible beneficial effects, principally through influence on microbial population of hindgut. Possible roles include inhibiting growth of intestinal pathogens and enhancing digestion. Although used widely and generally considered to be safe, their efficacy is doubtful and many products deliver less than the claimed number of viable organisms.

Prebiotics
Prebiotics differ from probiotics by being composed of nutrients that assist the growth of 'beneficial' microorganisms, rather than containing the microorganisms themselves. They consist mostly of non-digestible sugars and fibre. Efficacy uncertain but generally safe.

ASSESSING NUTRITIONAL PROBLEMS

An objective analysis is required when assessing any change in feeding practice or possible nutritional influence underlying a yard health problem. Formulation or detailed analysis of diet should be performed by a qualified nutritionist; however, basic investigations may be used to guide or monitor feeding practices.

History
- Determine whether the diet has changed in any respect (constituents/quantities) over the preceding months in response to perceived problems; previous diet may be more relevant to current clinical query.

Conducting a 'weigh-out'
- Measurement of total daily intake of all components of diet (concentrates, forage and supplements) as fed to an individual horse.
- Energy and nutritional values rely on weight (not volume).
- Observation of feeding practices.
- Subjective assessment of feed quality: discolouration of grains (possible fungal contamination)/rancidity of oil/spoiling of hay.
- Analysis (nutrients/dust/spores) of representative forage samples: useful but only relevant to individual batch.
- Comparison to previous yard data useful to identify any 'creep' in feeding practices.
- May permit simplification of diet through removal of components that are duplicated or have better quality/value alternatives.

Testing for nutritional imbalances
Homeostatic mechanisms generally maintain blood levels of electrolytes and nutrients within a tightly defined range so that important cellular functions continue uninterrupted regardless of fluctuations in nutritional status. Interpretation of blood analysis is therefore rarely straightforward. Testing for nutritional deficiencies is only useful if plasma concentration reflects total body store of a particular nutrient:
- Calcium/iron: plasma levels not affected by dietary intake.
- Potassium: plasma levels are a good measure of status but affected by dietary cation–anion balance.
- Copper: plasma levels only useful for long-term deficiency.
- Magnesium: plasma levels of little use to establish status.
- Selenium: blood selenium good measure of status.
- Vitamin E: assessment is problematic; measure serum α-tocopherol over several days.

POOR APPETITE/CONDITION

Optimal BWT in training varies between individuals. Horses that do not eat their full ration or fail to hold condition well during training are commonly encountered. Loss of appetite, or failure of appetite to keep pace with workload, may be a transient or persistent feature and can have several causes. The causes below should be considered.

'Overreaching'
Application of training/racing loads in excess of physical or temperamental capacity may lead to poor appetite and weight loss.

Teeth
A common cause of transient (few days) inappetence is shedding of deciduous premolar teeth ('caps') in late 2 to early 4 YOs (Chapter 5, p. 241). Loose caps are easily dislodged with forceps and immediate improvement in appetite should result. Rarely, laceration to tongue or cheek may cause oral pain: healing is rapid.

Gastric ulcers
Gastric ulcers are a common cause of reduced feed intake. The onset of clinical signs is typically concurrent with increased workload. Presence/severity can only be determined by gastroscopy. Treatment usually results in improved appetite/condition within days/weeks (Chapter 6, p. 255).

Parasites
Parasites are rarely the cause of poor condition in horses in training (Chapter 6, p. 260) but should be considered in new arrivals/young stock.

Feed quality
Palatability may be affected by feed quality and, to some extent, by individual appetite for salt. Grains do not spoil under normal storage conditions, but oils may suffer from rancidity and additives to processed feeds or hay may affect palatability. Oil rancidity can be determined by peroxide value. Mycotoxins can diminish appetite and laboratory analysis of grain/concentrate and hay rations may be considered.

Fillies

Feed intake of fillies is sometimes depressed during oestrus ('in season'), particularly during the transitional phase in late winter/early spring when workload is also increasing. Trial use of altrenogest or other methods to control oestrus behaviour may be beneficial (Chapter 7, p. 266).

Management

It is important to determine whether weight loss is absolute or relative to increased workload/energy expenditure, and if reduced/inadequate feed intake is responsible. Uneaten feed may represent over-feeding of energy-dense ration (rather than necessarily reflecting inadequate appetite). Some horses are simply unable to balance the rigours of training with a normal racing diet. The equine gastrointestinal system has evolved to accommodate many small grazing 'meals' of roughage and the small stomach size limits the ability to deal with large infrequent meals. Strategies to improve feed intake include:

- Smaller meals at more frequent intervals.
- Increase energy density through addition of vegetable oil (may permit reduction of weight/volume required).
- Provide good quality hay: poorly digestible fibre is retained for longer in hindgut and may depress appetite.
- May be appropriate in limited circumstances to use medication to improve appetite/assist weight gain. Limited anecdotal support for short-acting oral anabolic medication (ethyloestrenol); use subject to regulatory approval.

Once common causes of poor appetite have been ruled out, medical investigation may be warranted (infection/inflammatory bowel disease/tumours). Tests include blood analysis, ultrasonography and biopsy. Persistent and uncontrollable weight loss should prompt referral to a diagnostic facility.

FEEDING FOR PERFORMANCE

Carbohydrate loading

Unlike in people, carbohydrate 'loading' offers no advantages to racehorse performance and indeed carbohydrate overload is more likely to cause detrimental effects such as diarrhoea, colic or (rarely) laminitis. Feed intake should be determined by immediate needs rather than attempting to build up 'reserves' for future use. (See also Chapter 15, p. 333.)

Pre-race feeding

The body's response to a meal is for blood insulin levels to rise to assist with uptake of glucose from blood to muscle. High insulin levels have a detrimental effect on performance; however, this 'glycaemic response' varies between feeds and is influenced by many factors. Some dehydration also occurs in the immediate period after feeding. The optimum timing of pre-race meals is a poorly researched area; the general advice is that large glycaemic meals should be avoided. A small meal of concentrate/grain may be fed 4–5 hours pre-race, and withdrawal of forage on race day is recommended. Tapered reduction of forage intake (to ≤1% BWT) over the 3 days leading into a race may be beneficial to reduce gut fill/water retention (thereby reducing BWT); hays with greater digestibility are preferable in this pre-race period.

CHAPTER 15
ERGOGENIC AIDS

OVERVIEW

An ergogenic aid is any external factor beyond normal training that can enhance physical performance (speed, strength or endurance). It can refer not just to pharmaceutical agents but to training aids and nutritional manipulations. Scientific support for the most commonly used ergogenic aids (human and equine) is sparse due to difficulties associated with measuring performance; as a result many are considered theoretically advantageous but unproven.

Ergogenic aids should always be viewed in the context that physical, training and genetic factors account for the major part of any athletic performance. In certain circumstances, however, there may be a rationale for the use of some products or methods. Specifically these should be scientifically valid, not harmful and comply with regulatory requirements. Many ergogenic aids used in people are not necessarily applicable to equine use because of metabolic and physiological differences between the species. The main groups of ergogenic aids that have been applied to human and equine pursuits are discussed here, with particular emphasis on their validity for use in the racehorse; these can be split into two broad categories: nutritional and non-nutritional aids.

NUTRITIONAL AIDS

Nutritional ergogenic aids act through modification of a nutritional metabolic pathway to delay the onset of fatigue. Dietary manipulation or the provision of a key nutrient can lead to greater availability of stored energy or greater efficiency of energy production. When evaluating the merits of a nutritional supplement, consideration should be given to not just the potential efficacy of its active ingredient/s, but interactions with diet (possible toxicity through oversupplementation of certain nutrients) and the potential for contamination with prohibited substances. Popularity should not be taken as evidence of efficacy. As a general rule, nutritional supplements do not enhance performance in racehorses being fed an appropriately formulated diet.

Carbohydrate (glycogen) 'loading'
- Common practice in human endurance disciplines where duration of exercise is >90 minutes. High carbohydrate diet combined with exercise taper 1–4 days out from competition can boost muscle glycogen stores and delay onset of fatigue during event.
- Little rationale for use in horses: they have naturally high muscle glycogen content, and only very small (around 10%) increases are possible with dietary manipulation; also, a high-starch diet is associated with significant risks (colic, diarrhoea, laminitis).

- Horses: glycogen replenishment as an aid to recovery after intense exercise is more useful; it takes 2–3 days on a normal diet to correct the 20–25% depletion of muscle glycogen stores resulting from high-intensity exercise.

Amino acids (glutamine/glycine/tryptophan)
- Amino acid supplementation ('protein shakes') widespread in human sports.
- Proposed to build muscle mass in training; however, no significant ergogenic effect has been demonstrated in people or horses.
- Possibly beneficial in recovery phase following intense exercise.

L-carnitine
- Enzyme essential to cellular energy production through transport of long-chain fatty acids across inner mitochondrial membrane.
- Increased muscle concentration theoretically advantageous.
- Horses: supplementation (oral or intravenous) does not alter muscle carnitine content and therefore of no use.

Creatine
- Organic acid stored in muscle and derived from amino acids. Has a role in energy production within cell.
- Increasing muscle creatine content has an ergogenic effect (increased work capacity and peak strength) in human athletes.
- Horses: poor oral bioavailability (not a natural part of equine diet) limits use.

L-arginine
- Amino acid that is oxidized to nitric oxide (NO).
- Proposed mechanism: increased NO production in skeletal muscle, causing vasodilation/greater blood flow and improved tolerance to aerobic and anaerobic exercise.
- Little evidence to support use in fit athletes (or horses).

Ginseng
- Widely used herbal supplement in people.
- Reputed to increase stamina through unknown mechanisms.
- Little evidence to support use (people or horses).
- Prohibited substance in some jurisdictions.

Anti-oxidants
- High levels of reactive oxygen species are produced in skeletal muscle during intense exercise.
- Oral anti-oxidant supplementation is proposed to reduce oxidative stress and thereby improve muscle function.
- Consistently shown to have no effect either on performance or on prevention of muscle damage.

Beta-alanine
- Naturally occuring amino acid.
- Substrate for synthesis of muscle carnosine, an important intracellular buffer in type 2 skeletal muscle.
- Oral supplementation of β-alanine increases carnosine content of skeletal muscle in humans and horses.
- Ergogenic effect in human athletes: delayed fatigue and increased capacity for exercise (for exercise lasting >60 seconds).
- Horses: good bioavailability; biological rationale for use but clinical effect undetermined at present.

B vitamins
- Water-soluble vitamins essential for proper cell function.
- Thiamine/riboflavin/niacin/pantothenic acid have roles in muscle energy pathways.
- Folate and B_{12} have roles in cell synthesis and repair.
- Exercise increases requirements for some B vitamins.
- Thiamine (B_1) supplementation has been shown to delay fatigue (increases the anaerobic threshold) in some human athletic pursuits.
- Horses: little research available.

Other vitamin/mineral/electrolyte supplementation

- Supplementation over and above a well-balanced diet has not been shown to improve performance (people and horses).
- Little support for megadose supplementation; high doses of some vitamins can be harmful.

Sodium bicarbonate

- 0.3–1 g/kg BWT administered orally 2.5 hours pre-exercise reduces blood lactate acidosis and delays fatigue over middle-distance trips.
- 'Milkshaking': prohibited practice and enforced through established threshold for blood carbon dioxide (CO_2) concentration.
- Variation in blood levels of CO_2 can occur with exercise, frusemide administration and between individuals, but the established threshold at >1 hour post-race is robust.
- Diets containing sufficient quantities of bicarbonate or alkinizing agents have potential to result in positive test.

NON-NUTRITIONAL AIDS

Real/simulated high altitude training (hypoxic/hypobaric aids)

- Low oxygen tension has potential to stimulate production of RBCs, conferring potential advantage for later performance at sea level or as aid to acclimatization.
- Achieved by true altitude (>3,500 metres) or hypoxic/hypobaric conditions.
- Two main strategies: 'live low–train high' and 'live high–train low'.
- Live low–train high (train in hypoxia): does not improve performance at sea level and may be best suited to acclimatization.
- Live high–train low: may be the most beneficial ergogenic strategy but best achieved by spending >16 hours/day (preferably 20–22 hours/day) in hypoxia.
- Horses: little research but probable that short periods of hypoxia at rest (intermittent hypoxia units) have no effect.

Blood doping

- Misuse of certain techniques and/or substances to increase RBC mass, thereby increasing blood oxygen carrying capacity.
- May be achieved through direct transfusion of blood or through stimulation of increased RBC production.
- Autologous blood transfusions: boosting of 'race day' RBC numbers by reinfusion of autologous blood obtained 8–10 weeks prior to competition.
- Erythropoietin (EPO): peptide hormone originating from kidney cells that regulates the body's production of RBCs; is produced in response to hypoxia or anaemia and stimulates bone marrow to upregulate red cell production.
- Recombinant and biosimilar EPOs banned by sporting regulatory bodies.
- Development of other anti-anaemia therapies targeting alternative pathways to erythropoiesis stimulation in human medicine is leading to expanding opportunities for doping in human and equine sports; these 'erythropoiesis-stimulating agents' include orally bioavailable agents that activate the endogenous EPO gene, such as cobalt chloride.
- Potential for adverse side-effects including thrombotic/embolic disease, severe anaemia and death.
- Detection capability for emerging analogues is a constantly evolving field; in human sports there is increasing reliance on indirect methods such as longitudinal monitoring of biomarkers and haematological profile ('biological passport').
- Horses: limited available information on efficacy; however, as with other 'blood boosting' aids, ergogenic effect is likely to be of less importance than in humans due to naturally large splenic reserve of red cells.

Anabolic steroids

- Natural or synthetic derivatives of testosterone.
- Multiple anabolic effects including increased protein synthesis, increased lean body mass and reduced fat mass (partitioning), and enhanced recovery from injury.

- Use banned by most regulatory bodies.

Clenbuterol
- Beta-2 adrenergic agonist commonly used for treatment of equine respiratory disease.
- Demonstrable anabolic/partitioning effect in several species, although limited information available in horses.
- Any anabolic effect is likely to require prolonged administration.

Growth hormone
- Endogenous growth hormone is produced in the anterior pituitary gland.
- Multiple anabolic effects including increased protein synthesis, increased lean body mass and reduced fat mass (partitioning), increased power:mass ratio, enhanced cardiovascular function and recovery from injury.
- Perceived benefits from recombinant growth hormone doping in human sports exceed those determined scientifically.
- Testing for exogenous growth hormone in humans has good sensitivity and specificity.

Gene doping
- Non-therapeutic manipulation of genes or gene expression in order to improve athletic performance.
- Genes involved in muscle metabolism and key energy pathways (e.g. EPO, insulin-like growth factor-1, endorphin) are of most interest.
- Constantly evolving field in human athletics.

CHAPTER 16

BLOOD ANALYSIS

BLOOD CONSTITUENTS

The function of blood is largely to transport oxygen, nutrients, electrolytes and hormones to body organs and tissues, and to remove waste products from them. Blood has cellular (RBCs, WBCs, platelets) and plasma (water, electrolytes and plasma proteins) fractions.

Measuring these constituents can allow assessment of factors that might influence performance, such as the oxygen-carrying capacity of blood, hydration status and immune challenge. Haematology refers to the study of blood and biochemistry to the measurement of the enzyme, protein and electrolyte components of blood (*Table 16.1*).

Table 16.1 Haematology and biochemistry overview

CONSTITUENT	FUNCTION AND FEATURES	MEASURES AND INTERPRETATION
RBCs (erythrocytes)	Main cellular constituent of blood. Function: protein Hb binds and transports O_2. Produced in bone marrow. Circulation time: 155 days.	**Red cell count**: number of circulating RBCs per unit blood. **PCV**: percentage of blood as cells (primarily composed of RBC). Both red cell count and PCV may be elevated with sampling stress/splenic contraction. **MCV**: average size of RBCs. Indirect indicator of blood loss/cell age (cells become smaller as they mature). **MCHC**: amount of Hb in each RBC per unit size. Only relevant if decreased (anaemia); elevated levels indicate haemolysis of sample.
WBCs (leucocytes)	Cells with key roles in inflammation and immunity. Several types, all produced in bone marrow: • Neutrophils: first line of defence; ingest/destroy bacteria. Short (<24 hour) half-life. • Lymphocytes: B (plasma) cells produce antibodies; T cells involved in immune response. • Monocytes: precursors of macrophages. • Eosinophils: involved in allergic/hypersensitivity reactions.	**White cell count**: total circulating WBC count per unit blood. Raised with stress or infection. **'Differential'**: relative proportions of different WBC types in the sample; may allow differentiation of disease states but can also be influenced by excitement/stress and other factors such as recent corticosteroid use. Absolute cell counts of more importance than differential 'split'. **Neutrophil count**: increases with stress, bacterial (acute/chronic phase) or viral (acute phase) infections; decreases with excessive demand for neutrophils (severe acute infection, endotoxaemia). Persistently low counts seen with post-viral challenge. **Lymphocyte count**: reduced with acute viral infection; increases with chronic viral infection. **Monocyte count**: non-specific; raised with acute/chronic inflammation (particularly viral). **Eosinophil count**: non-specific; may be raised with allergic response/intestinal parasite burden.

(continued overleaf)

Table 16.1 *(continued)*

CONSTITUENT	FUNCTION AND FEATURES	MEASURES AND INTERPRETATION
Platelets	Main function: clotting; also have role in inflammatory/immune processes. Cell fragments produced in bone marrow from megakaryocytes. Circulation time: 4–7 days.	Low platelet counts usually due to clumping during sample processing (rather than clotting disorders).
Plasma proteins	**Albumin**: produced in liver; main function is as a transport/binding protein. **Globulins**: role in immune response.	**Total protein (albumin + globulins)**: elevated with dehydration or inflammation; decreased with severe protein loss (e.g. intestinal malabsorption). **Albumin**: mild decrease with chronic infection. **Globulins**: elevated with chronic infection.
Inflammatory markers	**Plasma fibrinogen and serum amyloid A**: acute phase plasma proteins produced by liver. Have roles in inflammatory response and clotting.	Acute phase protein levels allow interpretation of high/low WBC counts (inflammation or stress). **Plasma fibrinogen**: concentration increases with inflammation/dehydration. May take 1–2 days to rise in response to stimulus. **Serum amyloid A**: early rise (hours) in response to stimulus; peaks at ~48 hours and rapidly returns to normal after acute phase.
Muscle enzymes	Enzymes released into circulation from damaged muscle cells. **CK**: largely muscle specific. **AST**: less so as found in other tissues (including liver).	Allow interpretation of episodes of exertional rhabdomyolysis (severity and timing): differences in peak levels and plasma half-lives permit assessment of whether episode occurred within 24 hours (both elevated; CK higher than AST) or several days previously (higher AST). **CK**: short plasma half-life. Plasma levels peak at 4–6 hours. **AST**: longer plasma half-life. Plasma levels peak at 12–24 hours.
Liver function	**GGT**: enzyme found in bile ducts (also pancreas/kidney). Plasma half-life 3 days. **GLDH**: short half-life (14 hours). **ALP**: non-specific; found in liver, bone, intestine. **Bilirubin**: liver takes up, conjugates and excretes bilirubin. **Serum bile acids**: liver normally clears from circulation.	Elevations may indicate liver disease or insufficiency but are rarely specific for type of disease. **GGT**: moderate increases (with other liver enzymes normal) of no concern. Raised with cholestasis (acute hepatitis and cirrhosis); also with dantrolene sodium use and plant/fungal hepatotoxins. **GLDH**: specific for acute liver cell damage and indicator of ongoing damage. **ALP**: raised with chronic obstructive liver failure but non-specific. **Bilirubin**: rises in (unconjugated) bilirubin more likely to be due to inappetence or haemolysis than liver disease. **Serum bile acids**: raised with inappetence or hepatic insufficiency. Liver disease usually advanced before levels raised significantly, but good indicator of impaired function.
Kidney function	**Creatinine**: muscle breakdown product. **Blood urea nitrogen**: produced by liver as digestive product of protein. Both are waste products filtered out of the blood by kidneys.	Moderate increases in urea and creatinine seen with renal insufficiency; diagnosis of kidney damage/failure also requires urinalysis to differentiate from pre-renal (e.g. dehydration/circulatory shock) causes.

RBC, red blood cell; WBC, white blood cell; PCV, packed cell volume; Hb, haemoglobin; MCV, mean corpuscular volume; MCHC, mean corpuscular haemoglobin concentration; CK, creatine kinase; AST, aspartate aminotransferase; GGT, gamma-glutamyl transferase; GLDH, glutamate dehydrogenase; ALP, alkaline phosphatase

SAMPLING

- Technique and timing of blood collection and handling/storage of sample have the potential to affect results of haematological and biochemical analysis.
- Preferable to sample early morning (pre-exercise/feeding) or late afternoon (pre-feeding) to minimize effect of exercise, excitement and feeding. Haematological values return to baseline approximately 2 hours post exercise.
- Excitement of horse at sampling may cause splenic contraction and a resulting 'stress' profile (as for exercise): takes approximately 30 seconds to mobilize RBCs from spleen.
- WBC counts may be altered for up to 36 hours following racing/travelling.
- Blood tubes used are determined by tests required and preferences of receiving laboratory, but in general:
  - Haematology: EDTA.
  - Biochemistry: clotted (serum).
  - Plasma fibrinogen: sodium citrate.
- Delays in analysis may result in deterioration of sample and can affect both haematology and biochemistry results; cell rupture may alter red cell, enzyme and electrolyte figures.
- Cooling (4–8°C) of sample advised; avoid freezing or direct contact with icepacks. If delay is expected, separate serum from clotted samples.

EFFECTS OF TRAINING

Red blood cells
- Training stimulates an increase in total RBC numbers and haemoglobin.
- Rises in resting RBC count, PCV and haemoglobin concentration are modest and cannot be used to assess fitness.
- No link between RBC figures and racing performance.

White blood cells
- Training causes no alteration in total WBC counts or differential fractions.
- 'Reversed' neutrophil:lymphocyte ratio commonly seen in 2 YOs: likely to represent maturation of immune system rather than effect of training.

Biochemistry
- Training causes few changes to biochemistry values.
- Modest increase in serum GGT (in absence of other indicators of liver disease): not uncommon in healthy horses; may also result from drug use (dantrolene sodium) or stress/overtraining.

INTERPRETATION

Because of the horse's readily mobilized splenic reserve of blood cells, a venous blood sample is not necessarily representative of the whole-body status of many blood constituents. Relative proportions of circulating blood components may vary considerably with exercise, feeding and, sometimes, drug administration.

Haematology and biochemistry results are compared with recognized reference ranges of 'normal' values for age and stage of training. Reference ranges for some components may vary between laboratories depending on testing procedures and equipment. Reference ranges are population-based averages and individuals with non-conforming blood values in the absence of disease may be encountered. Reference ranges specific to the individual (if available) are of far greater use than population averages when determining the significance of values, particularly in relation to performance. Results of blood analyses should always be interpreted in the context of clinical presentation; the detection of a haematological or biochemical irregularity on routine sampling from an outwardly healthy animal may merit vigilance rather than intervention.

Health
- Blood analysis is most useful as a measure of health (not fitness).
- Permits detection of subclinical illness (through changes in inflammatory markers) and assessment of organ function.
- Inflammation/infection (bacterial or viral): typically raised WBC and neutrophil count plus raised acute phase proteins (viral challenge may lead to low WBC/neutrophil count in acute phase).
- Bacterial and viral infections may be differentiated by relative counts of neutrophils/lymphocytes in the post-acute phase.
- In the acute phase of severe infections (such as pleuropneumonia) WBC count may initially drop as white cells are sequestered to combat infection.
- Inflammatory profile is non-specific for location or type of disease but is good measure of severity and current status.

Fitness
- (See also Chapter 13, p. 322.)
- Reliable assessment of fitness through analysis of RBC figures is not possible.
- Increase in RBC count and PCV occurs through early training; however, figures vary between and within individuals and are highly labile with exercise, excitement and feeding due to splenic release and fluid shifts.
- Sampling immediately after exercise may give better indication of total circulating RBC counts.
- Measurement of plasma lactate concentration under controlled exercise conditions (treadmill) can be used to assess response to workload, but standardized protocol and horse-side testing essential.

Dehydration
- PCV and total protein are used as indicators of dehydration but may not reflect true status due to splenic contraction (RBCs) or gastrointestinal protein loss.
- In general: raised RBC count, PCV and total protein indicate dehydration.

Anaemia
- Anaemia is a decrease in the body's RBC mass, causing reduction in oxygen-carrying capacity of the blood.
- May be regenerative (due to blood loss or haemolysis) or non-regenerative (due to impaired production of red cells).
- True anaemia in horses in training is very rare; may occasionally result from blood loss.
- May take >24 hours for PCV and RBC count to drop after haemorrhage (due to compensatory release of cells from spleen).
- Following acute blood loss, PCV usually fully recovered by 1 month.
- Iron deficiency not a factor with balanced diets.
- EIA or piroplasmosis (Chapter 11, pp. 295 and 297, respectively) should be considered a possibility if anaemia is profound.

Musculoskeletal health
- CK/AST levels usually permit differentiation of muscular soreness/exertional rhabdomyolysis from potential skeletal injury (although concurrent exertional rhabdomyolysis may occur with some stress fractures).
- CK and AST blood levels 'peak' at different times; possible to determine approximate timing of episode of exertional rhabdomyolysis.
- Episode <24 hours prior to sampling: both enzymes elevated; CK higher than AST.
- Episode several days previously: both enzymes elevated, but AST higher than CK.
- Last episode 1–2 weeks previously: AST elevated, CK normal.

Electrolytes
- Circulating levels of electrolytes usually a poor indicator of total body status, as most plasma concentrations are held within tight range by homeostatic mechanisms to protect body functions.
- Urinary fractional electrolyte clearance ratios frequently permit better assessment than single serum assay.

CHAPTER 17

HERD HEALTH

BIOSECURITY

Although the racehorse population is highly mobile, continually mixing and housed intensively, the risk of serious disease transmission is generally considered to be low. This can be attributed to several factors: that horses attending races are by definition healthy enough for competition; that standards of husbandry in racing yards (including veterinary attendance and routine vaccination) are usually high; and that health testing and certification implemented by studs, public sales companies and border control authorities limit the spread of economically important diseases. When serious infectious disease does occur, however, the financial impact can be severe, and it is advisable for racing yard management to incorporate some basic biosecurity measures. These may include:

- Regular disinfection (steam cleaning followed by application of approved virucidal/bacteriocidal disinfectant) of horse transport and communal facilities.
- New arrivals from high-risk populations housed in isolation area (and exercised separately to core group) until health status established: period of 2–3 weeks is optimal (or until test results available).
- Vigilance for signs of disease (fever/nasal discharge/enlarged lymph nodes) in new arrivals.
- In the absence of an isolation facility, consider testing horses prior to/upon arrival to detect disease carriers (particularly *Streptococcus equi* serology [Chapter 11, p. 294]).

The risk of disease transmission (including respiratory disease and fungal skin infection) is greatest at times of year when high levels of population mixing occur, such as during and following autumn public sales. Vaccination programmes should take this into account and biosecurity measures (separation of new arrivals, disinfection of tack) used to minimize spread to resident horses nearing race targets.

Quarantine

Quarantine is the strict isolation of a group of horses in order to establish or maintain their health status prior to integration with a larger population. The two main circumstances in which racing yards may encounter quarantine are pre-export isolation prior to international shipping and quarantine within a yard in response to a suspected or confirmed infectious disease outbreak. Pre-export quarantine requirements are set out in the statutory regulations of the receiving country; typically, this form of isolation takes place on dedicated premises away from the normal operation of the training yard.

Quarantine procedures instigated within a yard due to a disease situation vary depending on the disease involved, extent of spread and practicalities determined by location and set-up of the yard. The most common diseases prompting quarantine in yards are neurological herpesvirus, strangles and infectious diarrhoea. Lengths of time required for quarantine, testing procedures and the rigour with which isolation is enforced are dictated by local codes of practice applicable to the disease in question (see Chapter 11, Infectious diseases). The goals are to limit spread to other horses or premises and to determine whether recovered horses are free from disease before release into the wider population. General principles relating to quarantine are discussed below.

Population at risk
- Initial action: divide yard population into risk groups; (1) horses with (or suspected to have) disease; (2) direct or close contacts of infected horses (physical contact or sharing facilities); and (3) low-risk group with no known contacts.
- Separate management of these groups with immediate effect, the goal being to move horses from in-contact group to low-risk group as they are cleared through testing.
- Appropriate testing procedures (blood sampling, nasopharyngeal or faecal swabbing) to determine exposure and infection status of all contacts. Testing may typically be conducted at weekly/bi-weekly intervals to allow for seroconversion and incubation periods.
- High vigilance to signs of disease within at-risk population.

Movements
- Depending on disease: all movements onto or off yard should cease from the time that disease is confirmed or strongly suspected, with a movement ban remaining in place until the disease status is confirmed. May have major impact on racing yard operations; however, the ramifications of (and liability for) not implementing a movement ban are far greater if infection spreads through racetracks or auction ring.
- In certain situations (particularly where there are few or no in-contacts) it is permissible to consider moving infected individual immediately off-site to a separate isolation facility, providing there is full disclosure to the receiving party. This may allow for more appropriate (and lower risk) management of an infected individual; most relevant for horses requiring hospital-based care (e.g. severe colitis). Important to follow through with movement ban, disease surveillance and testing in remainder of yard population.

Communication
- Communication with neighbouring yards and local trainers/breeders associations essential to enhance vigilance for disease and limit spread in locality, particularly when public training grounds are involved.
- In many jurisdictions there is a statutory requirement to notify national or state racing authority of suspected or confirmed infectious disease in training yard.
- Communication with yard staff and riders to combat misinformation and limit risk of spread to other horse populations.

Isolation procedures
- Inevitably involves some adaptation of 'textbook' procedures to the particular circumstances of yard.
- Infected horses should be housed >25 metres (100 metres for pre-export quarantine facilities) from other horses to minimize risk of airborne spread of disease.
- Isolation procedures should apply to exercise routes as well as stabling; if exercised on grounds accessible to other horses, a distance of at least 100 metres should be maintained.
- Isolation area should ideally have a separate water supply and waste bedding destroyed/removed in a manner that poses no risk of disease spread.
- Perimeter of isolation area should be clearly marked so that accidental entry by unauthorized personnel does not occur (may necessitate locking up after-hours).
- Designated staff to attend to horses in isolation area. These should be staff who have no other duties on remainder of premises for the duration of quarantine. If contact is required with non-isolation horses, this should take place before duties in isolation area are commenced (with no return later in day).
- Protective clothing/boots kept at and worn in isolation area; disinfectant foot baths (continually replenished) and hand wash at isolation perimeter to be used on entry and exit.
- Dedicated equipment (grooming, handling, riding) for isolation area, with no crossover of equipment to remainder of premises.
- Log-book to track entry of personnel and approved visitors (vets, farriers) to isolation area.

HOUSING AND AIR HYGIENE

Air quality
Air quality, measured by respirable particulate matter, can influence respiratory health. Inhalation of high concentrations of dust particles of a certain size (<5 μm diameter) has potential to cause respiratory inflammation or slow recovery from respiratory tract infections. In the stable environment, fungal spores are the major contributor to respirable dust; however, other organic particles and endotoxin may also have a significant impact on lower airway health. The concentration of these particles at any one time is determined by release of dust from feed and bedding, and its rate of clearance is determined by ventilation. In yards with good management and adequate ventilation, there is little difference in dust release rates between straw, wood shavings or paper bedding (although quality of straw and shavings can vary between suppliers).

Ventilation and housing
Stable and yard design have a major influence on air quality. Most racehorses are stabled either in loose boxes or in barns with shared airspace. There is some evidence that racehorses housed in loose boxes with sufficient ventilation are less prone to lower airway disease than those stabled in barns. Optimum ventilation rates when dust released from feed/bedding is not excessive should be ≥4 air changes/hour. In calm conditions loose boxes achieve good ventilation rates (6–7 air changes/hour) providing the top door is open (ventilation rates usually unsatisfactory with door closed). Barn ventilation is satisfactory even in still conditions with doors open at each end, although air quality varies with location within the barn (worse in middle and adjacent to doors). With the end doors shut, traditional barn ventilation is poor. Ventilation of barns is assisted by air movement caused by convection, with warm air exiting through ventilation spaces high in the walls or ceiling. Convection is less of a factor than in the more intensively managed housing of farm animals; however, insulation of walls and roof can improve its effectiveness and reduce the need for large ventilation inlets. Proximity of (and relationship of wind direction to) muck heaps and hay storage areas should also be considered when assessing a yard for respiratory hazards.

Minimizing respirable dust
Although adequate ventilation is an important factor in respiratory health, it does not always reflect air quality in the 'breathing zone' of the stabled horse. A large proportion of inhaled dust particles (including fungal spores) comes from hay/forage. Immersion of hay in water immediately prior to feeding can reduce this load by more than 90%; immersion for 5–10 minutes is sufficient, as nutrients are leached if forage is soaked for too long. Alternatively, haylage or steamed hay can be fed.

Yard management may be used to minimize inhaled dust loads. Dampening passageways before sweeping can reduce dust levels. When bedding is disturbed during cleaning out of a stable, the concentration of dust particulate matter in the air rises markedly. This effect is greatest with straw; however, regardless of bedding type the period of time around stable cleaning and laying down of new bedding is associated with poor air quality. Failure to remove soiled and wet bedding leads to rapid fungal growth and increased ammonia levels, which may cause respiratory irritation.

LOWER AIRWAY DISEASE

(See also Chapter 3, p. 222.)

The following points are relevant to the management of respiratory disease in racing yards:
- Lower airway inflammation/infection (characterized by increased tracheal mucus and coughing) is common and generally self-limiting.
- Causes are multifactorial and incompletely understood.
- Bacterial infection (either primary or secondary) is thought to play a large role in development and persistence of excessive tracheal mucus.
- Bacterial species involved are endemic in the normal population, therefore elimination of exposure is impractical.
- Viral infection is less important than bacterial infection.

Investigation
Onset of concern about a wider health problem in a yard is often insidious and may arise from increased frequency of coughing, 'dirty' endoscopy results or poor racetrack performances over a period of weeks.

Successful management should aim to minimize lost training days and economic cost. Appropriate treatment relies on the quality of information regarding prevalence and severity of respiratory disease:
- Background information: frequency of coughing/fevers/poor performers in recent weeks.
- 'Batch' scoping: best way to assess yard prevalence of lower airway disease; random sampling or entire group/s (coughing is an insensitive indicator of disease).
- Determine whether particular groups (e.g. 2 YOs) are most affected.
- Clinical, endoscopic and laboratory findings: generally (but not always) possible to determine whether respiratory disease has an infectious component or is primarily related to air hygiene.
- Blood sampling is of little use for the detection of respiratory disease.

Management
- Approach to treatment dictated by stage of season/extent and severity of disease/economic cost.
- Respiratory disease is common in yearlings/2 YOs during first months in training environment; at these times it is often preferable to restrict treatment to cases that do not resolve naturally (or to limit wider spread within yard).
- Treatment: either targeted at individual horses confirmed with respiratory disease (through endoscopy) or mass medication of target groups with high levels of disease.
- Mass medication: may be appropriate if guided by diagnostic work and administered responsibly; widely practised in farm animals to reduce morbidity associated with respiratory disease. May reduce shedding/transmission of bacterial pathogens and speed up yard recovery.
- 'Re-treats' (horses that fail to respond to initial course of medication) targeted for further investigation.
- Influence of continued exercise on persistence of lower airway disease has been poorly investigated: common advice is to refrain from fast work/racing while moderate–marked levels of excessive mucus are present in trachea.

- Routine endoscopy prior to race confirmation/declaration to establish respiratory health status of horses with race targets.
- Air hygiene problems should be addressed where practicable or if respiratory disease becomes a persistent concern.
- Immunostimulants: some evidence to support use of non-specific immunostimulants (inactivated *Propionibacterium acnes*/inactivated *Parapox ovis* virus) as adjuncts to conventional therapies; may assist recovery/reduce severity.

MUSCULOSKELETAL INJURIES

Unusually high rates or patterns of injury may prompt investigation of the overall musculoskeletal health of a yard. For meaningful conclusions to be drawn, assessment should be based on objective information rather than reaction to a recent injury cluster.

Quantifying injury rates
- Number and type of injuries over a set time period has to be determined and then assessed in the context of number of horses at risk.
- Minimum time period examined should be months/years, as prevalence of injury can fluctuate considerably through racing season.
- Injury incidence rate is best measured against the number of 'horse-training-days at risk'; however, calculating this figure (number of days training at different paces for each horse) is rarely possible in practice.
- More workable approach: analyse number of injuries in relation to average number of horses in work or yard.

Comparison of injury rates
- 'Normal' injury rates vary between training centres/types of racing and published research is limited.
- Disregarding sore shins, splints and accidental injury, approximately 20–25% of a yard population can be expected to sustain some form of musculoskeletal injury during a calendar year.

- Fracture rate in training is approximately 1/100 horse months (i.e. on average 1 fracture/month can be expected for every 100 horses in training). Accounting for irregular distribution throughout the year, this may equate to several fractures/month during high-risk periods.
- Availability of good records may allow comparison with previous seasons.

Analysis of injury types
- Patterns of injury vary between trainers/training centres and reflect many factors including training regime, track and horse and jockey variables.
- Flat race training: stress fractures involving the forelimb cannon, pelvis and tibia, osteochondral injuries of the fetlock and middle carpal joint and tendinitis predominate.
- Level of yard vigilance for early orthopaedic injury may be indirectly assessed by severity of stress injuries at time of diagnosis/detection: high incidence of 'end-stage' stress fractures (those requiring surgical repair or euthanasia) is indicative of poor detection or failure to react to early signs of injury.

Analysis of risk factors
- Trend towards greater incidence of hindlimb stress injuries with heavy use of uphill tracks (greater relative loading of hindlimbs).
- Risk of particular injuries varies with age profile; yard with a large proportion of 2 YOs might expect to have a greater incidence of sore shins, tibial stress fractures or proximal metacarpal lameness than a yard with predominantly older horses.
- Firm ground (turf) consistently associated with higher risk of fracture.

Minimizing injury rates
- (See also Chapter 1, Injury management and rehabilitation.)
- Reduction (but not elimination) of injury risk may be possible in many circumstances.
- Conditioning early in life (foal/yearling), nutrition and conformation may be associated with increased risk of particular injuries and should guide selection of yearlings.
- Chronic nutritional imbalances (particularly of calcium:phosphorus ratio) can lead to skeletal weakness and increase injury risk; this is usually readily determined through analysis of the yard diet.
- Inappropriate training goals/methods applied to late-maturing horses or those of particular physical types should be avoided.
- Stress fractures result from failure of skeletal repair processes to keep pace with workload. High stress injury rates may warrant consideration of longer intervals between fast exercise days or strategic use of low-intensity training periods to coincide with the peak risk (early fast-exercise) phase of training. Introduction of small cumulative training loads of fast exercise early in career, followed by a 'spell' rather than unbroken progression through to racing, may also be beneficial.

CHAPTER 18

TRANSPORT

OVERVIEW

Long-distance transport of racehorses by both road and air is commonplace. National legislation and international guidelines provide a framework for safe and humane movement of horses and for preventive measures to limit the spread of exotic diseases across national borders. Minimizing any negative effects of transport on athletic performance is also a key consideration for horses that are expected to race/train upon arrival at destination.

EFFECTS OF TRANSPORT

Factors such as individual temperament, route planning, transit conditions and expertise of travelling grooms are fundamental to the condition of a horse after the journey. Long-distance travel has the potential to detrimentally affect health in several ways.

Respiratory tract
- Restraining the head in a raised position for lengthy periods prevents natural drainage of respiratory secretions and contributes to bacterial colonization of lower airways.
- Quality of inhaled air (bacterial contamination and dust) is often poor during transport and particularly at times when air circulation is reduced, such as when vehicle is stationary (during plane refuelling stops).
- Breathing dry, cool air during air travel can dehydrate the respiratory tract mucosa and reduce mucociliary clearance of secretions.
- Overall effect of long distance travel (road or air) is a considerable bacterial challenge to the lower airways and impaired respiratory defences to deal with it.

Weight loss
- Regardless of temperament, most horses lose weight during transport.
- Due to the combination of reduced feed and water intake; also greater energy expenditure is required to maintain postural balance.
- Horses eat and drink less when in a moving vehicle.
- Road transport typically results in losses of 0.4–0.6% BWT/hour (around 3% for a 7-hour journey).
- Air transport losses typically total 3–5% of BWT.
- Rehydration after a flight is often rapid but BWT is slower to return to normal due to need to replenish gut fill.
- Speed of recovery is determined by temperament of horse (+/− previous travelling experience), amount of weight lost, duration of journey and environmental conditions at destination.
- Recovery time to normal BWT for air travel with 5% BWT loss can be >1 week.

Musculoskeletal system
- Considerable energy is expended in maintaining postural stability during both road and air transport.
- Wide-based stance with head and neck raised and more weight taken by hindlimbs for greater stability.
- Constant muscular effort can lead to very mild elevations in plasma concentrations of muscle enzymes (AST/CK).

Gastrointestinal system
- Reduced food/water intake, disrupted feed patterns and change of diet on arrival can affect hindgut flora.
- Subsequent effects on digestibility of feed and gut motility.
- Risk of developing colic.
- Effect on BWT may persist for weeks.

Blood profile
- Common to get mild inflammatory/dehydration changes in haematology profile in first 3 days following long journey.
- WBC count either normal or slightly raised (neutrophilia).
- +/− mild elevation in plasma fibrinogen concentration.
- RBC count and total protein figures reflect dehydration.

Jetlag and acclimatization
- 'Jetlag' in people is an alteration in the normal balance of circadian rhythms associated with the crossing of time-zones: manifested by sleep disturbances and flatness as well as athletic underperformance.
- Inadequately researched field in horses and validated recommendations for use of artificial lighting/shading to minimize possible effects do not currently exist.
- The horse's circadian rhythms are highly light-sensitive and may be influenced by exercise regimes, therefore a far more rapid adjustment to local time-zone than in people.
- Eastward travel across time zones ('phase advance') in the immediate pre-race period (<4 days) may have a potential ergogenic effect.
- Acclimatization to hot/humid climates appears to be relatively rapid with good management.

Shipping fever (Pleuropneumonia)
(See also Chapter 3, p. 233.)

Infrequent but regularly encountered condition in horses that have recently travelled long distances (greatest risk with journey times >20–24 hours), although can also be seen following shorter trips. Bacterial respiratory infection (most commonly *Strep. zooepidemicus*, *Pasteurella*) due to exposure to high bacterial loads in inspired air during transport and reduced clearance of respiratory secretions. Unless treated promptly and aggressively may progress to pleuropneumonia (life-threatening).

Signs
- Reduced feed and water intake.
- +/− fever.
- Increased respiration rate +/− cough.
- +/− nasal discharge.
- Depression/lethargy, sometimes profound.

Diagnosis
- Blood analysis: inflammatory profile.
- Auscultation of chest: increased lung sounds dorsally, absent/muffled lung sounds ventral fields may indicate development of pleuropneumonia.
- Ultrasonography: detection of pleural fluid accumulation.

Management
- Aggressive broad-spectrum antibiotic and anti-inflammatory therapy (see Chapter 3, p. 234.)

Prognosis
- Good prognosis for full recovery with prompt and aggressive treatment.

VETERINARY MANAGEMENT FOR LONG-DISTANCE TRANSPORT

Pre-departure
- Pre-departure health and identification checks +/– disease testing protocols as required by receiving country/state.
- Important to ensure respiratory health during immediate period prior to travel; rectal temperature monitored daily and any cough/nasal discharge investigated/treated.
- Pre-shipment weighing useful to allow determination of weight lost during transit.
- Normal diurnal BWT variation: lowest early morning before feeding or immediately post exercise; highest in evening after feeding.
- If a new diet (forage/concentrate ration) is to be used at destination, gradual introduction over several weeks prior to travel is advantageous.
- Maintenance of appetite during/after travel may be assisted by administration of anti-ulcer medication (omeprazole); should commence >1 week prior to departure.
- Prophylactic use of antibiotics does not reduce risk of bacterial colonization of the lower airways and is not recommended.
- Limited evidence that use of immunomodulators (*Parapox ovis* virus/*Propionibacterium acnes*-derived products) in period leading up to travel may be beneficial.
- Care required when planning orthopaedic medications in immediate pre-travel period: corticosteroids can depress appetite, suppress immune system and produce haematological changes similar to those seen with illness. NSAID administration should be avoided for 2–3 days pre- and post-travel in order not to mask pyrexia or early signs of shipping fever.

Post-arrival
- Monitoring food/water intake during transit and after arrival guides need for fluid replenishment.
- Weighing is useful to determine loss of BWT and allows estimation of likely dehydration.
- Fluid administration if BWT loss is >5%.
- Nasogastric intubation is acceptable for mild deficits; IV isotonic fluids for larger deficits or more rapid replenishment.
- Twice-daily monitoring of rectal temperature for at least 1–2 weeks post arrival.
- Blood analysis if any depression/inappetence/fever is observed.

PART 4
APPENDICES

- **APPENDIX 1** — Normal clinical parameters
- **APPENDIX 2** — Drug administration reference table
- **APPENDIX 3** — Guide to best practice for humane destruction in emergency situations
- **APPENDIX 4** — Blood reference ranges

APPENDIX 1
NORMAL CLINICAL PARAMETERS

Celsius–Fahrenheit conversion chart	
°C	°F
36.9	98.5
37.2	99.0
37.5	99.5
37.8	100.0
38.1	100.5
38.3	101.0
38.6	101.5
38.9	102.0
39.2	102.5
39.4	103.0
39.7	103.5
40.0	104.0
40.3	104.5
40.6	105.0

Resting heart rate: 28–36 bpm

Maximal heart rate (HR_{max}) at exercise: 200–240 bpm

Resting respiration rate: 8–12/minute

Rectal temperature: 37.2–38.3°C (99–101°F)

APPENDIX 2
DRUG ADMINISTRATION REFERENCE TABLE

DRUG	DOSAGE (BWT)	ROUTE	FREQUENCY
Antibiotic drugs			
Cefquinome sulphate	1–2 mg/kg	IM or IV	q24h
Ceftiofur sodium	2.2 mg/kg	IM or IV	q24h (or12h)
Doxycycline	10 mg/kg	PO	q12h
Enrofloxacin	7.5 mg/kg	PO	q24h
	5 mg/kg	IV	q24h
Gentamicin sulphate	6.6 mg/kg	IV or IM	q24h
Metronidazole	25 mg/kg	PO	q12h
Marbofloxacin	3.5–4 mg/kg	PO	q24h
Oxytetracycline hydrochloride	5 mg/kg	IV	q24h (or 12h)
Procaine benzyl penicillin	12 mg/kg	IM	q24h
Trimethoprim–sulphonamide	15–30 mg/kg	PO	q12h
Anti-inflammatory drugs			
Acetylsalicylic acid (aspirin)	10 mg/kg	PO	q12–24h
Flunixin meglumine	1.1 mg/kg	IV	q24h
	1.1 mg/kg	PO	q24h
Ketoprofen	2.2 mg/kg	IV	q12–24h
Meloxicam	0.6 mg/kg	PO	q12–24h
	0.6 mg/kg	IV	q12–24h
Phenylbutazone	2.2–4.4 mg/kg	PO	q12h
	2.2–4.4 mg/kg	IV	q12h
Suxibuzone	3.3–6.6 mg/kg	PO	q12h
Morphine	0.02–0.2 mg/kg	IV	(single)
Pethidine	0.4–2.0 mg/kg	IM	q24h
Dexamethasone	0.1 mg/kg	IV	q24–48h
Prednisolone	0.2–4.4 mg/kg	PO	q12–24h
Respiratory drugs			
Frusemide	0.5–1.0 mg/kg	IV	Pre-exercise
Clenbuterol	0.8–1.6 µg/kg	PO	q12h
	0.8 µg/kg	IV	q12h
Dembrexine	0.3–0.5 mg/kg	PO	q12h

(continued)

DRUG	DOSAGE (BWT)	ROUTE	FREQUENCY
Potassium iodide	10–40 mg/kg	PO	q24h
Sodium iodide	100 mg/kg	IV	q24–72h
Gastric ulcer drugs			
Omeprazole	2–4 mg/kg	PO	q24h
Ranitidine	6.6 mg/kg	PO	q8h
Cimetidine	16–20 mg/kg	PO	q8h
Miscellaneous orthopaedic drugs			
Dantrolene sodium	1–4 mg/kg	PO	Pre-exercise
Tiludronate	1 mg/kg	IV	(Single)
Sedative drugs			
Acepromazine	0.02–0.06 mg/kg	IV	As required
Detomidine	0.004–0.02 mg/kg	IV	As required
Xylazine	0.2–0.8 mg/kg	IV	As required
Butorphanol	0.01–0.04 mg/kg	IV	As required
Inhaled respiratory drugs			
Beclomethasone	500–3750 µg (total)	MDI	q12–24h
Fluticasone	2000 µg (total)	MDI	q12h
Ipratropium bromide	2–4 µg/kg	MDI	q12h
Salbutamol	360–720 µg (total)	MDI	q12–24h

BWT, bodyweight; IM, intramuscular; IV, intravenous; PO, per os (by mouth); MDI, metered dose inhaler (inhaled); q, each/every.

APPENDIX 3
GUIDE TO BEST PRACTICE FOR HUMANE DESTRUCTION IN EMERGENCY SITUATIONS

In the case of suspected but not definite grounds for immediate euthanasia a second opinion should be sought before proceeding.

CONDITION	IMMEDIATE DESTRUCTION	PROGNOSIS: PASTURE	PROGNOSIS: ATHLETIC
Skeletal			
Pastern fracture: non-comminuted	No	Good	Good–guarded
Pastern fracture: comminuted, one intact strut	No	Guarded	Guarded–poor
Pastern fracture: comminuted, no intact strut	Yes	Poor–hopeless	Poor–hopeless
Condylar (Mc3/Mt3) fracture:	No	Good	Good–guarded
Condylar (Mc3/Mt3) fracture: compound + comminuted	Yes	Poor–hopeless	Poor–hopeless
Compound long bone fracture	Yes	Poor–hopeless	Poor–hopeless
Humeral/radial/tibial/femoral fracture: displaced	Yes	Poor–hopeless	Poor–hopeless
Third carpal bone fracture	No	Good	Good–guarded
Multiple carpal/tarsal bone fractures (+ carpal/tarsal instability)	Yes	Poor–hopeless	Poor–hopeless
Pelvic fracture: standing	No	Good	Good–guarded
Pelvic fracture: recumbent	Yes	Poor–hopeless	Hopeless
Pedal bone fracture	No	Articular: good–guarded Non-articular: good	Articular: good–guarded Non-articular: good
Navicular bone fracture	No	Good–guarded	Guarded–poor
Soft tissue			
SDFT tendonitis	No	Good	Good–guarded
SDFT rupture (below carpus)	No	Good–guarded	FL: guarded–poor HL: good
SDFT rupture (musculotendinous junction)	Yes	Poor	Hopeless
SDFT rupture (bilateral)	Yes	Poor	Hopeless
Complete breakdown of suspensory apparatus	No	Guarded–poor	Hopeless
Partial laceration of SDFT/DDFT +/− suspensory ligament	No	Good	FL: guarded–poor HL: good
Complete laceration of SDFT	No	Good	FL: guarded–poor HL: good
Complete laceration of SDFT+ DDFT	No	Fair–good	Poor

(continued)

CONDITION	IMMEDIATE DESTRUCTION	PROGNOSIS: PASTURE	PROGNOSIS: ATHLETIC
Complete laceration of SDFT, DDFT + suspensory ligament	Yes	Very poor	Hopeless
'Slipped' tendon (displacement of SDFT from point of hock)	No	Good	Good–poor
Synovial sepsis (acute/chronic)	No	Acute: good Chronic: poor	Acute: good–guarded Chronic: poor
Neurological			
Spinal fracture + hindlimb paralysis/paresis	Yes	Hopeless	Hopeless
Recumbent non-responsive: post trauma	Yes (+ 2nd opinion)	Hopeless	Hopeless
Wobbler syndrome (grade 1–3)	No	Good–guarded	Good–guarded
Wobbler syndrome (grade 4)	No	Guarded–poor	Poor–hopeless
Wobbler syndrome (grade 5)	Yes	Poor–hopeless	Poor–hopeless

FL, forelimb; HL, hindlimb; Mc3/Mt3, third metacarpal/metatarsal; SDFT, superficial digital flexor tendon; DDFT, deep digital flexor tendon.

Modified from Appendix II of the BEVA/Equine Group of Veterinary Ireland document "*A Guide to Best Practice for Veterinary Surgeons When Considering Euthanasia on Humane Grounds*" (reprinted 2009).

APPENDIX 4
BLOOD REFERENCE RANGES

TEST	ABBREVIATION	RANGE	UNITS
Total red blood cells (erythrocytes)	RBCs	8.6–11.7	$\times 10^{12}/l$
Packed cell volume	PCV	0.34–0.45	l/l
Haemoglobin	Hb	12.8–16.6	g/dl
Mean cell volume	MCV	37–43	fl
Mean cell haemoglobin concentration	MCHC	35.9–38.8	g/dl
Mean cell haemoglobin	MCH	13.7–16.2	pg
Total white blood cells (leucocytes)	WBCs	5.5–11.0	$\times 10^{9}/l$
Segmented neutrophils	Segs	3.9–6.0 (42–64%)	$\times 10^{9}/l$
Lymphocytes	Lymphs	2.3–4.4 (28–46%)	$\times 10^{9}/l$
Monocytes	Monos	0.2–0.56 (2–6%)	$\times 10^{9}/l$
Eosinophils	Eos	0–0.3 (1–3%)	$\times 10^{9}/l$
Platelets	Plts	127–206	$\times 10^{9}/l$
Total protein	TP	58–67	g/l
Albumin	Alb	35–40	g/l
Globulin	Glob	21–29	g/l
Plasma fibrinogen	Fib	1.4–3.0	g/l
Serum amyloid A	SAA	0	mg/l
Aspartate aminotransferase	AST	<400	iu/l
Creatine kinase	CK	<400	iu/l
Lactate dehydrogenase	LD	430–917	iu/l
Gamma glutamyl transferase	GGT	12–47	iu/l
Glutamate dehydrogenase	GLDH	3–12	iu/l
Serum alkaline phosphatase	SAP	277–672	iu/l
Intestinal alkaline phosphatase	IAP	64–171	iu/l
Urea	Urea	3.8–6.4	mmol/l
Creatinine	Creat	110–167	µmol/l
Glucose	Glu	3.4–5.9	mmol/l
Total bilirubin	TBili	13–39	µmol/l
Direct bilirubin	DBili	4–15	µmol/l
Bile acids	BAcids	0–8	µmol/l

Modified from Beaufort Cottage Laboratories' reference ranges for 2- and 3-YO Thoroughbred racehorses.

INDEX

Note: Page numbers in *italic* refer to tables

abscess
    cheek/lip 252–3
    injection site 187
    subsolar 36–8
    tooth root 243–4
accessory carpal bone 108, 109
    fracture 122, 123
accessory ligament
    DDFT (AL-DDFT/inferior check ligament) 92, 93
        injury 101–2
    SDFT (AL-SDFT/superior check ligament)
        desmopathy 134
        desmotomy 26
acclimatization 350
acepromazine
    dose/frequency *357*
    exertional rhabdomyolysis 191, 192
    laminitis 47
    laryngeal function 208, 311
acetabulum 168, 169
    fracture 174–6
acetylsalicylic acid (aspirin) *19*, 238, *356*
'Achilles' tendon bundle 137, 148
acupuncture 29
aerobic metabolism 317
African horse sickness (AHS) 298
age, and risk of injury 4
air quality 345, 349
air transport 349, 350
albumin *338*, *360*
alkaline phosphatase (ALP) *338*, *360*
alpha-2 agonists 258, *357*
altitude training, real/simulated 335
altrenogest 266, 332

amino acid supplementation 334
aminocaproic acid *232*
anabolic steroids *18*, 335–6
anaemia 340
anaerobic metabolism 317
'anaerobic threshold' 323
antacids 257
antebrachiocarpal joint 108, 109, 114
    fracture/fragmentation 110, 111, *119*
antibiotic-associated diarrhoea 261, 262
antibiotics
    administration table *356*
    eye infections 246, 247
    lower airway disease 228
    topical 278–9
anti-fibrinolytics *232*
antifungal medication 248, 249
    topical 281
anti-inflammatory medications
    administration table *356*
    misuse/overuse 5
    topical 20, 30, 277
    see also non-steroidal anti-inflammatory drugs (NSAIDs)
anti-oxidants 328, 334
antiprotozoal drugs 297
antispasmodic agents 260, 263
antiviral medication 274
aortic regurgitation *235*
appetite 331–2
    travel 351
arboviral encephalitis 275–6
L-arginine 334
articular windgalls 52
articulating process joints (APJs/facet joints) 179
    arthropathy 183–4
aryepiglottic folds 201
    axial deviation 212–14

    collapse 207
arytenoid cartilages 201, 202
    paralysis 205
    ulceration/chondritis 218–19
arytenoidectomy, partial 210
aspartate aminotransferase (AST) 191, *338*, 341
    exertional rhabdomyolysis 191
    reference range *360*
Aspergillus spp. 247, 249
aspirin *19*, 238, *356*
astringents, topical 10
ataxia 271–2, *273*
atheroma, nasal 253
athletic potential
    and conformation 313
    genetics 315
atrial fibrillation (AF) *236*, 237
atrial premature complexes (APCs) *236*
atrioventricular block, second-degree *236*
atrioventricular regurgitation *235*
atropine sulphate 247
autologous biological products (regenerative therapies) *18*
autologous blood transfusion 335
autologous conditioned serum (ACS) *18*
avocado/soybean lipids *20*
avulsion injuries
    proximal sesamoid bone 82, 83
    proximal suspensory ligament origin 100
    skull base 188

Babesia caballi 297
bacitracin 246, 247
back
    applied anatomy 180
    examination 180
    saddle sores 189–90
    spinal stress injury 183–4

back pain 180
  causes 169, 177–8, 184
Bacteroides spp. 233
BAD, *see* branchial arch defects
balancers (feed) 328
bandage 'bow'/'bind' 13–14
barley 329
barn stabling, ventilation 345
bar shoe 36, 42, 45
beclomethasone *357*
benzimidazoles 260
beta-alanine 334
betamethasone, intra-articular *17*
bicarbonate 335
biceps brachii muscle 125
biceps femoris 168
biceps tendon 124–5
  tenosynovitis 130–1
bicipital bursa 124, 125
  septic tenosynovitis 130–1
bile acids, serum *338*, *360*
bilirubin *338*, *360*
bioflavonoids *232*
'biological passport' 335
biosecurity measures 226–7, 295, 343–4
biotin 35, 330
bismuth subsalicylate 262
bisphosphonates 69, 103, 120, 139, 193, 196
  actions *19*
  administration table *357*
  use/efficacy *19*
bit injuries 244
'bleeding', *see* exercise-induced pulmonary haemorrhage (EIPH)
'blisters' 30
blood analysis
  blood constituents *337*–*8*
  effects of training 339
  effects of transport 350
  fitness assessment 322
  interpretation 340–1
  nutritional imbalances 331
  pre-purchase examination 306
  reference ranges 340, *360*
  sample collection/storage 339
blood collection 339
blood doping 335
blood urea nitrogen (BUN) *338*
blood volume, total circulating 317

body weight (BWT)
  and fitness 323
  loss 331–2
  and transport 349
boils and 'runners' 279–80
bone
  adaptation to load/stress 3, 318, 319
  sequestrum 10, 11
'bone islands' (enostosis-like lesions) 194–6
bone spavin 138–40
bone spurs
  carpal bones 116–17, *308*
  lower hock 139, *309*
Bordetella spp. 227
box walking 291
brachytherapy, interstitial 285
bran 330
branchial arch defects (4-BAD/6-BAD) 219–20
breeze-up sales 312–13
bronchoalveolar lavage 231
brushing injuries 12
Burkholderia mallei 299
butorphanol *357*
B vitamins 334

calcaneus 136, 137
calcinosis circumscripta 289
cannon bone, *see* metacarpal/metatarsal bone, third (Mc3/Mt3)
canter, training speeds 319–20
capped elbow 134, 135
capped hock 145–7
capsaicin 30
carbazochrome *232*
carbohydrates 327
  'loading' 332, 333–4
  overload 46
carbon dioxide (CO_2) 335
cardiac arrhythmias 236–7
  fatal 239
cardiopulmonary failure 239
cardiovascular system 317
  disorder 235–9
  and fitness 318, 322
L-carnitine 334
carpal canal 108
carpal sheath, tenosynovitis 120–2
carpal valgus 314
carpometacarpal joint 108, 109, 119

carpus ('knee')
  applied anatomy 108, 109
  conformation 108, 115, 314
  examination 108–9
  fractures 122, 123, *358*
  lameness/injuries 109–19
  management and prognosis 118–19
  pre-purchase radiography findings and significance *308*
  protocols *307*
  road wounds 9
cartilage 15, 16, 319
  repair 16
  structure 15
Caslick's vulvoplasty 268
castration 268, *269*
  cryptorchid 270
cataracts *305*
cefquinome sulphate *356*
ceftiofur sodium *356*
cellulitis 278
Celsius–Fahrenheit conversion chart 355
cereals 329
  overfeeding 327
cervical spine injuries 8, 180–1
cervical stenotic myelopathy (wobbler syndrome) 271–3
chaff 329
check ligament
  inferior (AL-DDFT) 92, 93
    injury 101–2
  superior (AL-SDFT)
    desmopathy 134–6
    desmotomy 26
cheek, abscess 252–3
'chip' fracture
  carpal bones 110–12
  fetlock 70–2
chiropractic *28*
chlorhexidine 278
'choke' (oesophageal obstruction) 262–3
chondroitin sulphate *20*
chorioretinopathy *305*
cimetidine *257*, *357*
circadian rhythms 350
clay/smectite 262
clenbuterol 228, 336, *356*
Clostridium spp. 233, 261
cobalt chloride 335

coffin joint (distal interphalangeal joint) 31–2, 43
Coggins test 296
cold therapy 25, 28
colic 258–60, 291
collagen necrosis nodule 285
collapse, fatal 239
coloboma *305*
colonic impaction *259*
comatose horse 8
common digital extensor tendon 32, 108
computed tomography (CT)
  acetabular fracture 175
  dentition of 2.5 YO 241
  ethmoidal haematoma 250
  keratoma 48
  proximal sesamoid bone fracture 84
concentrates 327, 329
  overfeeding 327
condition
  loss 331–2
  see also body weight
condylar fracture (Mc3/Mt3) 59–64
  concurrent sesamoid bone fracture 84
  euthanasia guide *358*
  prevention 6
condylar stress reaction 66–9
conformation
  assessment 313–14
  carpus 108, 115, 314
  changes with maturity 314
  corrective surgery 314
  foot 32
  hock/hindlimb 138, 149, 314
conjunctivitis 246
contagious equine metritis (CEM) 296–7
cool-down 322
corn (bruised foot) 32–3
corneal oedema *305*
corneal stromal abscess 247–8
corneal ulceration 246–7, *305*
Cornell collar 212
corpora nigra *305*
corticosteroids
  dose/frequency *356*
  joint disease (intra-articular) *17*, 78
  joint disease (systemic) *19*

laminitis risk *17*, 46
  topical 10
  urticaria 283
coughing 222, 227
counter-irritation 30
cracked heels (pastern dermatitis) 278
creatine 334
creatine kinase (CK) 191, *338, 341, 360*
creatinine *338, 360*
crib-biting 258, 291
cricoarytenoideus dorsalis 202
cricoarytenoideus lateralis 207
cruciate ligaments 153
  injuries 166
crude protein (CP) 327
cryotherapy (freeze firing) 30
cryptorchid (rig) 268–70
Culicoides midges 288, 298
curb 149–50
cyathostomes 260, *261*
cysts
  dermal inclusion (nasal atheroma) 253
  dermoid 288
  pharyngeal 220–1
  see also subchondral bone cysts

Damalinia equi 287
dantrolene sodium 191, 339, *357*
DDSP, *see* dorsal displacement of the soft palate
deep digital flexor tendon (DDFT) 32, 92, 93
  accessory ligament (AL-DDFT) 93
  injury 101–2
  hindlimb 136, 137
  injury in foot puncture 38
  radial head tearing 120, 122
dehydration
  blood analysis 340
  diarrhoea 261, 262
dembrexine 228, *356*
dental malalignment 243
dentistry 241–4
dermal inclusion cyst (nasal atheroma) 253
dermatitis
  Culicoides hypersensitivity (sweet itch) 288
  harvest mite 286–7

  pastern (mud fever/cracked heels) 278–9
  saddle region 189–90
dermatophilosis (rain scald/rain rot) 282
Dermatophilus congolensis 282
dermatophytosis (ringworm) 280–2
dermoid cysts 288
deslorelin 266
desmotomy
  accessory ligament of SDFT 26
  medial patellar ligament 166
detomidine 208, 258, *357*
detraining 320
developmental orthopaedic disease, *see* osteochondrosis
dewormers 260
dexamethasone
  dose/frequency *356*
  intra-articular *17*
  urticaria 283
diarrhoea 260–2
DICOM (Digital Imaging and Communications in Medicine) 308
Digital cushion 31
dimethyl sulphoxide (DMSO) 30, 238
diminazene aceturate 297
dioestrus 265
dirt tracks 5, 324, 325
disinfectants 227
distal interphalangeal joint (DIPJ) 31–2, 43
distal intertarsal (DIT) joint 136, 137
  arthritic changes 138–40
distal phalanx (P3/pedal bone) 31
  cysts 42–4, *310*
  fracture 40–2, *310*
  proliferative modelling *310*
  'reverse rotation/inclination' 34, 35
  rotation/sinking 47
  septic osteitis 39–40
distal sesamoidean ligament (DSL), desmopathy 90–1
diuretics *232, 233, 356*
dorsal displacement of the soft palate (DDSP) 210–12
  intermittent 206

dorsal metacarpal disease (sore/bucked shins) 102–3
dorsal osteochondral disease (Mc3/Mt3) 73–4
dorsal spinous processes (DSPs) 180
    fractures 186–7
    impingement 181–3
dorsal splint (Kimzey Leg Saver) 7
dourine 298–9
doxycycline *356*
drinking, excessive 265
DSPs, *see* dorsal spinous processes

Eastern equine encephalitis 275–6
echocardiography 315
effusion
    carpal sheath 120, 121, 122
    fetlock 52
    shoulder/elbow joints 125
EIPH, *see* exercise-induced pulmonary haemorrhage
elbow
    anatomy 124, 125
    capped 134, 135
    fracture stabilization 7
    kick wound 14
    osteochondrosis 133–4
electrocardiogram (ECG)
    arrhythmias 237
    heart scores 315
    training monitors 321
electrolytes 328, 330, 341
    assessment 341
electrotherapy *29*
ELISA 295, 296
encephalitis, arboviral 275–6
endoscope, disinfection 226–7
endoscopy
    lower airway disease 222–5, 345, 346
    overground/treadmill 206–7
    pre-purchase examination 311
    resting 203–6, 217, 220, 221, 311
    video 311
endotoxaemia 46, 237
enilconazole 249, 281
enostosis-like lesions ('bone islands') 194–6
enrofloxacin *356*
Enterobacter spp. 233
eosinophilic collagen necrosis 285

eosinophils *337*, *360*
epaxial muscles 180
epiglottic entrapment 214, 215
epiglottic retroversion 214–16
epiglottis 201, 202
    size/flaccidity 311
epiglottitis 220
epistaxis 210, 222, 229
    ethmoidal haematoma 250
EPO, *see* erythropoietin
equine herpesvirus (EHV) 227, 273–4, 293–4
    EHV-1 273–4
    EHV-4 293
    management and prevention 294
    neurological form 273–4, 293, 294
    respiratory 294
    transmission 294
equine infectious anaemia (EIA/'swamp fever') 295–6
equine influenza 293
equine protozoal myeloencephalitis (EPM) 274–5
equine viral arteritis (EVA) 295
ergogenic aids
    definition 333
    non-nutritional 335–6
    nutritional 333–5
erythrocytes, *see* red blood cells
'erythropoiesis-stimulating agents' 335
erythropoietin (EPO) 335
Escherichia coli 233
ESWT, *see* extracorporeal shock-wave therapy
ethmoidal haematoma 250–1
ethylene oxide sterilization 227
euthanasia
    at track 6
    guide to best practice *358–9*
exercise
    injury prevention 5–6
    joint disease 16
    rehabilitation programmes 22, 27
exercise-induced pulmonary haemorrhage (EIPH) 229–32
    causes 230
    diagnosis 231
    management 231–2

    risk factors 210, 227, 230–1
exercise physiology 317–19
exertional rhabdomyolysis ('setfast') 190–2, 341
    diagnosis 191
    management 191–2
exhaustion 8
extensor tendons 32, 108
extracorporeal shockwave therapy (ESWT) 69, 82, 88, 99, 100, 101, 103
    description *28*
    use and clinical effect *28*
eye disease 246–8
eye examination, pre-purchase 304, *305*

facet joints 179
    arthropathy 183–4
faecal egg count (FEC) 260
fatalities
    causes 4, 60, 239
    rates 4, *5*
fatigue 317
fats, diet 191–2, 327, 330
feeding 327
    and colic 258
    exertional rhabdomyolysis 191–2
    gastric ulcers 255, 257
    individual strategies 327
    key nutrients 327–8
    pre-race 332
    radial physitis 123
    rehabilitation 24
    supplements 328, 330, 333–5
    transport 350, 351
    see also nutrition
feed intake, strategies to improve 332
feeds
    mould contamination 329
    quality 331
feed types 329–30
female reproductive system 265–8
femoropatellar joint (FPJ) 152, 153
femorotibial joints 152, 153
    medial (MFTJ) osteochondrosis lesions 160–3
fenbendazole 260
fetlock
    anatomy 50–2

dorsal osteochondral disease
    (overextension injury) 73–4
examination 52
fractures
    'chip' 70–2
    condylar 6, 59–64
    proximal phalangeal (pastern)
        52
    sesamoid bones 82–7
    stabilization 7
interference injury 12–13
osteochondrosis 74–8
radiographs
    flexed dorsopalmar 6
    pre-purchase 307
    radiological abnormalities in
        sales yearlings 309
    road wounds 9
sesamoiditis 79–82
subchondral bone cyst 77–8
synovitis 69–70
fibre (nutrition) 328
fibrinogen, plasma *338*, *360*
fibrinolytic drugs 238
fillies
    feed intake 332
    in-foal 266–7
    oestrus 265–6
firing *26*, 30
'fissure' fracture
    carpal bones 113, *118*
    condylar 60–3
fitness
    and blood analysis 340
    testing 322–3
FLAIR nasal strip *232*
flexion tests 304
fluid administration, after travel
    351
flunixin meglumine 247, 258, *356*
fluorescein staining 247, 248
5-fluorouracil 285
fluticasone *357*
folliculitis, bacterial 280
foot
    anatomy 31–2
    bruised (corn) 32–3, 37
    conformation/uneven sized 314
    examination 32
    penetration/puncture 38
    pre-purchase radiography 307
    radiological abnormalities in
        sales yearlings *310*

subsolar abscess 36–8
foot balance
    assessment 32
    dorsopalmar 33–5
foot support, laminitis 47
forage 192, 327, 329
fractures
    acute management 6–8
    carpal bones 122, 123, *358*
    causal factors 3
    cervical vertebrae 8, 180–1
    'chip' 70–2, 110–12
    distal phalanx/pedal bone 40–2
    euthanasia guidelines *358–9*
    fetlock
        'chip' 70–2
        condylar 6, 59–64
        proximal phalangeal
            (pastern) 52–8
        stabilization 7
    'fissure' 60–3, 113, *118*
    jaw 245–6
    lateral malleolus 145
    Mc3/Mt3 condylar 59–64
    navicular bone 44–5
    pelvis 169–76
    proximal phalanx (pastern) 52–8
    proximal sesamoid bones 82–7
    rates in training 347
    ribs 185–6
    scapula 127–9
    shoulder joint 131–3
    splint bones 103
    tarsal bones 141–3
    tibial tuberosity 167
    withers 186–7
    see also stress fractures
frog 31
    thrush 48–9
frusemide *232*, *356*
fungal infections
    eye 247–8
    skin 280–2
Fusarium spp. 247
Fusobacterium necrophorum 49

gait abnormalities
    stringhalt 151–2
gallop, training speeds *320*
gamma-glutamyl transferase
    (GGT) *338*, *339*, *360*
ganglion, lateral hock 149
'gargle' 203, 211

gas sterilization 227
gastric ulcers 255–7, 331
    causes and risk factors 255
    treatment *257*, *357*
gastrocnemius tendon 137
gastroscopy 255–7
gene doping 336
genetics
    and athletic potential 315
    and laryngeal paralysis 208
genotype testing 315
gentamicin sulphate *355*, *356*
GGT, *see* gamma-glutamyl
    transferase
gingival disease 243
ginseng 334
girth 'gall' 277
glanders 299
globulin *338*, *360*
glucosamine *18*, 20
glucose, blood levels *360*
glutamate dehydrogenase
    (GLDH) *338*, *360*
glutaraldehyde 227
gluteal muscles 168
glycaemic response 332
glycogen 333–4
going 4, 324–5
GoingStick 325
gonadotropin-releasing hormone
    (GnRH) 266
GPS tracking 321
granulation tissue 10
grasses 323, 329
green-lipped mussel *20*
growth hormone 336
growth plates, closure 108
guttural pouches 202, 295

haemarthrosis, idiopathic
    recurrent 197
haematoma 196–7
    ethmoidal 250–1
Haematopinus asini 287
haemoglobin (Hb) *360*
haemorrhage
    ilial fractures 170, 172
    nostrils 210, 222, 229, 250
    post castration *269*
    see also exercise-induced
        pulmonary haemorrhage
        (EIPH)
'hamstring' muscles 168, 169

harvest mite dermatitis 286–7
hay 329, 332
haylage 329
heart murmurs 235–6
heart rate 317
   colic 258
   fitness testing 322
   maximal at exercise 317, 355
   normal resting 317, 355
'heart scores' 315
heart size 315
heat therapy 28
heels
   collapsed/flat 33–5
   cracked 278
   overreach injury 11–12
herbal extracts, diuretics 232
hill work 320
hip
   acetabular fracture ('knocked-down hip' 174–6
   anatomy 169
histamine receptor antagonists 257
hives (urticaria) 282–3
Hobday (ventriculectomy) 209
hock, see tarsus
hoof–pastern axis 34
hoof–pedal bone relationship 33, 34
hoof wall
   growth 31, 35
   quarter crack 35–6
human chorionic gonadotropin (hCG) 270
humerus 124
   stress fracture 125–7
hurdle racing 5, 60
hyaluronic acid (HA)
   intra-articular 18
   systemic 19, 20
hyoid apparatus 202
hyoscine butylbromide 258, 263
hyperbaric oxygen therapy (HBOT) 29
hyperkeratosis, linear 286, 287
Hypochoeris radicata 151
hypoxic/hypobaric aids 335

iliac artery 169
ilium 168
   stress fractures 169–73
imidocarb dipropionate 297
imiquimod cream 285

immobilization, injury rehabilitation 22
immunostimulants 229, 346, 351
inflammatory markers 338
influenza virus 227
in-foal filly/mare 266–7
inguinal infection (lymphangitis) 193–4
injection abscess/reaction 187
injuries
   causes 3
   fatal 4, 5, 60
   joints 16–20
   management on track 6–8
   minimizing 5–6, 347
   rates of 4, 5, 346–7
   risk factors 4–5
   risk management/prevention 5–6, 347
insecticidal agents 287, 288
insulin levels 332
interference injuries 11–14
interleukin-1 receptor antagonist (IRAP) 18
intersex disorders 270
intertrigo 288, 289
intervertebral sagittal ratio 272, 273
intra-articular therapies 17–19
intralesional injection 26
intrauterine devices 266
ipratropium bromide 357
iris, disorders 305
ischium 168
isolation procedures 344

Japanese encephalitis 275–6
jaw fractures 245–6
'jetlag' 350
joint capsule 15
joint lavage 15
joints
   anatomy 15–16
   injury and repair 16
   management of disorders 16–20
   pain 16
   synovial infections 15
joint supplements 20
JPEG images 308
jugular vein, thrombosis/thrombophlebitis 237–9
jump racing 5, 60, 239
juvenile pharyngitis 217

juvenile tendinitis 96–7

keratitis 305
keratolytics 278, 281
keratoma 47–8
ketoprofen 356
kick wounds 14
kidney function 338
Kimzey Leg Saver 7, 63
'kissing spines' 181–3
knee, see carpus
'knocked down hip' 173–4

lactate
   blood 323, 340
   muscles 317
lactate dehydrogenase 360
laminitis 46–7
   corticosteroid-induced 17, 46
   Obel grading 46
laryngeal dysplasia 219–20
laryngeal function
   assessment 203–6
   grading 204, 205, 206
   relationship between resting and exercising 208–9
laryngeal hemiplegia (recurrent laryngeal neuropathy) 205, 208–10
laryngeal reinnervation 210
laryngeal tie-forward 212
laryngoplasty, prosthetic ('tie-back') 209–10
larynx
   anatomy 201–2
   pre-purchase examination 311
   ultrasonogaphy 312
laser therapy 26, 29
lateral malleolus, fracture 145
lecithin 257
lens, luxation 305
leucocytes, see white blood cells
lice 287–8
ligaments
   response to training 318
   wounds 10–11
   see also specific ligaments
lime sulphur 281
linear keratosis 286, 287
linseed meal 330
lip, abscess 252–3
liver function tests 338
longissimus dorsi 180

Index

lower airways 222–34
   anatomy 222
   assessment 224–6
   disease 227–9
   yard-wide 345–6
   mucus 222, 223
lumbar vertebrae 179, 180
lumbosacral junction 177–8, 180
lumbosacral pain 177–8
lung radiography 231
lung sounds 233
lupins 330
lymphadenopathy, submandibular 251–2
lymphangitis 193–4, 278
lymphocytes *337*
lymphoid tissue, nasopharynx 217

macrocyclic lactones 260
magnesium sulphate *259*
maize 329
male reproductive system 268–70
mandible fractures 245–6
manipulative therapy *28*
marbofloxacin *356*
massage *28*
mastitis 267
mean cell volume (MCV) *337, 360*
mean corpuscular haemoglobin concentration (MCHC) *337*
meloxicam *356*
menace reflex 304
menisci 153
   tears 166
menthol 30
metabolic pathways 317
metacarpal/metatarsal bone, third (Mc3/Mt3/cannon) 92–107
   applied anatomy 92, 93
   condylar fracture 59–64
   dorsoproximal stress fracture 143–5
   osteochondral disease 73–4
   stress reactions/fractures 105–7
   supracondylar lysis 72
   transverse fracture 64–5
methylprednisolone acetate (MPA), intra-articular *17*
methylsulphonylmethane (MSM) *20*
metritis, contagious equine (CEM) 296–7
metronidazole *356*

miconazole 248, 281
Microsporum spp. 280
'milkshaking' 335
mineral oil *259*
minerals 328
mirror, stable 291
mitral regurgitation *235*
monocytes *337, 360*
morphine *356*
moulds 329
moxidectin 260
'mucoactive' agents 228
mucosal protectants *257*
mucus, lower airway 222, 223
mud fever (pastern dermatitis) 278–9
multifidus muscle 180
murmurs, *see* heart murmurs
Murray Valley encephalitis 275–6
muscle
   fatigue 317
   glycogen 333–4
   response to training 318
muscle enzymes 191, *338, 341*
muscle fibres 318, 319
muscle wastage 125, 132, 166, 176
mycotoxins 329
myectomy, strap muscles 212
myeloencephalopathy, EHV-1 273, 274
myostatin gene 315

nail bind ('quicked hoof') 38–9
nasal bleeding 210, 222, 229, 250
nasal discharge 222, 249
nasal passages, anatomy 201
nasal strips *232*
nasogastric tubing, colic *259*
nasolacrimal (tear) duct 252
nasopharyngeal swab 293
natamycin 248
natural behaviour of horses 291
navicular bone
   bipartite *310*
   fracture 44–5
navicular bursa, pathology 32
neck
   anatomy 179–80
   examination 180
   fractures 8, 180–1
neomycin 246, 247
Neorickettsia 261
Neospora hughesi 274

neurological examination, acute injury 8
neuromuscular electrical stimulation (NMES) *29*
neutrophils *337, 360*
nitazoxanide 275
nitric oxide (NO) 334
'nits' (lice eggs) 287
non-steroidal anti-inflammatory drugs (NSAIDs) *19*, 255, *356*
noseband, crossed 212
nostrils 201
   atheroma 253
   wounds 244–5
nuchal ligament 180, 188
nutrition
   assessment of problems/imbalance 330–1
   ergogenic aids 333–5
   imbalances 331, 347
   key nutrients 327–8
   poor appetite/condition 331–2
   see also feeding

oats 329
Obel grading (laminitis) 46
oesophageal obstruction ('choke') 262–3
oestrone sulphate 270
oestrus 265–6
   control/suppression 266
   feed intake 332
   transitional 266
offset ('bench') knee 314
oils
   feeding 191–2, 327, 330
   rancidity 331
omega-3 fatty acids *232*, 330
omeprazole *257, 357*
optic disc atrophy *305*
orthophthalaldehyde 227
osseous cyst-like lesions (OCLs), *see* subchondral bone cysts
osteoarthritis (OA) 16
   intra-articular therapies 17–19
   nutraceuticals (joint supplements) 20
   pain 16
   systemic medications 19
osteochondral fragments ('chips')
   carpal bones 110–12
   fetlock 70–2

osteochondroma, distal radius 120, 121
osteochondrosis 192–3
  causes and risk factors 192
  common sites 192
  diagnosis 193
  elbow joint 133–4
  fetlock 74–8
  history and clinical signs 192
  management 193
  pedal bone 42–4
  prevalence and significance for training 306, *308–10*
  shoulder joint 130
  stifle 160–3, *310*
  tarsus (hock) 140–1
osteochondritis dissecans (OCD) 192, 193
  common sites 192
  diagnosis 193
  fetlock 74–6
  management 193
  stifle 163–4
over-at-the-knee 314
overloading/overextension syndrome (fetlock) 70, 72, 73
'overreaching' (training) 319, 320, 331
overreach injuries 11–12
oxygen therapy, hyperbaric (HBOT) *29*
oxygen utilization 202–3, 317, 318
oxytetracycline hydrochloride *356*
oxytocin 263, 266

packed cell volume (PCV) *337*, 340, *360*
paddock turnout, rehabilitation 22
palatal displacement/instability 210–12
palatopharyngeal arch, rostral displacement 219
palatoplasty, tension 212
palmar nerve, trauma 13
palmar/plantar condylar osteochondral disease (POD) 66–9
papillomatosis ('warts') 283–4
Parapox ovis virus-derived products 229, 346, 351
parasites, intestinal 260, *261*, 331
parrot mouth 243

pastern, *see* proximal phalangeal bone
pastern boot 134, 135
pastern dermatitis (cracked heels/mud fever) 278–9
pastern joint, *see* proximal interphalangeal joint
Pasteurella spp. 227, 233
patella 153
  locking 165–6
patellar ligament, desmotomy 166
PCR tests 294
pectin *257*
pectoral muscles 124
pedal bone, *see* distal phalanx
pedal osteitis, septic 39–40
pelvic fractures
  acetabular/pubic 174–6
  euthanasia guidelines *358*
  ilial wing/shaft 169–73
  rehabilitation 24
  tuber coxa 173–4
  tuber ischium 174
pelvis
  anatomy 168–9
  examination 169
  symmetry 169, 173, 174
pentosan polysulphate *18, 19*
performance (causes of poor)
  EIPH 231
  laryngeal function 208
  musculoskeletal disorders 169, 178, 184, 185
  palatal displacement/instability 211
  tracheal mucus 227
periosteum, injury 10
peritarsal infection 193–4
peritonitis, post-castration 269
pethidine *356*
pharyngeal collapse, dorsal 216
pharyngeal cysts 220–1
pharyngeal lymphoid hyperplasia (juvenile pharyngitis) 217
pharyngeal ostium 202
pharynx, anatomy 202
phenylbutazone 255, *356*
physical therapies 16, 28–30
pinworms *261*
piroplasmosis 297–8
plant oil, intrauterine 266
plasma proteins *338*

platelet-rich plasma (PRP) *18*
platelets *338*
  reference range *360*
pleural fluid 233
pleuropneumonia 233–4, 350
  management 233–4
pneumovagina 267–8
POD, *see* palmar/plantar condylar osteochondral disease
poll injuries 188
polydipsia, *see* psychogenic polydipsia
polymyxin B 246, 247
polysulphated glycosaminoglycans (PSGAGs) *19*
polyuria/polydipsia 265
ponazuril 275
potassium, intake 192
potassium iodide 228, *357*
poultice, foot 33, 38
prebiotics 330
prednisolone 283, *356*
pregnancy 266–7
premolar 'caps' 241–2
pre-purchase examination 303
  airway function 311–12
  conflict of interest 303
  physical examination 304–6
  public auctions 312–13
  radiography 306–10
  ultrasonography 311
probiotics 262, 330
procaine benzyl penicillin, dose/frequency *356*
prodromal injury, condylar fracture 60–3
prognosis, categorization 21
Propionibacterium acnes-derived products 229, 346, 351
protein
  nutritional requirements 327
  total *360*
proton pump inhibitors *257*
protozoal myeloencephalitis, equine (EPM) 274–5
proud flesh 10
proximal interphalangeal joint (PIPJ/pastern joint)
  involvement in P1 fracture 54
  osteoarthritis 78–9
  radiological abnormalities in sales yearlings *309*
  subchondral bone cyst 77

proximal phalangeal bone (P1/
    pastern)
  anatomy 50–2
  conformation 314
  fractures 52–8, *358*
proximal sesamoid bones (PSBs)
    51
  changes in SLB desmopathy 88,
    89
  fracture 82–7
  radiological abnormalities in
    sales yearlings *309–10*
  sesamoiditis 79–82
PRP, *see* platelet-rish plasma
pruritus
  harvest mite dermatitis 286
  sweet itch 288
  tail 286
Pseudomonas spp. 247
psychogenic polydipsia 265
pubis 168
  fracture 174–6
public auctions
  conditions of sale 304
  vetting 312–13
pulmonary haemorrhage
  acute fatal 239
  see also exercise-induced
    pulmonary haemorrhage
    (EIPH)
pulsed magnetic field therapy *26,
    29*
puncture wounds 10
pyrantel 260

quadriceps femoris 165
quarantine 343–4
quarter crack 35–6
quinidine sulphate 237

radial physitis 123
radiography
  digital images 308
  pre-purchase 306–10
radius
  distal growth plate closure 108
  distal subchondral bone injury
    119–20
  stress fracture 129–30
'rain scald'/'rain rot'
    (dermatophilosis) 282
ranitidine *257, 357*
reciprocal ('stay') apparatus,

hindlimb 137, 153, 165
recumbent horse 8
recurrent laryngeal neuropathy
    (RLN) 205, 208–10
red blood cells (RBCs) 317
  anaemia 340
  effects of training 339
  functions and features *337*
  measures *337*
  reference ranges *360*
  techniques to increase mass 335
  tracheal wash 231
reflexes, injured horse 8
regenerative therapies *18*
rehabilitation 21–30
  exercise 22–3, 27
  monitoring 24
  nutrition 24
  physical therapies 28–30
  stress fractures 23–4
  tendon injuries 24–30
reproductive system
  female 265–8
  male 268–70
respiration rate 322, 355
respiratory diseases, *see* lower
    airways, disease; upper airway
    disease
respiratory drugs 356–7
respiratory health 345, 350, 351
respiratory noises 203, 211
respiratory system 318
retinal detachment *305*
rhinitis, fungal (mycotic) 249–50
rib fractures 185–6
rice bran 330
rig (cryptorchid) 268–70
ringworm (dermatophytosis)
    280–2
road wounds 9
Robert Jones bandage 7, 63
roundworms (ascarids) *261*
'runners' 279–80

sacroiliac joints 168–9
sacroiliac pain 169, 177–8
saddle sores 189–90
salbutamol *357*
Salmonella spp. *261, 262*
sand tracks 324
Sarcocystis neurona 274
sarcoids 284–5
scalping injury 13

scapula
  anatomy 124–5
  stress fracture 127–9
sedative drugs *357*
  and laryngeal function 208, 311
seedy toe 45
semimembranosus 168
semispinalis capitis tendon,
    avulsion 188
semitendinosus 168
serum amyloid A *338, 360*
sesamoid bones, *see* navicular bone;
    proximal sesamoid bones
sesamoidean ligament, distal
    (DSL), desmopathy 90–1
sesamoiditis 79–82
  clinical signs 80
  diagnosis 80–1
  management and prognosis
    81–2
  prevalence and significance 82,
    309–10
'setfast', *see* exertional
    rhabdomyolysis
shear stress, hoof/track 4
shipping fever (pleuropneumonia)
    233–4, 350
shoeing
  bruised foot 33
  dorsopalmar foot balance 34
  pedal bone fracture 42
  prevention of interference
    injuries 12, 13
  quarter cracks 36
  white line disease 45
shoulder joint
  anatomy 124–5
  examination 125
  osteochondrosis 130
  supraglenoid tuberosity fracture
    131–3
'sickle hock' conformation 138,
    314
sildenafil *232*
sinoatrial (SA) node 236
sinusitis 248–9
sinus lavage 248
skin wounds 9–10
skull base fractures 188
SLB, *see* suspensory ligament
    branch
slings 22
slipped tendon 150–1

sodium bicarbonate 335
sodium iodide 228, *357*
soft palate 202
soft palate displacement/instability 210–12
sore shins (dorsal metacarpal disease) 102–3
soybean meal 330
speedy cuts 13
spinal column
    applied anatomy 179–80
    movement 180
    stress injury 183–4
spinal cord compression 271, 272
spinal injuries 8
    cervical 8, 180–1
    euthanasia guidelines *359*
spleen 317, 322
splint bones (Mc/Mt2/4) 92
    fractures 103, 104, 105
splints (metacarpal/metatarsal exostosis) 103–5
sprint distances 317
stable rest 22
stabling
    air hygiene 345
    and stereotypic behaviours 291
stanazolol *18*
staphylectomy 212
Staphylococcus spp. 247
Staphylococcus aureus 15
starch, dietary 327, 333
staying distances 317
stay (reciprocal) apparatus, hindlimb 137, 153, 165
stem cell therapy *18, 26*
stereotypic behaviours ('stable vices') 265, 291
stifle
    anatomy 152–3
    examination 153
    locking patella 165–6
    osteochondrosis 160–4, *310*
    pre-purchase radiography *307*
    radiological abnormalities in sales yearlings *310*
    synovial spaces 153
    tibial tuberosity fracture 167
    trauma 166–7
strangles 294–5
streptococci, beta-haemolytic 247
Streptococcus equi 294
Streptococcus pneumoniae 227

Streptococcus zooepidemicus 227, 267
stress fractures
    causes 3
    classification 23
    diagnosis 23
    dorsal cortical (Mc3/Mt3/cannon) 107
    dorsoproximal articular, Mt3 143–5
    humerus 125–7
    ilium 169–73
    monitoring healing 24
    palmar cortical (Mc3/cannon) 105
    patterns/high rates of 347
    pelvis 169–73
    radius 129–30
    rehabilitation 23–4
    scapula 127–9
    tibia 153–60
stringhalt 151–2
strongyles 260, *261*
subchondral bone cysts (OCLs) 192
    common sites 192
    diagnosis 193
    elbow 133
    fetlock 77–8
    pastern joint 77
    pedal bone 42–4
    shoulder 130
    stifle 160–3, *310*
    treatments 193
subchondral bone injury, distal radius 119–20
subepiglottic cysts 221
submandibular lymphadenopathy 251–2
sucralfate *257*
sudden death, exercise-related 239
sugar beet pulp 330
superficial digital flexor tendon (SDFT) 24
    accessory ligament (AL-SDFT) desmopathy 134–6
    desmotomy *26*
    applied anatomy 92, 93
    disease ('tendinitis') 92–6
    rehabilitation 24–30
    examination 92
    fetlock 52
    hindlimb 137
    subluxation (slipped tendon) 150–1

    insertional branch tendinitis 91–2
    'juvenile' tendinitis 96–7
supplements
    joint support 20
    nutritional 328, 330, 333–5
supraglenoid tuberosity, fracture 131–3
supraspinous ligament 180
suspensory ligament
    forelimb desmopathy 97–9
    hindlimb desmopathy 99–100
    origin avulsion fracture 100–1
suspensory ligament branch (SLB) 52
    desmopathy 80, 82, 86–90
suxibuzone 255, *356*
'swamp fever' (equine infectious anaemia) 295–6
sweat, electrolyte loss 328
sweet itch 288
swimming 22, 321
synechiae, ocular *305*
synovial fluid 16
synovial membrane 15
synovial sepsis 15
synoviocentesis 15
synovitis
    chronic proliferative ('villonodular') 72–3
    fetlock 69–70
synthetic surfaces 4–5, 324, 325
systolic ejection murmur *235*

tail rubbing 286
talus 137
tapeworms 258, 260, *261*
tarsal synovial sheath 136, 137, 147
    effusion (thoroughpin) 147
tarsometatarsal (TMT) joint 136, 137
    arthritic changes 138–40
tarsus (hock) 136–52
    applied anatomy 136–7
    capped 145–7
    central tarsal bone fracture 142–3
    conformation 138, 149, 314
    curb 149–50
    examination 138
    lateral extensor tenosynovitis/ganglion 149
    osteoarthritis (bone spavin) 138–40

osteochondrosis 140–1, *309*
pre-purchase radiography *307*
radiological abnormalities in sales yearlings *309*
slipped tendon 150–1
third tarsal bone
    fracture 141–3
    wedge-shaped 141, *309*
thoroughpin/false thoroughpin 147–8
Taylorella equigenitalis 296
teeth 241–4
    malalignment 243
    poor feeding/condition 331
    premolar 'caps' 241–2
    routine rasping 241
    'wolf' 242
temperature
    normal rectal 355
    Celsius–Fahrenheit conversion chart 355
tendinitis
    'juvenile' 96–7
    SDFT 91–6
tendinous windgall/windpuff 52
tendon injuries
    acute phase management 25
    additional therapies 26
    classification 25
    euthanasia guidelines *358*
    lacerations 10–11
    rehabilitation 24–30
    see also specific tendons
tendon knock 13–14
tendons, response to training 318
tendon splitting 26
tenosynovitis
    biceps tendon/bursa 130–1
    carpal sheath 120–2
testes 268–70
tetracyclines 246, 247
tetrahydropyrimidines 260
Theileria equi 297
thermocautery
    palatal displacement 212
    tendon injuries 26
thoracic vertebrae
    anatomy 180
    dorsal spinous process fracture 186–7
    dorsal spinous process impingement 181–3
thoracolumbar fascia 180

thoracolumbar spine, stress injury 183–4
thoroughpin 147
    false 147–8
thrombophlebitis, septic 238, 239
thrombosis, jugular vein 237–9
thrush 48–9
tibia
    anatomy 152
    examination 153
    fractures
        rehabilitation 24
        stabilization 7
    stress 153–60
    tuberosity 167
tibiotarsal joint 137, *309*
tick-borne disease 297
'tie-back' 209–10
'tie-forward' 212
tiludronate *19*, *69*, *196*, *357*
TMT, *see* tarsometatarsal joint
toe-out conformation 314
tongue, wounds 244
tongue-tie 212
tooth root abscess 243–4
tracheal blood 224, *225*, 231
tracheal lavage (tracheal 'wash') 225–6, 228
    laboratory analysis 228, 231
    sample grading *225*
tracheal mucus 22, *223*
    and EIPH 227
    and performance 227
    treatment 228
tracheostomy, semi-permanent 210
track
    design/geometry 5, 324
    injury management 6–8
    maintenance 324–5
    surfaces and conditions 4–5, 324–5
training
    bone remodelling 3
    cool-down 322
    detraining 320
    GPS tracking/ECG monitors 321
    injuries 3, 4
    injury prevention 5–6
    'overreaching' 319, 320, 331
    physiological adaptations 318–19

programme elements 319
speeds 319–20
warm-up 322
tranexamic acid *232*
transcutaneous electrical nerve stimulation (TENS) 29
transport 349–51
    effects of 349–50
    injured horse 7–8
    veterinary management 351
treadmill endoscopy 206–7
treadmill exercise 22, 23, 320–1
treadmill field test 323
triamcinolone acetonide (TA) *17*
Trichophyton spp. 280
tricuspid regurgitation *235*
trimethoprim–sulphonamide *356*
Trombicula autumnalis 286–7
trot, training speeds *320*
Trypanosoma equiperdum 298
tuber coxa 168
    fracture 173
tuber ischium 168, 169
    fracture 174
tuber sacrale 168
turf tracks 5, 323–4
    maintenance 324–5
'tying-up', *see* exertional rhabdomyolysis

ultrasonograms
    pre-purchase examination 311
ultrasound, therapeutic 26, 29
uphill tracks/training 69, 154, 320, 347
upper airway
    anatomy 203
    endoscopy 203–7, 311–12
    overground/treadmill 206–7
    resting 203–6
    resistance/obstruction 202–3
upper airway disease
    arytenoid ulceration/chondritis 218
    axial deviation of aryepiglottic folds 212–14
    complex collapse 216
    epiglottic entrapment 214, 215
    epiglottitis 220
    infections 248–50
    laryngeal dysplasia 219–20
    palatal displacement/instability 210–12

upper airway disease – *contd*
    pharyngeal cysts 220–1
    pharyngeal lymphoid
        hyperplasia 217
    recurrent laryngeal neuropathy
        208–10
urea *338, 360*
urinary tract infections 265
urination, excessive (polyuria) 265
urine specific gravity 265
urovagina 267–8
urticaria 282–3
uveitis *305*

vaccination
    arboviral encephalitis 276
    EHV 274, 294
    immunocontraceptive 266
    influenza 293
    strangles 295
vagina
    urine pooling (urovagina)
        267–8
    'windsucking' (pneumovagina)
        267–8
valacyclovir 274
vasodilatory drugs *232*
Venezuelan equine encephalitis
    275–6
ventilation, stables/barns 345
ventricular premature complexes
    (VPCs) *236*
ventricular septal defect *235*
ventriculectomy ('Hobday') 209
ventriculocordectomy 209
vertebrae, anatomy 179
vetting
    public auctions 312–13
    see also pre-purchase
        examination
vibration therapy *29*
viral infections 273–6
vision testing 304
vitamin C *232*
vitamins 328, 334–5
vocal cords 201
voriconazole 248

walking exercise 22
warm-up 322
warts (papillomatosis) 283–4
water deprivation testing 265

water intake 265, 351
    excessive (polydipsia) 265
water treadmill 22, 321
weaning 291
weaving 291
'weigh-out' (nutrition) 331
weight loss 331–2
    chronic diarrhoea 261, 262
    transport 349, 351
Western equine encephalitis
    275–6
West Nile virus 275–6
wheat bran 330
white blood cells (WBC/
    leucocytes)
    effects of training 339
    function and features *337*
    and health 340
    measures *337*
    reference ranges *360*
white line 31
    disease ('seedy toe') 45
    haemorrhage 33
'winded' horse 8
windgalls 52
windsucking (behaviour) 258, 291
windsucking (pneumovagina)
    267–8
wind testing 203, 311
witch hazel 30
withers, fractured 186–7
wobbler syndrome 271–3, *359*
wolf teeth 242
woodchip surfaces 324
wound dressings, and exercise 10
wounds
    cleansing/irrigation 9
    interference injuries 11–14
    kicks 14
    nostril 244–5
    poll 188
    skin 9–10
    stifle 166–7
    synovial infection 15
    tendon/ligament 10–11
    tongue 244

xylazine *357*

yard management
    air quality 345
    and stereotypic behaviours 291

yearlings
    conformation assessment 313–14
    genetic selection 315
    'juvenile' tendinitis 96–7
    public auction vetting 312
    radial physitis 122–3
    radiological abnormalities 139,
        160, 163, 308, *309–10*
    sesamoiditis 79, 82
    SLB desmopathy 86
    see also pre-purchase
        examination

zinc sulphate 10